Towards Prescribing Practice

Towards Prescribing Practice

Edited by
JOHN McKINNON
MSc, PG Dip, BA (Hons), RGN, RNT, RMN, RHV
University of Lincoln

John Wiley & Sons, Ltd

Copyright © 2007   John Wiley & Sons Ltd, The Atrium, Southern Gate, Chichester,
West Sussex PO19 8SQ, England

Telephone   (+44) 1243 779777

Email (for orders and customer service enquiries): cs-books@wiley.co.uk
Visit our Home Page on www.wiley.com

Designations used by companies to distinguish their products are often claimed as trademarks. All
brand names and product names used in this book are trade names, service marks, trademarks or
registered trademarks of their respective owners. The Publisher is not associated with any product or
vendor mentioned in this book.

This publication is designed to provide accurate and authoritative information in regard to the subject
matter covered. It is sold on the understanding that the Publisher is not engaged in rendering
professional services. If professional advice or other expert assistance is required, the services of a
competent professional should be sought.

Other Wiley Editorial Offices

John Wiley & Sons Inc., 111 River Street, Hoboken, NJ 07030, USA

Jossey-Bass, 989 Market Street, San Francisco, CA 94103-1741, USA

Wiley-VCH Verlag GmbH, Boschstr. 12, D-69469 Weinheim, Germany

John Wiley & Sons Australia Ltd, 42 McDougall Street, Milton, Queensland 4064, Australia

John Wiley & Sons (Asia) Pte Ltd, 2 Clementi Loop #02-01, Jin Xing Distripark, Singapore 129809

John Wiley & Sons Canada Ltd, 6045 Freemont Blvd, Mississauga, ONT, L5R 4J3

Wiley also publishes its books in a variety of electronic formats. Some content that appears in print
may not be available in electronic books.

Anniversary Logo Design: Richard J. Pacifico

Library of Congress Cataloging in Publication Data

Towards prescribing practice / edited by John McKinnon.
      p.   ;   cm.
   Includes bibliographical references and index.
   ISBN-13: 978-0-470-02843-8 (pbk. : alk. paper)
   ISBN-10: 0-470-02843-2 (pbk. : alk. paper)
   1. Drugs—Prescribing. I. McKinnon, John.
   [DNLM: 1. Patient Care—methods.   2. Prescriptions, Drug.
   QV 748 T737 2007]
   RM138.T69 2007
   615′.1—dc22   2006025189

British Library Cataloguing in Publication Data

A catalogue record for this book is available from the British Library

ISBN-10: 0-470-02843-2
ISBN-13: 978-0-470-02843-8

Typeset in 10/12pt Times by Integra Software Services Pvt. Ltd, Pondicherry, India
Printed and bound in Great Britain by TJ International Ltd, Padstow, Cornwall
This book is printed on acid-free paper responsibly manufactured from sustainable forestry in which
at least two trees are planted for each one used for paper production.

"To my loved ones, loyal friends and colleagues. They know who they are."

Contents

List of Contributors

THE EDITOR

John McKinnon MSc, PG Dip, BA (Hons), RGN, RNT, RMN, RHV

John is a senior lecturer in nursing at the Faculty of Health, Life and Social Sciences, University of Lincoln. John was a practising nurse for over 20 years across a range of specialties in adult, mental health nursing and health visiting. Following this he was a nurse specialist in child protection before becoming a lecturer. He studied at Sheffield Hallam University, obtaining a BA (Hons) in Health Care Practice and afterwards an MSc in Health Care Education. He is currently a doctoral student with the International Institute for Education Leadership. He was a prescribing academic lead for two years, taught an undergraduate nursing therapeutics module, and continues to lecture on public health and concordance on the non-medical prescribing programme. In addition he has co-authored regional guidance for medical supervisors.

John's other interests include public health, children's rights and intuitive knowing in practice, on which he presented a paper to an International Nursing Conference in Finland in 2000.

CONTRIBUTORS

Clare Allen MA, BSc (Hons), RHV, RGN

Clare is specialist associate in learning at the NHS Institute for Innovation and Improvement. She is a nurse practitioner and health visitor and was formerly a senior lecturer and programme lead for public health nursing and the MSc Primary Care at the University of Derby. She is currently studying for her PhD at the University of Sheffield.

Linda Bray MSc, BA (Hons), RGN, DN

Linda is a Macmillan Clinical Nurse Specialist in Palliative Care in East Lincolnshire. She has 15 years' service as a community practitioner and served as a PCG Board nurse in the late 1990s.

Dr Ruth Goldstein PhD

Ruth is responsible for clinical governance in medicines management for a Derbyshire PCT. She is a qualified pharmacist and was involved in the development of the National Service Framework for Older People. Her doctorate was concerned with issues of concordance among the older population.

Yvonne Hopkins MSc, PG Cert, BA, RGN, RNMH

Yvonne is senior manager for cancer and palliative care within East Lincolnshire. During the 1990s she was a Macmillan Nurse in Hull and went on to become the Regional Nurse Specialist for Palliative Care. During this time she received national recognition for her work in quality management within East Yorkshire.

Stuart Kennedy BSc (Hons), Dip Nursing, RMN

Stuart has been a mental health practitioner for 16 years and was one of the first mental health nurses in the country to become a prescriber. He was a contributing author for a resource pack for carers of people with dementia.

Ian Loveday MSc, PG Cert, BA (Hons), RN

Ian is an emergency care practitioner for Derby City Primary Care Trust. He was formerly a senior lecturer and programme lead for MSc Critical Care at Sheffield Hallam University and remains an associate lecturer there. A former clinical skills educator in accident and emergency, Ian is a facilitator for the RCN faculty of emergency nursing and has formed close links with paramedic practitioners.

Richard Pilbery BSc (Hons), BMed Sc (Hons), SYAS, IHCD

Richard is a Lecturer-Practitioner in Paramedical Studies at Sheffield Hallam University and is currently part of a pilot scheme concerned with calls to older people. He is a graduate of the University of Bristol and the University of Sheffield and is a member of the Faculty of Prehospital Care affiliated to the Royal College of Surgeons.

Ruth Reilly M Med Sci, BA, PGCE, RGN, RNT, HV, RHV

Ruth Reilly has been a practising nurse, health visitor and educationalist in excess of thirty years. Specialising in developing and teaching of post-registration programmes, including a nurse prescribing programme, she recently collaborated in the curriculum development of a new public health focused BSc (Hons) degree in adult nursing. Ruth has teaching and research interests in clinical governance, biological sciences and mentorship.

Joanne West MSc, BPharm (Hons), Pharm Dip

Jo is lead pharmacy lecturer on the Non-Medical Prescribing Programme at the University of Lincoln. She has been a practising pharmacist for over 20 years, is currently consultant pharmacy prescribing adviser to East Midlands Ambulance Trust and has held a number of offices with the Royal Pharmaceutical Society of Great Britain. She is a graduate of King's College London and the University of Nottingham.

Acknowledgements

Dr David Brandford, Chief Pharmacist, Derbyshire Mental Health Trust

Dr Adam Britton, Senior Researcher for Wildlife International, Darwin, Australia

Dr Peter Calveley, General Practitioner, Lincoln

Petra Clarke, Non Medical Prescribing Academic Lead, University of Lincoln

Steven Davidson, Nurse Consultant, Queen's Medical Centre, University Hospital Nottingham

Jayne Dunnett, Senior Community Physiotherapist, West Lincs PCT

Timothy Earnshaw, State Registered Paramedic with the Helicopter Medical Emergency Service, East Midlands Ambulance Service

Colin Hardman, Senior Pharamacist, United Lincolnshire Hospital Trusts

Dr Jennifer Hartman, Consultant Psychiatrist (Older People), Derbyshire Mental Health Trust

Dr Roslyn Kane, Senior Lecturer in Nursing, University of Lincoln

Roma Kennedy, Senior Nurse, Leicester City West PCT

Markallen Healthcare Publishing Ltd, London

Professor Philip Routledge, Therapeutics and Toxicology Centre, University of Cardiff

Vicky Shilton, Pharmacist, United Lincolnshire Hospital Trust

Neil Short, Clinical Nurse Specialist Alcohol Problems, North Derbyshire Alcohol Team

Rachael Spencer, Senior Lecturer in Nursing, University of Lincoln

Finally I would like to thank my wife Tina for all her patience and support.

1 Understanding Basic Pharmacology

JOHN McKINNON

This chapter provides an introduction to the fundamental principles of pharmacology. Many nurses and allied health professionals approach this aspect of their prescribing studies with a sense of dread, believing it to be an area of knowledge that is unknown to them. However, the fundamental principles of pharmacology are linked to the same anatomical and physiological knowledge base that underpins many other areas of health-care practice.

As we journey through the different phases of the pharmacokinetic cycle – absorption, distribution, metabolism and elimination – examine how drugs effect their action and consider the different types of adverse drug events, a functional rather than a mathematical approach will be taken to enable the reader to grasp these principles whether or not they have a background in clinical chemistry.

Pharmacology forms a significant part of prescribing practice. It is important for prescribers to be able to construct a profile of any given drug and judge its suitability for treating any patient in their care. The starting point for this process is the *British National Formulary*, which is published every six months and is available in an electronic version online. It is structured in sections, each dealing with a different drug group and providing the specific dosage, contraindications, anticipated side effects and dose formulation for each drug. Supplements also provide instruction on prescription writing, drug licensing and monitoring.

Adherence on the part of the prescriber to drug-specific guidance in the *British National Formulary* (BNF) is essential. For the prescribing student, familiarisation with the structure and layout of the BNF is a preliminary study task that will prove beneficial. Good prescribing practice also recognises the place of collaborative working with the pharmacist where there is any doubt about prescribing issues.

To begin with some definitions, *pharmacology* is a broad term used to describe the study of drugs from their origins, chemical structure and administration to their absorption, distribution, actions, metabolism and excretion. There are other terms defining parts of this that we will mention briefly and with which you

Towards Prescribing Practice. Edited by J. McKinnon.
© 2007 John Wiley & Sons, Ltd.

will become better acquainted as you continue to learn and use them with confidence.

Pharmacokinetics relates to drug concentrations in body tissues and fluids, and the physiological processes that influence those concentrations over time. (In other words, what the body does to the drug.) This can be divided into absorption, distribution, metabolism and excretion.

Pharmacodynamics relates to the fundamental action of a drug on a physiological, biological or molecular level. (In other words, what the drug does to the body.)

Therapeutics is the branch of pharmacology concerned with the use of drugs to produce a desired clinical response in an individual.

ABSORPTION

Looking at the membrane of a cell (Figure 1.1) can teach us a great deal about the properties that drugs must have to be effectively absorbed by the body. The bilayer is so called because it is made up of a double layer of phospholipids arranged so that the water-loving (hydrophilic) positively charged heads face outwards towards the aqueous environment, either intracellular or extracellular, and the lipid-loving

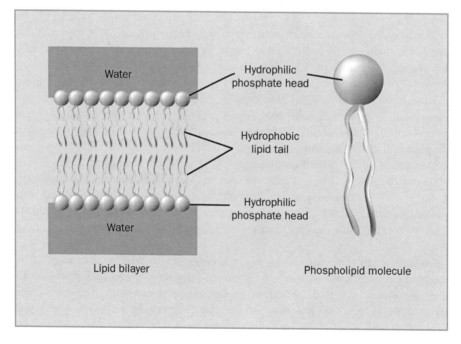

Figure 1.1 Structure of a cell membrane. Reproduced by permission of MA Healthcare. (See also colour plate 1).

(lipophilic) tails face inwards away from the aqueous environment. Over 45 % of the cell membrane is made up of lipid (Seeley et al., 2000).

Therefore the first three properties of a drug are ideally:

1. *Lipid solubility*, to diffuse easily across membranes.
2. *Water solubility*, to dissolve easily in aqueous solutions.
3. Possession of a *neutral or negative charge* so as not to be repelled by the positive charge of the external bilayer.

When a drug is dropped into oil and water, the proportion of the drug that dissolves in lipid is called the lipid *partition co-efficient*. In drug design a delicate balance must be struck between lipid and water solubility. If this is not done, the oral route will be less viable: highly lipid-soluble drugs will have delayed or failed absorption because of their reduced capacity to dissolve in the aqueous fluid of the gastrointestinal tract. Similarly, highly water-soluble drugs will not permeate the lipid bilayer of the gastrointestinal wall.

The *size of a drug molecule or molecular weight* is also relevant. The smaller the molecular weight, the more easily the drug is absorbed across membrane barriers. The degree of acidity or *pH* also plays a part as some drugs are more 'at home' and therefore more easily absorbed in an acid environment than in an alkaline or base one or vice versa. Many drugs exist as weak acids or as weak bases and the pH of their container compartment will influence the degree of ionisation that takes place and therefore membrane solubility (Rang et al., 2000).

Theoretically then, when an acidic drug such as aspirin is given orally, we might expect most of it to be absorbed in the stomach; this is not what happens in practice. This is because it can normally be predicted that passive diffusion of a molecule down a concentration gradient will take place at a faster rate across a large surface area than a small surface area. The greater surface area of the small intestine, comparable to that of a singles tennis court (Figure 1.2), facilitates the greater amount of absorption. The quality of *local blood supply* also powers absorption. A patient with congestive heart failure, for example, will have relatively poor absorption of oral drugs. *Peristalsis* inhibits absorption; *food* delays it. For this reason oral drugs should always be taken one hour before or two hours after food unless otherwise instructed. An example of an exception to this rule is ibuprofen, which should be taken with food to protect the stomach lining from damage.

DISTRIBUTION

Once in the bloodstream, some drugs are carried in the plasma as solutes, but many drugs to a greater or lesser extent bind to plasma proteins. The three-dimensional shape of the protein molecule is what makes it ideal for this purpose. When

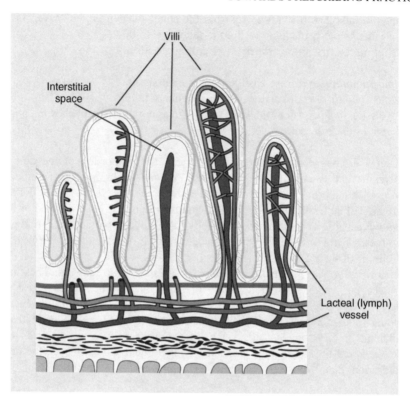

Figure 1.2 Structure of small intestinal wall, showing large surface area. Reproduced by permission of MA Healthcare. (See also colour plate 2).

drugs are bound to plasma proteins they are essentially inactive. It is the 'free' or 'unbound' drug that is active. The drug that is bound to plasma is automatically released as the free drug leaves the circulation and enters target tissues. Under normal circumstances the percentage of the drug in a bound state and that in a free state remains constant. This predictable homeostatic pattern is useful to pharmacists who are seeking to calculate viable and safe dosages (Greenblatt et al., 1982). However, problems can occur when drugs are displaced prematurely. This can happen in a disease such as liver failure, where excess bilirubin competes for binding space and the bound drug is displaced. The result is excess unbound drug in the bloodstream, which may lead to toxicity or an undesirably high clinical response (Downie et al., 1995).

Drugs that are administered orally are absorbed via the gastrointestinal tract and carried by the hepatic portal circulation to the liver. One of the functions of the liver is to change the chemical structure of drugs to allow easy disposal by the body. This role of the liver in relation to drug distribution in the body is called *hepatic first pass*. In the case of some drugs the liver is very efficient in rendering the drug ineffective and such a drug is said to have a *high hepatic first pass*. For this reason, some drugs such as glyceryl trinitrate would be completely ineffective if given orally and must be administered by another route (e.g. sublingually, subbuccally or transdermally) so that they have the opportunity to act on the body before reaching the liver (Murphy and Carmichael, 2000; Mcleod, 2003). Other drugs such as pethidine and propranolol must be given in much higher doses when administered orally than if given intravenously in order to compensate for their high first-pass metabolism (Pond and Tozer, 1984; Young and Koda-Kimble, 1995).

SPECIALISED CAPILLARY BEDDING

THE BLOOD–BRAIN BARRIER

In most parts of the body capillary walls are one cell thick, making for easy passage of substances across the semi-permeable barrier. There are three exceptions to this. The first is the blood–brain barrier (BBB) (Figure 1.3).

The blood–brain barrier exists to protect brain tissue from potentially harmful substances that may be present in the blood. It is present throughout the brain and spinal cord, except the floor of the hypothalamus and the area postrema.

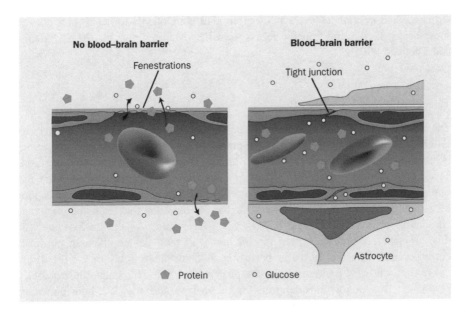

Figure 1.3 Blood–brain barrier. Reproduced by permission of MA Healthcare. (See also colour plate 3).

The fenestrations found in the endothelial tissue of the capillary bed else-where in the body are absent in the Circle of Willis. Instead of this, tight junctions are in place between the endothelial cells, which means that effec-tively materials in the bloodstream must transverse two membranes and, of course, the cytoplasm of the endothelium to reach cerebral tissue. This altogether more substantial structure is supported by foot-like processes of glial cells called astro-cytes.

Although special transport systems are in place to facilitate passage of nutrients such as glucose, only drugs that are highly lipid soluble may cross this barrier. This is an advantage for clinicians seeking to use drugs that would be damaging to the central nervous system, as these drugs cannot cross the BBB. However, practitioners need to bear in mind that the BBB may not be as fully developed in infants and is less efficient in the elderly. It is a disadvantage for clinicians seeking to treat infections of the central nervous system, as antibiotics such as penicillin cannot penetrate the BBB. An exception to this would be severe meningitis, when the meningeal BBB may be damaged and some antibiotics are able to pass across the compromised buffer.

In the face of a fully functioning BBB, antibiotics must be given intrathecally (into the cerebral spinal fluid). Intrathecal injection is, however, a difficult procedure in view of the lack of room for manoeuvre and the close proximity of neural tissue that is vulnerable to damage (Tortora and Grabowski, 2003).

Since the beginning of the twenty-first century, researchers seeking to advance the treatment of conditions such as Alzheimer's disease have been experimenting with attached substances such as ascorbic acid components to act as carriers for some drugs, facilitating transfer across the BBB (Manfredini et al., 2002; Egleton and Thomas, 2005).

THE PLACENTAL BARRIER

The second exception is the *placental barrier* (Figure 1.4). This is not nearly as efficient as the BBB because the prime purpose of the structure of chorionic tissue is to allow maximum possible access to the maternal circulation for nutrition. Tree-like structured placental villi extending and carrying fetal blood from the umbilical cord originating in the amniotic sac are immersed in the maternal pool of blood present in uterine tissue. The barrier between the fetal and maternal circulation at any given time is less than wafer thin. As the surface area of this structure progressively increases in line with fetal development to permit a corresponding increase in tissue perfusion, it therefore follows that most drugs enjoy similarly easy passage across the placental barrier. This helps illustrate why pregnancy is a major consideration for prescribers and why a whole appendix in the BNF is dedicated to this subject. Groups of antibiotics that inhibit cell division (e.g. co-trimoxazole) are among the many drugs that are contraindicated in pregnancy.

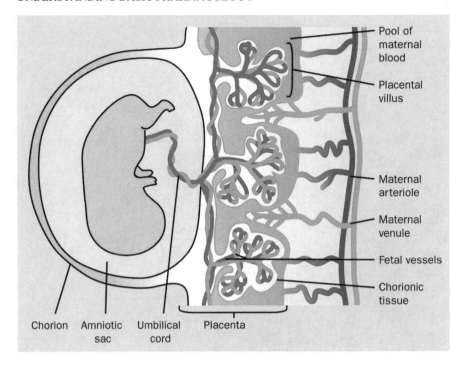

Figure 1.4 The placental barrier. Reproduced by permission of MA Healthcare. (See also colour plate 4).

THE BLOOD–TESTICULAR BARRIER

The third area of specialised capillary bedding is the *blood–testicular barrier*. Relatively little is known about this barrier, but it seems that the Sertoli cells (Figure 1.5) play a major part in safeguarding spermatogenesis. Sertoli cells form tight junctions with each other and the inner luminal surface of the seminiferous tubules. They encase the developing spermatocytes as they mature into sperm and prevent substances detrimental to spermatogenesis, such as antibodies, from passing from the blood to the tubular compartment. As with any other protective barrier, it is not totally impregnable. It has recently been shown that the chemical lindane can cross the testicular barrier and cause damage to spermatogenesis (Silvestroni et al., 1997).

DRUG RECEPTORS

A *drug receptor* is the site of drug action where the molecular event occurs that leads to a therapeutic response. This, like the term pharmacology, is a broad concept, because receptors can take a variety of forms. The majority are complex macromolecular proteins such as enzymes or hormones. However, certain drugs

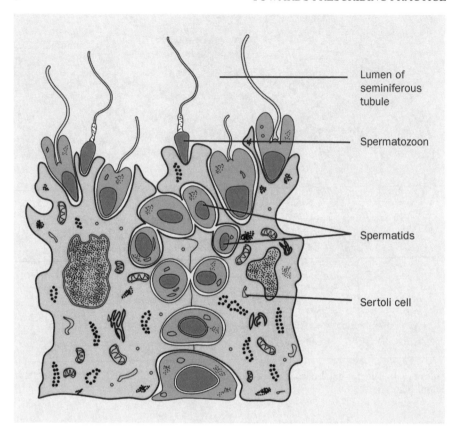

Figure 1.5 The blood–testicular barrier. Reproduced by permission of MA Healthcare. (See also colour plate 5).

can bind to non-protein substances such as nucleic acids. We can recall from our discussion of the distribution phase of pharmacokinetics that the three-dimensional shape of plasma proteins makes them natural binding sites during drug distribution. For the same reason, most drug receptors have a protein component. The meaning of the term drug receptor should help us see that drugs do not themselves bring about a therapeutic response. Rather, they work by enhancing, blocking or diminishing the body's extracellular and intracellular mechanisms. In this process the drug receptor acts as a catalyst; that is, a third-party facilitator of a reaction that changes both the participants in the molecular event, the enzyme within the receptor and the substance binding with it, without changing itself.

Receptors are located within the channel proteins embedded in the membranes of cells. Receptors are also located in the intracellular environment to act as junctions in message-conduction pathways. A substance that binds with a receptor is known as a *ligand*. There are a number of ways in which a ligand is identified by and able to bind with a receptor. For example, some receptors are gated by an electrical charge or voltage gated. Here, the rate of ionic conductance is altered by the ligand (e.g. cardiac muscle tissue). In other cases the ligand sets a biochemical chain of events in motion that manipulates intracellular function. This is known as ligand gating. A receptor site may also bear glycoprotein pendant chains as markers to attract the appropriate ligands (Figure 1.6). This latter method is common in the immune system and is also the way an oocyte attracts sperm in the reproductive process (Seeley et al., 2000).

In order to be accepted, a drug must therefore deceive the receptor by resembling the appropriate ligand, rather like the wrong key can sometimes be placed in a lock. Drugs can broadly be categorised by their roles of action. Those that stimulate receptors are *agonists*. Those that diminish the message normally transmitted by receptors are *antagonists*. Antagonists may also be described as acting competitively when they 'compete' with the relevant ligand for the same receptor site. This is called *competitive inhibition*. Antagonists may also act non-competitively by binding to an alternative receptor site and compromising the ligand signal from there. This is called *non-competitive inhibition* (Figure 1.7).

A bronchodilator such as salbutamol is an example of an agonist as it selectively stimulates the Beta 2 receptors located in the smooth muscle of the bronchioles. The vasodilator nifedipine is an example of a calcium antagonist as it blocks the

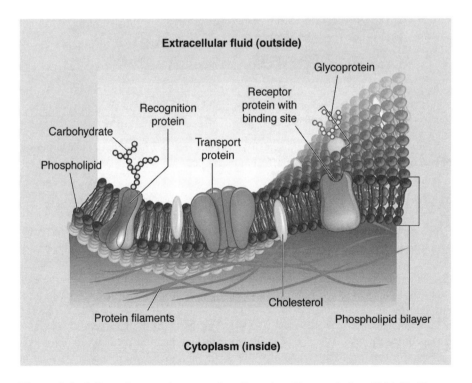

Figure 1.6 Cell membrane and receptor sites. Reproduced by permission of MA Healthcare. (See also colour plate 6).

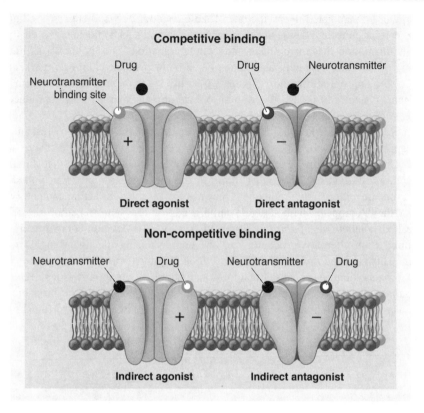

Figure 1.7 Competitive and non-competitive inhibition. Reproduced by permission of MA Healthcare. (See also colour plate 7).

calcium channels of vascular muscle. The more selective drugs are in their targeting of receptors, the less likely side effects are to occur.

METABOLISM AND ELIMINATION

Drug metabolism is the first stage of drug clearance and describes the means by which a drug is chemically altered to facilitate elimination from the body. Many drugs are essentially lipophilic to permit effective absorption. Were they to remain in this state, they would either be reabsorbed in the renals or the gut, with undesirable or even toxic consequences. Alternatively, the more hydrophilic drugs will often pass through the body unchanged. Some drugs are actually designed to take advantage of this process and in such cases it is the drug metabolite that exerts the greater therapeutic response. When this is the case the medication actually administered is termed a *prodrug*. An example of this is the antianxiolytic diazepam, which is metabolised to nordazepam and oxazepam, both of which are active substances (Lin and Lu, 1997).

Although the main organ of metabolism is the liver, metabolic properties are present in most body cells. This is particularly the case in lung tissue, which explains why some drug metabolites are exhaled. It is, of course, this route of elimination that makes measurement of blood alcohol levels by breathalyser possible. Widespread metabolic tissue distribution in the body also explains why drugs can be excreted in the host's sweat, saliva and tears in addition to the host's urine and faeces. This is the second stage of clearance.

The *cytochrome P450 enzymes* exist within endoplasmic reticulum of liver and other body cells in a sufficiently wide range of varieties to enable them to metabolise a correspondingly wide range of drugs. They achieve this by:

- *Oxidation*, in which the positive charge of the drug molecule is increased.
- *Reduction*, the addition of an oxygen atom to the drug molecule.
- *Hydrolysis*, the breakdown of the drug molecule through the addition of water.
- *Conjugation*, the coupling of the drug molecule with an acid making for greater water solubility.

Oxidation, reduction and hydrolysis are known as phase one metabolism. Conjugation constitutes phase two metabolism. Essentially the outcome of both phase one and phase two reactions is an increase in the hydrophilicity of a drug, which facilitates excretion by the kidneys.

Most drugs follow *first-order kinetics*, where the rate of metabolism and elimination is related to the level of plasma concentration. Here an increase in the plasma concentration of the drug leads to stimulation of synthesis of cytochrome P450 enzymes, often called *enzyme induction*. A minority of drugs follow *zero-order kinetics*, in which metabolism is not related to the rate of plasma concentration but takes place at a constant rate. This is often the case when drugs such as alcohol are taken in excess and *enzyme saturation* takes place. Put simply, first-order kinetics is rather like a supermarket queue that as it increases in length leads to other checkouts being opened and customers being processed at a faster rate. Zero-order kinetics is like a supermarket checkout queue that regardless of length is served by the same number of checkouts.

In the kidneys, drugs of a low molecular weight are eliminated by glomerular filtration (Figure 1.8). Further secretion takes place in the proximal tubule. Here carriers exist to remove both bound and unbound drug through the creation of a concentration gradient that favours dissociation and passage from the capillary bed into the tubular lumen. Reabsorption also takes place in the tubules by active and passive diffusion. Drugs that are lipophilic are normally reabsorbed. Drugs that are unionised in a low pH medium such as urine but ionised in a higher pH medium such as plasma will be partially reabsorbed by means of a phenomenon known as ion trapping. Here the pH of the new compartment of the translocated molecule – that is, the blood – ensures that the drug compound is ionised and cannot permeate back from whence it came (Brody et al., 1998; Rang et al., 2000).

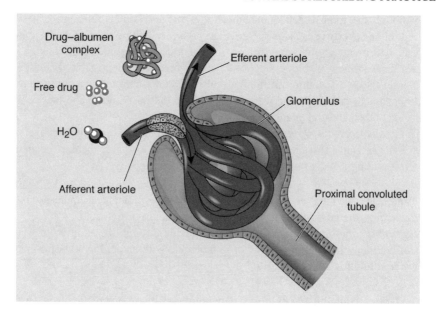

Figure 1.8 Glomerular filtration of drugs of low molecular weight. Reproduced by permission of MA Healthcare. (See also colour plate 8).

These reabsorption mechanisms underline the value of phase one and phase two metabolism to irreversible elimination of a drug from the body (Brody et al., 1998; Seeley et al., 2000).

PLASMA CONCENTRATION

Sustaining drug serum plasma levels within the range in which a therapeutic agent is simultaneously safe and effective is a major part of good medicines management. Clearance is the singularly most important parameter, but there are a number of others that deserve consideration.

THERAPEUTIC INDEX

The margin of safety within which drug treatment is delivered and sustained is called the *therapeutic index (TI)*. The TI is calculated by dividing the plasma level above which the drug becomes toxic, the maximum safe concentration (MSC) or *toxic threshold*, by the level below which the drug is ineffective, the *subtherapeutic threshold* or minimum effective concentration (MEC) (Figure 1.9). When this ratio is 2.0 or less the drug in question is said to have a narrow therapeutic index and must be used in conjunction with strict regular monitoring of plasma levels. The cardiac drug digoxin (Gibbs et al., 2000), the antibiotic gentamicin (Sorger et al.,

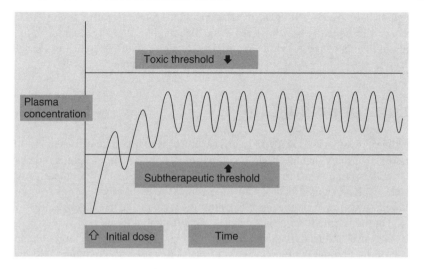

Figure 1.9   The therapeutic index. (See also colour plate 9).

1999) and the mood stabiliser lithium carbonate (Jefferson, 2002) are all examples of drugs with a narrow TI.

HALF LIFE

The *half life* $(t_{\frac{1}{2}})$ is the time taken for the drug's plasma concentration to decrease by half. This means that 500 mg of a drug with a half life of four hours entering the bloodstream at 9 a.m. has a plasma concentration of 250 mg by 1 p.m. and 125 mg by 5 p.m. A *steady state concentration (SSC)* is a plateauing drug plasma level achieved when the amount of drug eliminated per dose interval is equal to the dose of that interval. A good rule of thumb is that drug plasma levels reach a therapeutic level after four or five half lives from the time of the initial dose and that doses should be given with every passing half life in order to sustain an SSC. In Figure 1.9 the SSC is represented by the wave form, with maintenance doses being given at the low points of the configuration. In the example given above repeat doses would be given every four hours.

   Knowledge of the half life and TI of a drug is important when calculating the recommended dosage and frequency of administration, because a drug with a long half life and a narrow therapeutic index may only be given once a day. In contrast, a drug with a short half life and a broad therapeutic index may be given several times per day. In some cases, the drug half life is so short that an initial 'loading dose' of twice the maintenance dose is given to ensure a higher initial plasma concentration level and that maximal therapeutic effect is attained quickly. For example, in cases where a patient has a severe infection and the drug of choice has a sufficiently broad TI, a loading dose may be given to accelerate clinical response time. The individual half life of a drug also helps calculate total clearance time if there is a need to subsequently administer a drug that might adversely interact with any plasma remnants of the previous agent. This explains why adherence to an agreed medication schedule is vital for effective treatment (Downie et al., 1995).

VOLUME OF DISTRIBUTION

The volume of distribution (Vd) is a measurement of the extent to which a drug is dissolved throughout the body's compartments. In a man weighing 70 kg, the total blood volume is 5 litres and the total fluid volume of body compartments is 40 litres. A blood sample is taken at 'time zero' (the point at which the drug enters the bloodstream) and if plasma concentration is found to be significantly lower than the administered dose, it is assumed that substantial tissue perfusion has taken place. Because of the hypothetical nature of the estimation, the term 'apparent' volume of distribution is often used. Some drugs that are very lipophilic will have a greater binding affinity to adipose tissue and therefore their overall Vd may appear to be in excess of total body fluid volume (Brody et al., 1998).

Table 1.1   Learning exercise

1. Choose any one drug commonly used in your practice.
2. List your working knowledge of this drug in practice, including dosage range, formulation and route of administration.
3. Construct a pharmacological profile of the drug including absorption, half life, volume
   of distribution and elimination route. Describe the drug's therapeutic action at receptor
   level and explain any contraindications and side effects.
4. Justify your practical working knowledge of the drug using the profile you have
   constructed.

THE RELATIONSHIP BETWEEN PARAMETERS

All pharmacokinetic parameters should be seen as relating to one another. Although clearance and volume of distribution are independent in their function, they have a direct impact in health and disease states on the half life and margin of therapeutic safety. Hepatic and renal disease both compromise clearance and can increase the half life of drugs. Increased absorption also increases the volume of distribution. Drug interactions are also relevant. Digoxin is one of many drugs that when inter-acting with others at different points in the pharmacokinetic cycle may have its volume of distribution and peak plasma concentration adversely altered, with toxic results (Haji and Movahed, 2000).

AGE

EARLY LIFE

Children cannot be treated as linear adults in terms of prescribed dosage. The *British National Formulary for Children* should be adhered to when prescribing medicines for children and adolescents. The age ranges identified against which to prescribe for the young (neonate, infant, child and adolescent) reflect the variance in the pace of growth during a specific time period (National Prescribing Centre, 2000).

Absorption

The pH gradient of a young child's alimentary tract is not as steep as in adulthood and the rate of gastric emptying varies a great deal in infants of under 6 months. Peristalsis is also slower. This can lead to higher levels of drug absorption. Peripheral perfusion and muscle mass are lower in the young, which can compromise absorption from an injection site. A child's topical surface area is proportionately larger and skin thinner, which results in greater absorption of topical agents.

Distribution

The higher body water content associated with the early years of life means that there will overall be a lower concentration of a drug at intracellular and receptor levels. Adipose tissue acts as a bank for residual drug and, as children have less body fat content, the pharmacodynamic response is likely to be swifter and more potent.

Metabolism and Elimination

Drug potency in neonates is also increased by the reduced plasma protein concentration and consequently higher levels of unbound active drug. The development of the cytochrome P450 enzymes continues until 3 years old. This, together with the fact that glomerular fitration and renal perfusion rates are reduced in infants, means that hepatic and renal clearance of drugs is less efficient in the very young, leading to longer half lives of administered medication, greater pharmacological effect and potential toxicity (National Prescribing Centre, 2000; Walker and Edwards, 2003).

ADVANCED AGE

Absorption

Gastric emptying, reduced mesenteric blood flow, reduced peripheral perfusion and skeletal muscle mass are all characteristic of advanced age. While overall the resultant pattern is one of slowed absorption from the gut and injection sites and therefore a delayed therapeutic response, there are some exceptions to this rule.

Delayed gastric emptying may mean that enteric coated medication intended for absorption in the gut may be absorbed earlier in the stomach. Also changes in bowel habit, not uncommon in old people, may interfere with the enterohepatic cycle (Heath and Scofield, 1999; National Medicines Information Centre, 2000).

Distribution

Old people have reduced intracellular fluid levels, an indication of increased concentration of drug at the receptor sites with enhanced effects. Increased levels of adipose tissue in the older patient predispose lipid-soluble drugs to a longer half life. Reduced plasma protein concentration means that more unbound active drug is present at any one time. On the other hand, a more sluggish systemic circulation results in slower 'bulk flow' transport of therapeutic agents (Heath and Scofield, 1999).

Metabolism and Elimination

Reduced hepatic perfusion would appear to be more responsible for reduced hepatic clearance in old age than enzymatic changes. While there is considerable variation among individuals, the overall tendency in the older population is one of decline in glomerular filtrate rate and tubular function. This, together with reduced renal blood flow, means that the risk of drug toxicity and overdose is increased (Heath and Scofield, 1999; Walker and Edwards, 2003).

Prescribing Implications for Older People

Receptor Sensitivity

The ageing process is known to produce drug receptor changes that appear to cause increased sensitivity to some drugs. These changes include a decrease in the number of receptors, reduced receptor affinity for specific ligands and the reduced response of target tissues (Department of Health, 2001).

Cognition

There is evidence (discussed in more detail in Chapter 2) to suggest that older people are not as forgetful and easily confused as previously thought and that many retain judgement, skill and independence throughout life. Nevertheless, cognitive centre changes mean that such problems are incidental to old age and that individual assessment, dosage and dose titration are required. Regular evaluation and review are also important to measure progress and address any practical difficulties arising from the prescribed regimen. Anticholinergics, H_2 antagonists and beta-blockers are examples of drugs that can cause confusion in the elderly and should be used with caution.

Cardiovascular Stability

Altered orthostatic circulatory response means that drugs that reduce sympathetic nervous activity such as barbiturates, benzodiazepines, antihistamines and morphine are more likely to cause hypotension in older people. The same applies to agents that block adrenoreceptors, such as trycyclic antidepressants and phenothiazines. Some anti-Parkinsonian drugs also fall within this category.

Postural Control

Increased corrective movement aimed at sustaining balance is required of many old folk. Consequent prospects of prolonged complicated recovery from injury caused by falls means that hypnotics and tranquillisers are contraindicated in this age group, as they can exacerbate problems with postural control. The fragmented sleep patterns that often characterise this time of life also make the use of hypnotics unsound in older people, as they merely induce sleep rather than sustain it.

Body Temperature Regulation

The problems sometimes experienced by the old relating to thermoregulation make inadvisable the prescribing of drugs that have a sedatory effect leading to vasodilation. Benzodiazepines, tricyclic antidepressants and opiods all meet this description. Even the moderate consumption of alcoholic beverages with or without drugs should be viewed with caution for the same reasons.

Visceral Muscle Function

Altered visceral muscle function occurs in old age. Medicines that directly or indirectly affect muscle tone may cause unnecessary discomfort and distress to older patients. Loop diuretics may exacerbate episodes of incontinence in patients with genito-urinary problems. Anticholinergic drugs have been known to cause urinary retention in older men. Reduced motility of the gut means that constipation as a documented side effect of opiates, trycyclic antidepressants and anticholinergic drugs is more likely to occur if prescribed for older people (Heath and Scofield, 1999; Walker and Edwards, 2003; Curtis et al., 2004).

Safe and effective prescribing behaviour is all the more challenging when treating groups who are vulnerable or who have special needs. Health advice that provides alternative and less risk-laden strategies to medicine is always an important part of the consultation. This is discussed in Chapter 4.

ADVERSE REACTIONS: PATHOGENESIS AND TREATMENT

Concern over public safety in the face of increasing adverse drug events means that pharmacovigilance has become a key part of the prescribing practitioner's armoury in the drive for optimum medicines management (NPC and National Primary Care Research and Development Centre, 2002; Walker and Edwards, 2003). The Audit Commission (2002) reported an increase in the number of patients suffering adverse drug events, adding that this resulted in extended hospital stays, increased professional deployment and an additional cost to the NHS of over £1 billion.

An adverse drug event or reaction has been defined by the World Health Organization as 'any response to a drug which is noxious and unintended, and which occurs at doses normally used in man for prophylaxis, diagnosis, or therapy of disease or for the modification of physiological function' (Consultant Council for International Organizations of Medical Sciences, 1993: 45). However, this definition has been criticised as failing to include the reactions occurring as a result of human error. For many, a more comprehensive definition might simply be 'an undesirable response to a therapeutic agent'.

CLASSIFICATION

According to Rawlins and Thompson (1977), adverse reactions can be broadly divided into two types: A and B. Type A reactions are related to the pharmacokinetics of a drug and are therefore predictable when these are known. Many such adverse drug events result from interaction with other agents at different points in the pharmacokinetic process. They are dose related and, while morbidity and incidence are high, mortality is usually low and the effects of the reaction subside when the drug is withdrawn. Type B reactions are largely unpredictable and individual to the patient. Such reactions also take place at different points in the pharmacokinetic process, but instead of being dose related have their roots in the patient's genetic make-up. Mortality is high.

Aronson and Ferner (2003) proposed a new classification system for adverse drug reactions based on dose responsiveness, time course and susceptibility. While this can be recommended to the prescribing student as a valuable multidimensional tool for practice, Rawlins and Thompson's system is used here as it facilitates a better understanding of the processes at work.

Predisposing Factors

Polypharmacy by virtue of increased risk of synergistic interaction predisposes the patient to an adverse drug event (National Prescribing Centre, 1999). However, it should be remembered that multiple drug therapy is usually in place to treat multiple disease states, which may also affect pharmacokinetics. The very old and the very young are also susceptible and women are at greater risk, although it is uncertain why this is so. Genetic and familial factors also play a part (Walker and Edwards, 2003).

Type A

The rate and extent of absorption are influenced by gastrointestinal motility, gut pH and conjugation. It follows, therefore, that drugs that increase gastric emptying such as metoclopramide will consequently increase the absorption of some other medicines. H_2 antagonists such as ranitidine alter the gut pH to the extent that absorption of some drugs by passive diffusion is reduced. In a process known as chelation, the tetracycline group of antimicrobials binds with trivalent and divalent ions, including calcium and iron found in dairy products and antacids, resulting in poor absorption. Therapeutic plasma levels will be affected accordingly (Rang et al., 2000; Walker and Edwards, 2003).

The key role played by plasma protein binding, discussed earlier, may be disrupted through drug displacement, either where drugs such as aspirin and warfarin compete for binding sites or in hepatic disease where raised levels of bilirubin can also cause displacement of bound agents. The consequence of this is increased potency of a prescribed drug at the site of action beyond what has been planned, although in the absence of other mechanisms the effect is usually transient (Sellers, 1979; Brown, 1999).

Drugs may also affect metabolism by inducing (in the case of drugs such as phenytoin) or inhibiting (in the case of erythromycin) cytochrome P450 enzymes. The metabolism of other drugs that are in concurrent use may also be affected (Cupp and Tracy, 1998; Yamazaki et al., 2001). Drugs with a narrow therapeutic index are the most likely participants in such interactions, as the margin of safety between ineffectiveness and toxicity is so small. Alternative therapies used in conjunction with prescribed, pharmacy-only or general sales list medicines can also cause adverse reactions. St John's Wort and some formulations of ginseng have been known to adversely effect the metabolism of warfarin (Greenblatt and Von Moltke, 2005).

In the *British National Formulary*, potential interactions and contraindications such as this are always listed alongside any given drug to help guide safe and effective prescribing.

Type B

The unpredictable nature of type B reactions is explained only by idiosyncrasy. Genetic disposition and host factors such as underlying disease processes have been known with hindsight to be responsible. It is also thought that environmental factors may also be at work in some cases. Allergies in the shape of drug hypersensitivity require further categorisation.

Drug Hypersensitivity Reactions

Hypersensitivity occurs when a parent drug or drug metabolite alone or in combination with a hapten acts as an antigen stimulating the immune system into action. The idiosyncratic and unpredictable nature of drug hypersensitivity reactions mean that their place in Rawlins and Thompson's classification is within the type B category. The greater the molecular weight and chemical complexity of a drug, the more likely it is to be independently immunogenic. Streptokinase is one example of such a compound. Drugs with a smaller molecular weight (less than 1,000 daltons) need to conjugate with a protein to stimulate the immune system. This can only take place following re-exposure of the host to a metabolite, parent drug or related substance. It can therefore be defined as an immune response to a therapeutic agent in a sensitised patient. Although the purpose of the immune system is to protect the body from potentially harmful organisms that have been absorbed, the response may be so disproportionate as to damage adjacent tissue. This is a localised reaction. Much less common is the situation in which the immune cascade powers a systemic reaction that is potentially fatal to the host. This is more likely to occur if the antigen is administered parenterally. Such a systemic reaction is termed anaphylaxis. Drug hypersensitivity accounts for around 5–10% of all adverse drug reactions (Riedl and Casillas, 2003).

Gell and Coombs (1975) classified hypersensitive reactions and their categories are used here to help explain the background pathology. However it should be remembered that such classification is artificial. In the world of clinical practice, these demarcation lines are often blurred and some drug reactions will present with symptoms of more than one type or with symptoms that do not strictly fit any one (Riedl and Casillas, 2003).

Type I IgE Hypersensitivity   IgE hypersensitivity is an allergic reaction. It has also been called immediate hypersensitivity (Brody et al., 1998) because of the speed of its onset. A drug or hapten-conjugated agent, once absorbed, stimulates B lymphocyte cells to produce large numbers of IgE antibodies. This is done by activating the T helper cells to produce cytokines, which in turn recruit mast cells, basophils and macrophages. The antibodies bind to the antigens and inactivate them. Following this neutralisation process, the excess antibodies bind to mast cells in the tissues and basophils in the plasma via the Fc receptors on the cell surface (Figure 1.10). The half life of membrane-bound IgE is substantially longer than serum IgE. This is the point at which the antigen becomes known to the immune system. It is as if a photograph has been taken of the invasive substance that permits recognition by the body should it ever be exposed to the antigen again (Kumar et al., 2003). Such 'priming' or sensitisation of the mast cells directly predisposes the host to type I drug-specific hypersensitivity.

Re-exposure to the same antigen sets in motion the same sequence of events regardless of the length of the interim time period. The newly reintroduced antigens crosslink the mast cell IgE antibodies and initiate a series of intracellular messages that result in degranulation, consisting of two distinct waves of mediator release (Figure 1.11). The first wave includes histamine, which causes increased vascular permeability, vasodilation, bronchoconstriction and increased secretion of mucus. The second wave of mediators is much more potent than the first. The cell membrane phospholipids produce arachidonic acid, which sets up two metabolic pathways: the

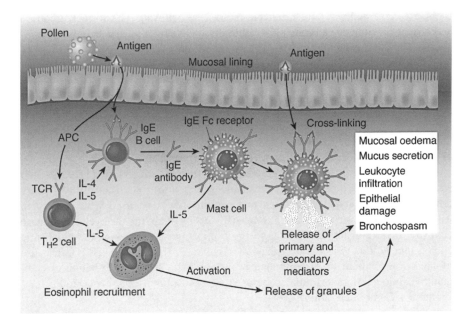

Figure 1.10 Type I hypersensitivity: excess antibodies bind to mast cells in the tissues. Reproduced by permission of MA Healthcare. (See also colour plate 10).

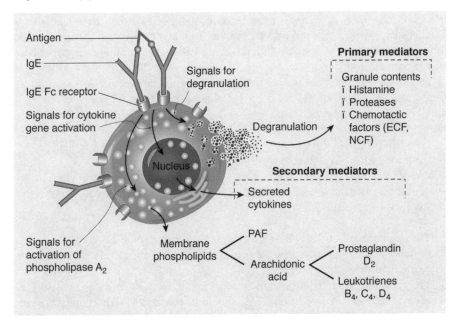

Figure 1.11 Type I hypersensitivity: antigens initiate a sense of intracellular messages. Reproduced by permission of MA Healthcare. (See also colour plate 11).

5-lipoxygenase pathway and the cyclo-oxygenase pathway. The former produces leukotrienes, which drive bronchial smooth muscle contraction and vascular permeability. The latter produces prostaglandins and thromboxanes, which together cause bronchospasm, more histamine secretion and platelet aggregation, and stimulate pain receptors. All products of mast cell granulation are also chemotactic; that is, they recruit other immune cells such as eonisophils and neutrophils.

There are two phases to an allergic reaction with two corresponding sets of clinical symptoms. The initial response takes place 5–30 minutes following re-exposure of the host to the allergen and lasts approximately one hour. The second phase takes place 2–8 hours later and lasts for several days.

IgE hypersensitivity is the mediator route for the onset of asthma (Taylor, 1998) and the detail of its pathogenesis explains why non-steroidal anti-inflammatory drugs (NSAIDs) such as ibuprofen and aspirin should be used with caution in patients suffering from this condition. NSAIDs act by inhibiting the cyclo-oxygenase pathway, diverting greater impetus to the 5-lipoxygenase pathway and enhancing leukotriene production (Baud et al., 1987; Funk, 2001; Kimball, 2004). The use of such drugs should be discontinued in patients who show exacerbation of asthmatic symptoms. Paracetamol can be used as a substitute (Rang et al., 2000; Joint Formulary Committee, 2006).

B-lactam antibiotics have been shown to produce type I hypersensitivity in some patients (Solensky, 2003). Also since Nutter (1979) noted topical reactions to latex, the use of latex gloves among healthcare professionals has increased dramatically as a result of regulatory advice on the prevention of HIV transmission (Department of Health, 1998). It is perhaps not surprising, then, to find that there has been a parallel increase in type I IgE hypersensitivity to the latex proteins absorbed in the lubricant powder of latex gloves (Charous et al., 1994). An alarming example of how such hypersensitivity may develop by introduction via the respiratory airways is evident in the fact that skin contact in such cases is not a prerequisite to absorption. Lubricant powder propelled into the surrounding air when gloves are removed may be inhaled by others (United States Food and Drug Administration Center for Devices and Radiological Health, 1997).

Type I hypersensitivity can also be induced by pollen, dust, animal hair and by certain foods such as peanuts, seafood and eggs (Kimball, 2004).

In anaphylaxis, the patient will present with respiratory distress characterised by bronchospasm and laryngeal oedema, severe abdominal cramps and hypotensive shock. First-line treatment is:

1. The maintenance of the patient's airway and administration of oxygen.
2. Positional management of blood pressure by laying the patient in the supine position and elevating their feet.
3. The intramuscular administration of adrenaline 500 micrograms (0.5 ml adrenaline injection 1 in 1,000). This should be repeated at five-minute intervals until viable cardiovascular stability is achieved.
4. Discontinuation of the allergenic agent and the patient educated about avoiding allergens.

Intravenous corticosteroids are sometimes used to suppress and minimise the effects of phase two of type I reactions (Joint Formulary Committee, 2006).

Type II IgG and IgM Hypersensitivity In IgG and IgM hypersensitivity the drug molecule binds to the surface of a blood cell, inducing antibody production. On subsequent exposure, the drug–protein complex bound to the antibody induces complement fixation, leading to cell death. This occurs in one of two ways:

1. Complements C5–9 form the membrane attack complex (MAC), a doughnut-shaped complex that embeds itself in the blood cell, creating a channel through the surface membrane. This 'hole-punching' technique causes osmotic flux and the cell swells and bursts. This is osmotic lysis (Figure 1.12).
2. The antibody-bound drug–protein complex becomes coated in opsonins or fragments of complement C3b. This makes the complex chemotactic to macrophages and therefore susceptible to phagocytosis. This is opsonization (Figure 1.13).

Haemolytic anaemia, agranulocytosis or thrombocytopenia can occur as a result of type II hypersensitivity. Incompatible blood transfusions and rhesus incompatibility (Sandler and Sandler, 2004), quinine and methyldopa (Daniels and Calis, 2001) have all been recorded as catalysts of this type of reaction.

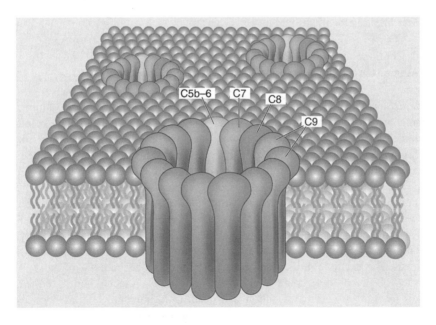

Figure 1.12 Type II hypersensitivity: the membrane attack complex. Reproduced by permission of MA Healthcare. (See also colour plate 12).

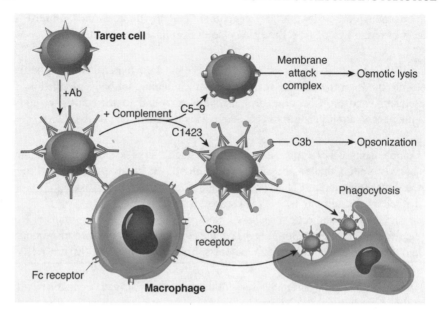

Figure 1.13 Type II: hypersensitivity: drug protein complex induces complement fixation. Reproduced by permission of MA Healthcare. (See also colour plate 13).

First-line treatment is:

1. Discontinue the causative therapeutic agent.
2. Administer parenteral corticosteroids (Riedl and Casillas, 2003).

Type III (Immune Complex Mediated) Hypersensitivity Circulating antibodies interact with the therapeutic agent while it is still in the plasma. The resultant immune complexes cannot easily be managed by phagocytes and deposit themselves in the blood vessel walls and base membranes. This activates the complement system. Complements C3–5 initiate mast cell degranulation and recruit neutrophils. This consequently causes increased vascular permeability. Depending on their size, immune complexes deposit themselves in the blood vessel walls or in subepithelial tissue. Neutrophils release lytic enzymes, which cause tissue damage (Figure 1.14).

The number of immune complexes and the extent of the immune deposit spread dictates the size of the reaction, which may range from inflammation to tissue necrosis. For example, a localised reaction may occur at the point of entry. This is often observed some hours after administration of a vaccine and is termed an arthus reaction. A systemic reaction will result from immune complex deposits in the synovial membrane joints and the glomerular tissue of the renals.

The type III hypersensitivity clinical manifestation, Steven–Johnson syndrome, has been traced to administration of sulphonamides. The anti-convulsant phenytoin, antisera (Daniels and Calis, 2001), the anti-hypertensive hydralazine (Riedl and

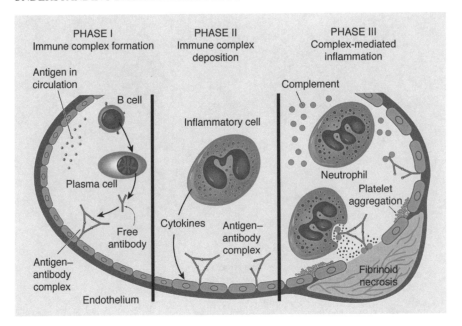

Figure 1.14 Type III hypersensitivity. Reproduced by permission of MA Healthcare. (See also colour plate 14).

Casillas, 2003) and the ACE inhibitor captopril (Schatz et al., 1989) have also been linked to type III hypersensitivity reactions.

The treatment of choice is similar to that for type II hypersensitivity (Riedl and Casillas, 2003).

Type IV (Cell-Mediated) Hypersensitivity Cell-mediated hypersensitivity occurs mainly in the skin. It is said to be cell mediated because it is facilitated by sensitised T cells rather than antibodies. A local area of erythema can be detected after 8–12 hours, but produces a full inflammatory response after 24 to 72 hours. This slow onset has earned this reaction the title of 'delayed onset hypersensitivity'.

A drug antigen in combination with skin proteins interacts with T lymphocytes leading to production of cytokines that attract basophils, which in turn produce macrophages, resulting in tissue damage (Figure 1.15).

Sulphonamide administration can result in type IV hypersensitivity (Cribb et al., 1997); photosensitivity arising from treatment with anti-psychotic drugs is another example of delayed-onset hypersensitivity (Warnock and Morris, 2002). Some substances can produce a type IV hypersensitivity through mere contact in some people. Nickel allergy is an example of contact sensitisation (Rahilly and Price, 2003). Latex features here as it does in IgE hypersensitivity, but in the case of type IV it is not the latex proteins that provoke the reaction but the chemicals used in processing (Wyss et al., 1993; Sommer et al., 2002). The increase in occupational health hazards encountered in the use of latex gloves has led to their replacement with vinyl gloves where possible in many healthcare settings.

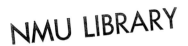

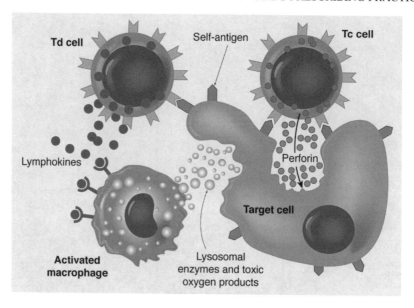

Figure 1.15 Type IV hypersensitivity. Reproduced by permission of MA Healthcare. (See also colour plate 15).

Besides discontinuation of the causative drug in question, recommended treatment for this reaction is the use of topical corticosteroids (Riedl and Casillas, 2003).

Table 1.2 Learning exercise

1. List the 20 most commonly used drugs in your practice.
2. Cross-reference your list with the BNF and identify side effects and contraindications.
3. Identify drugs that have a narrow therapeutic index, or cause enzyme induction or enzyme inhibition.
4. Identify those patients within your prescribing remit who are most vulnerable to adverse drug events and profile the diverse evidence base for this.
5. Review the medication profile of a patient in a vulnerable group.

Reproduced by permission of MA Healthcare.

CONCLUSION

No one prescriber in any profession has a comprehensive knowledge of every drug. Most are familiar with a few dozen that they regularly prescribe. Once a basic working knowledge of pharmacology is in place, continuing professional development in this field should be directed by reflective practice towards the specialist field in which the practitioner prescribes in order to maintain competence. This is where in-depth therapeutic knowledge finds its place.

GLOSSARY

Agonist: a drug that stimulates receptors.

Antagonist: a drug that diminishes the message normally transmitted by receptors.

Antigens: large molecules of 10,000 daltons or more that stimulate adaptive immunity.

Complement: a group of 20 plasma proteins that increase vascular permeability, stimulate histamine, activate kinins, lyse cells, promote phagocytes, attract neutrophils, monocytes, macrophages and eosinophils.

Drug receptor: the site of drug action where a molecular event occurs.

Half life: the time taken for the drug's plasma concentration to decrease by half.

Haptens: small molecules capable of combining with a protein carrier and acting as an antigen.

Histamine: an amine released from mast cells, basophils and platelets. Histamine causes vasodilation and smooth muscle contraction, increases vascular permeability and attracts eosinophils.

Leukotrienes: a group of lipids produced by mast cells and basophils that causes prolonged smooth muscle contraction (especially in the bronchioles), increases vascular permeability and attracts neutrophils and eosinophils.

Ligand: a substance that binds with a receptor.

Mast cells and basophils: The 'production factories' of the immune system, those derived from bone marrow. As granulocytes, their cytoplasm contains mediators that when stimulated power up the immune response. Although similar in their structure and function, mast cells are widely found in tissue, particularly near blood vessels and nerves, while basophils are mainly blood borne.

Metabolism: the means by which a drug is chemically altered to facilitate elimination from the body.

Prodrug: a drug that produces a metabolite that exerts a greater therapeutic response than the parent drug.

Subtherapeutic threshold: the level below which the drug is ineffective.

Therapeutic index: the margin within which drug treatment is delivered and sustained in a safe but effective dosage range.

Therapeutics: the branch of pharmacology that is concerned with the use of drugs to produce a desired clinical response in an individual.

Toxic threshold: the plasma level above which a drug becomes toxic.

Voltage gated: a ligand's access to bind with a receptor is allowed or prevented by an electrical charge.

Volume of distribution: a measurement of the extent to which a drug is dissolved throughout the body's compartments.

APPENDIX: DRUGS AND NUMERACY

by Petra Clarke, University of Lincoln

VOLUME MEASUREMENTS

1 litre = 1000 millilitres (ml)

WEIGHT MEASUREMENTS

1 gram (g) = 1000 milligrams (mg)

1 milligram = 1000 micrograms (mcg, microg orμg)

1 mcg = 1000 nanograms

LENGTH MEASUREMENTS

1 metre (m) = 100 centimetres (cm)

1 cm = 10 millimetres (mm)

CONVERTING FROM LITRES TO MILLILITRES (I.E. NO. 1000 TIMES BIGGER)

When multiplying by any factor of ten, the decimal point should be moved to the **right**, so when converting to values that are 1000 times greater the decimal point needs to move 3 places to the right, e.g. 0.5 litres = 500 ml

CONVERTING FROM MICROGRAMS TO MILLIGRAMS (I.E. NO. 1000 TIMES SMALLER)

When dividing by factors of ten, the decimal point should be moved to the **left**, so when converting to values that are 1000 times smaller the decimal point needs to move 3 places to the left, e.g. 5000 mcg = 5 mg

CALCULATING A DRUG DOSE FROM THE AVAILABLE STRENGTH OF A DRUG

Exercises such as this are made easier by translating all the figures involved (those of the prescribed dose and those of the drug strength held in stock) into the same unit of measurement.

1. The prescribed dose is 300 micrograms. The dose in stock is 0.1 milligrams. To convert 0.1 mg to micrograms the decimal point is moved 3 places to the right:

$$0.1 \text{ mg} = 100 \text{ micrograms}$$

2. On administration the prescribed dose should be divided by the dose in stock:

$$\frac{\text{Prescribed dose}}{\text{Dose in stock}} = \text{number of tablets administered:}$$

$$\frac{300 \text{ micrograms}}{100 \text{ micrograms}} = 3 \text{ tabs}$$

3. Within prescribing, you should familiarise yourself with the different strengths and formulations of individual drugs:

$$\frac{\text{Amount you need}}{\text{Amount of drug within formulation}} = \text{Amount to prescribe}$$

Tablets or capsules are straightforward:

$$\frac{\text{Dosage you want}}{\text{Dosage per tablet}} = \frac{1000 \text{ mg}}{500 \text{ mg}}$$

$$\frac{1\text{g paracetamol}}{500 \text{ mg tablets}} = \text{Two tablets}$$

Suspensions are slightly different. Again you need to ensure you are working both figures in the same measurement, but also consider the amount of liquid it is in:

$$\frac{\text{What you want}}{\text{What you've got}} \times \text{What it's in}$$

$$\frac{1\text{g paracetamol}}{250 \text{ mg/5ml}} \times 5\text{ml} = \frac{1000 \text{ mg}}{250 \text{ mg}} \times 5 \text{ ml} = 20 \text{ ml}$$

THE USE OF BODY WEIGHT IN DRUG CALCULATIONS

Body weight may be used in the calculation of dosage for children or adults and this will be expressed as mg/kg. For a child who weighs 15 kg the medication ibuprofen has a daily dose of 20 mg/kg and this is to be administered three times daily. The calculation would be:

$$\frac{\text{Daily drug dose} \times \text{patient weight} = \text{daily amount} \div \text{individual doses}}{20 \text{ mg} \times 15 \text{ kg} = 300 \text{ mg} \div 100 \text{ mg} \times 3}$$

Therefore if the oral suspension is 100 mg/5 ml, the amount prescribed would be (100 mg) 5 ml three times a day.

THE AMOUNT TO SUPPLY

The supply amount is very important when prescribing, as it can have an effect on concordance and time management. A 28-day quantity is accepted as best practice, however you should take note of the different pack size of medications, especially if more than one drug is being prescribed. One way around providing un-equivalent quantities is to prescribe weekly or monthly; the pharmacist is then able to decide the easiest option. Also, ensure that an appropriate amount is given, for example a prescription of two tablets to be taken four times a day, supply 24 would be inappropriate (not to mention expensive) for a long-term condition. 112 or 224 would be a more reasonable option.

GENERAL SAFETY TIPS

1. There is a difference in terms of bioavailability between different forms of drugs, so remember that a tablet can have a different active ingredient to liquid, which can be different again to an injection or suppository.
2. Be familiar with modified-release preparations and ensure the correct dosing schedule is adhered to.
3. Remember, if writing a prescription that can be termed 'as required' you should stipulate the minimum dose interval.
4. Be sure that the number of pills prescribed matches the duration of treatment.
5. Do not assume that the pharmacist will advise your patient about side effects and precautions.
6. If reviewing a patient and changing medication, do not forget to cross off original medication.
7. Try not to rely on your memory.
8. Beware of interruptions (distractions) while writing prescriptions; this is a major cause of prescription error.
9. Ensure safety by good team communication.
10. If in doubt – do not prescribe it!

REFERENCES

Aronson, JK & Ferner, RE (2003) Joining the DoTS: New approach to classifying adverse drug reactions. *British Medical Journal* **327**(7425): 1222–1225.

Audit Commission (2002) *A Spoonful of Sugar*. London: Audit Commission Publications.

Baud, L, Perez, J, Denis, M & Ardaillou, R (1987) Modulation of fibroblast proliferation by sulfidopeptide leukotrienes: Effect of indomethacin. *Journal of Immunology* **138**(4): 1190–1195.

Brody, TM, Larner, J & Minneman, KP (1998) *Human Pharmacology, Molecular to Clinical* (3rd edition). St Louis, MO: Mosby.

Brown, AM (1999) Drug interactions that matter. *Pharmaceutical Journal* **262**(7035): 325–327.

Charous, BL, Hamilton, RG & Yunginger, JW (1994) Occupational latex exposure: Characteristics of contact and systemic reactions in 47 workers. *Journal of Allergy and Clinical Immunology* **94**(1): 12–18.

Consultant Council for International Organizations of Medical Sciences (1993) Establishing requirements for the use of terms for adverse drug reactions (ADR). *Maternal Medicine Policy* **25**: 45–6.

Cribb, AE, Pohl, LR, Spielberg, SP & Leeder, JS (1997) Patients with delayed-onset sulfonimide hypersensitivity reactions have antibodies recognizing endoplasmic reticulum luminal proteins. *Journal of Pharmacology and Experimental Therapeutics* **282**(2): 1064–1072.

Cupp, MJ & Tracy, TS (1998) Cytochrome P450: New nomenclature and clinical implications. *American Family Physician* **57**(1): 107–116.

Curtis, LH, Ostbye, T, Sendersky, V, Hutchison, S, Dans, PE, Wright A & Woosely, RL (2004) Inappropriate prescribing for elderly Americans in a large outpatient population. *Archives of Internal Medicine* **164**(15): 1621–1625.

Daniels, CE & Calis, KA (2001) Clinical analysis of adverse drug reactions. *Pharmacy Update* September/October: 1–8.

Department of Health (1998) *Guidance for Clinical Healthcare Workers: Protection Against Infection with Blood Borne Viruses, Recommendations of the Expert Advisory Group on Aids and the Advisory Group on Hepatitis*. London: The Stationery Office.

Department of Health (2001) *National Service Framework for Older People*. London: The Stationery Office.

Downie, G, Mackenzie, J & Williams, A (1995) *Pharmacology and Drug Management for Nurses*. Edinburgh: Churchill Livingstone.

Egleton, RD & Thomas, PD (2005) Development of neuropeptide drugs that cross the blood brain barrier. *NeuroRX Journal* **2**(1): 44–53.

Funk, CD (2001) Prostaglandins and leukotrienes: Advances in eicosanoid biology. *Science* **294**(5548): 1871–1875.

Gell, PGH & Coombs, RRA (1975) Classification of allergic reactions responsible for hypersensitivity and disease. In P Gell, R Coombs & P Lachmann (eds) *Clinical Aspects of Immunology*. Oxford: Blackwell.

Gibbs, CR, Davies, MK & Lip, GYH (2000) ABC of heart failure; Management: Digoxin and other inotropes, betablockers, antiarrhythmics and antithrombitic treatment. *British Medical Journal* **320**(7233): 495–498.

Greenblatt, DJ & Von Moltke, LL (2005) Interaction of warfarin with drugs, natural substances and food. *Clinical Pharmacology* **45**(2): 127–132.

Greenblatt, DJ, Sellers, EM & Koch-Weser, J (1982) The importance of protein binding for the interpretation of serum plasma drug concentrations. *Clinical Pharmacology* **22**(5): 259–263.

Haji, SA & Movahed, A (2000) Update on digoxin therapy in congestive heart failure. *American Family Physician* **62**(2): 409–416.

Heath, H & Scofield, I (1999) *Healthy Ageing: Nursing Older People*. London: Mosby Harcourt.

Jefferson, JW (2002) Rediscovering the art of lithium therapy. *Current Psychiatry Online* **1**(12) www.currentpsychiatryonline.com/2002_lithium.asp [accessed June 26, 2006].

Joint Formulary Committee (2006) *British National Formulary* **52** September. London: British Medical Association and Royal Pharmaceutical Society of Great Britain.

Kimball, J (2004) Allergies. http://users.rcn.com/jkimball.ma.ultranet/BiologyPages/A/Allergies.html [accessed June 26, 2006].

Kumar, V, Cotran, RS & Robbins, SL (2003) *Basic Pathology* (7th edition). Philadelphia: Saunders.

Lin, JH & Lu, AYH (1997) The role of pharmacokinetics and metabolism in drug development and discovery. *Pharmacological Reviews* **49**(1): 403–449.

Manfredini, S, Pavan, B, Vertuani, S, Scaglianti, M, Compagnone, D, Biondi, C, Scatturun, A, Tanganelli, S, Ferraro, L, Prasad, P & Dalpiaz, A (2002) Design, synthesis and activity of ascorbic acid prodrugs of nipecotic, kynurenic and diclophenamic acids liable to increase neurotropic activity. *Journal of Medicinal Chemistry* **45**(3): 559–562.

Mcleod, HL (2003) Pharmacokinetics for the prescriber. *Clinical Pharmacology* **31**(8): 11–17.

Murphy, M & Carmichael, AJ (2000) Transdermal drug delivery systems and skin sensitivity reactions: Incidence and management. *American Journal of Clinical Dermatology* **1**(6): 361–368.

National Medicines Information Centre (Republic of Ireland) (2000) Prescribing in the elderly. *Bulletin* **6**(1) http://www.stjames.ie/ClinicalInformation/NationalMedicines InformationCentre/NMICBulletins/2000/PrescribingintheElderlyVolume6Number12000/ [accessed June 26, 2006].

National Prescribing Centre (1999) Signposts for prescribing nurses: General principles of good prescribing. *Prescribing Nurse Bulletin* **1**(1): 1–4.

National Prescribing Centre (2000) Prescribing for Children. *MeRec Bulletin* **11**(2): 5–8.

National Prescribing Centre & National Primary Care Research and Development Centre (2002) *Modernising Medicines Management. A Guide to Achieving Benefits for Patients, Professionals and the NHS.* Liverpool NPC.

Nutter, AF (1979) Contact urticaria to rubber. *British Journal of Dermatology* **101**(5): 597–598.

Pond, SM & Tozer, TN (1984) First-pass elimination. Basic concepts and clinical consequences. *Clinical Pharmocokinetics* **9**(1): 1–25.

Rahilly, G & Price, N (2003) Nickel allergy and orthodontics. *Journal of Orthodontics* **30**(2): 171–174.

Rang, HP, Dale, MM & Ritter, JM (2000) *Pharmacology* (4th edition). Edinburgh: Churchill Livingstone.

Rawlins, MD & Thompson, JW (1977) Pathogenesis of adverse drug reactions. In DM Davies (ed.) *Textbook of Adverse Drug Reactions.* Oxford: Oxford University Press.

Riedl, MA & Casillas, AM (2003) Adverse reactions: Types and treatment options. *American Family Physician* **68**(9): 1781–1790.

Sandler, SG & Sandler, DA (2004) Transfusion reactions. www.emedicine.com/med/topic2297.htm [accessed June 26, 2006].

Schatz, PL, Mesologites, D, Hyun, J, Smith, GJ & Lahiri, B (1989) Captopril-induced hypersensitivity lung disease. An immune-complex-mediated phenomenon. *Chest* **95**(3): 685–687.

Seeley, RR, Stephens, TD & Tate, P (2000) *Anatomy and Physiology.* Boston: McGraw-Hill.

Sellers, EM (1979) Plasma protein displacement interactions are rarely of clinical significance. *Pharmacology* **18**(5): 225–227.

Silvestroni, L, Fiorini, R & Palleschi, R (1997) Partition of the organochlorine insecticide lindane into the human sperm surface induces membrane depolarization and Ca^{2+} influx. *Biochemical Journal* **321**(3): 691–698.

Solensky, R (2003) Hypersensitivity reactions to ß-lactam antibiotic. *Clinical Review of Allergy and Immunology* **24**(3): 201–219.

Sommer, S, Wilkinson, SM, Beck, MH, English, JS, Gawkrodger, DJ & Green, C (2002) Type IV hypersensitivity reactions to natural rubber latex: Results of a multicentre study. *British Journal of Dermatology* **146**(1): 114–117.

Sorger, JI, Kirk, PG, Ruhnke, CJ, Bjornson, SH, Levy, MS, Cockrin, J & Tang, P (1999) Once daily, high dose versus divided low dose gentamicin for open fractures. *Clinical Orthopaedic Journal* **366**(1): 197–204.

Taylor, AJN (1998) Asthma and allergy. *British Medical Journal* **316**(7136): 997–999.

Tortora, GJ & Grabowski, SR (2003) *Principles of Anatomy and Physiology* (10th edition). New York: John Wiley & Sons Ltd.

United States Food and Drug Administration Center for Devices and Radiological Health (1997) *Medical Glove Powder Report.* http://www.fda.gov/cdrh/glvpwd.html [accessed June 26, 2006].

Walker, R & Edwards, C (eds) (2003) *Clinical Pharmacy and Therapeutics* (3rd edition). Edinburgh: Churchill Livingstone.

Warnock, JK & Morris, DW (2002) Adverse cutaneous reactions to antipsychotics. *American Journal of Clinical Dermatology* **3**(9): 629–636.

Wyss, M, Elsner, P & Wuthrich, B (1993) Allergic contact dermatitis from natural latex without urticaria. *Contact Dermatitis* **28**(3): 154–156.

Yamazaki, H, Komatsu, T, Takemoto, K, Saeki, M, Minami, Y, Kawaguchi, Y, Shimada, N, Nakajima, M & Yokoi, T (2001) Decreases in phenytoin hydroxylation activities catalyzed by liver cytochromal P450 enzymes in phenytoin treated rats. *Drug Metabolism and Disposition* **29**(4): 427–434.

Young, YY & Koda-Kimble, MA (eds) (1995) *Applied Therapeutics: The Clinical Use of Drugs.* Vancouver: Applied Therapeutics.

2 Patient-Centred Planning and Concordance

JOHN McKINNON

'*Writing a prescription is easy but to come to an understanding with people is hard.*'

'A country doctor', in *The Kafka Project* by Mauro Nervi
(trans. Ian Johnston of Malaspina University College in Naraimo, BC, Canada)

Most books have a defining chapter, a point at which keynote values are established as pivotal to the subject in hand. In this case we hold that patient-centred planning and concordance are those values. This should not be read in any way as diminishing the worth of the other areas of knowledge pertinent to prescribing. Instead, individualised and concordant approaches are held to be pivotal in that they provide essential support for optimum and effective mosaic use of those expert skills and understandings that provide acumen in therapeutics. Without them the goals and aspirations of prescribing practice would be hollow. The practitioner who cannot recall the precise pharmacokinetics of a drug may consult a reliable current source of such information. The prescriber who is faced with an ethical conflict may take advice from an appropriate authority. On the other hand, the practitioner who is knowledgeable in pharmacology, aware of their accountability, informed by a contemporary evidence base but yet somehow in want of patient-centred principles will manifest practice that is both disabled and unsafe. In this way, patient centredness and concordance have primacy.

In this chapter theory will be solicited to demonstrate the relevance of patient-centred planning as a mindset for the prescribing situation. Concordance will be defined and shown to be an evolving concept resulting from reflection on research in therapeutics and psychology, together with allied social change and the rights of patients to self-determination. The implications for the rights of children and older people will also be discussed. The positive relationship between patient-centred planning and concordance will be explored and we will see that other desirable facets of practice can be viewed as pre-packaged subsidiaries to individualised care as a paramount concept.

Towards Prescribing Practice. Edited by J. McKinnon.
© 2007 John Wiley & Sons, Ltd.

DEFINING PATIENT-CENTRED PLANNING

In recent years the government has emphasised that patients should be placed at the core of care planning (Department of Health, 1998). This approach has been underlined by the stated preference for individualised prescribing modes (Department of Health, 2003). So the question arises: what is patient centred care and how is its absence sometimes made conspicuous in prescribing?

We have all at some point in our lives left a surgery or clinic with a prescription in our hand yet believing that our concerns had not been heard, acknowledged or addressed. In such cases it is likely that patient-centred planning was missing from the prescribing episode. Patient-centred planning is not a model or protocol, though some excellent patient-centred models exist; nor is it encapsulated in any decision-making tree, though some frameworks and pathways may facilitate this. Rather, patient-centred planning is a mindset, an attitude, an approach to practice that recognises the uniqueness of each individual and values their perspective on their care as an essential key to engineering improved health status and enhancing the quality of prescribing. In Chapter 7, Clare Allen discusses a variety of facilitative models and approaches to guide practice in this way. Here, however, we are concerned with the nature and substance of patient centredness and how it informs and promotes other working concepts that are closely related to the prescribing process.

THE MYTHOLOGY OF UNIVERSAL PATIENT-CENTRED CARE

The frequency with which the term appears in the literature might lead us to believe that patient-centred planning is well enshrined within healthcare practice. However, there is evidence to suggest that this is far from the case.

Rubin (1996) found that the experienced nurses making up the sample group of her study were experts in the clinical conditions of their patients, but when asked to recall or articulate the patient as an individual their knowledge base was deficient. Schwartz (2000) argued that paternalism superseded patient choice in many hospital procedures and professional practices. Redfern's work (1996) has shown that individualised patient care is often limited because of a number of factors. These include low staffing levels, impoverished skill mix, a rapid throughput of large, high-dependency patient populations, a lack of administrative support, the nature of ward organisation and a lack of commitment by nurse leaders and individual nurses to patient-centred planning as an ideal. She further comments that in some clinical settings, nurses claimed that patient-centred planning was practised when in fact only lip service was paid to individualised care.

This latter point confirms the impression gained by my experience of work submitted for assessment on the prescribing programme. Not infrequently, an

A4 plan of care inserted in the appendices of a reflective journal or mere token use of politically correct jargon is presented as evidence of patient-centred planning.

IDENTIFYING THE CONSTITUENTS OF THE INDIVIDUAL PATIENT PERSPECTIVE

GOOD HISTORY TAKING

> 'I should have written everything down before I went in there. Your mind goes blank so quickly. He latched on to the fact that I'm having difficulty sleeping and after that he seemed to stop listening. I didn't get the chance to talk about anything else. He was too busy looking at his watch.'

Good history taking is essential for effective prescribing behaviour and allowing the patient to tell their story in their own way is essential to good history taking (National Prescribing Centre, 1999; Epstein et al., 2000). For example, interrupting or non-empathic body language automatically conveys the impression to the patient that the practitioner's agenda is more important than theirs. Whether or not this is the correct interpretation matters little. When a patient feels interrogated or unheard rather than consulted, the information threshold between patient and practitioner rises. Consequently, the information-gathering process necessary for problem framing, accurate diagnosis, effective treatment and prescribing behaviour is incomplete. The idea that this process can be abbreviated for the sake of economy of time is actually false economy of care. Inadequate patient profiling and an overall subjective approach to care planning may result in at best poorly focused treatment and the patient making costly return visits because of unmet needs, or at worst unwanted drug interactions and adverse reactions. Good history taking therefore has a phenomenological approach at its heart.

THE 'HUMANISED' SITUATION

The pathway to identifying the perspective that shapes the patient's concerns is 'skill gated'. The clinical environment is foreign ground to patients to such an extent that it may even affect healthcare professionals when in the patient role. In order to establish the ground for individualised care, the situation must be 'humanised'. In any episode of care practitioners must first use their interpersonal skills to implicitly or explicitly identify themselves as the patient's friend and advocate in what may appear a cold, authoritative or even hostile environment. This reduces the patient's feelings of vulnerability and thaws their self-expression, releasing details that might otherwise have remained hidden. This process by which practitioners help a patient feel sufficiently 'at home' in a care setting to predispose them to openness has been called the preservation of 'personhood' (Benner et al., 1996: 21).

THE PATIENT'S INTERPRETATIONS, BELIEFS AND CONCERNS

'I brought him here today because I believed it's the right thing to do, but now I'm here I'm not so sure. I know all the experts say it's safe, but if it's safe why are all these parents saying it caused their children's autism? I can't help thinking my child might be the one to suffer a reaction.'

There is now compelling evidence to show that there is no connection between the MMR (measles, mumps and rubella) vaccine and either autism or Crohn's disease (Miller, 2003; Seagroatt and Goldacre, 2003). Previous research that appeared to show a connection has been discredited (Murch et al., 2004). Yet the UK has yet to enjoy a return to herd immunity. This is a frustrating situation for healthcare professionals who have worked hard to meet government immunisation-uptake targets and promote the safety of the MMR vaccine together with the benefits it affords to children and by extension to non-rubella-immune pregnant women. In the light of such endorsements, the practitioner may therefore view the degree of vacillation portrayed above on the part of a parent as incomprehensible. However, to do so is to fail to own the parent's perspective. The patient's beliefs, regardless of how fanciful they may seem, have been shown to be the prime motivator behind healthcare choice (Horne and Weinman, 1999). The situation as it is interpreted by the patient and the concerns it generates must be permitted to aid care planning.

Practitioner advice is but one of many variables affecting the decision making of patients. The media have been accused of generating public hysteria over the MMR vaccine by delivering an unbalanced and negative picture of its safety record (Jackson, 2002). The Internet has arguably resulted in a more informed rather than a better informed public, who have no way of checking the accuracy and neutrality of the information they download. Cultural and subcultural communities and groups form powerful internal and external lobbies to achieve their vision of desirable behaviour. The criteria for such behaviour may have underpinning values and beliefs quite distinct from those in which public health medicine is couched. They may include local folklore that time has fused into fact. Such lobbies exert pressure on the choices of individuals and instil doubt in the face of what might to a professional appear cogent evidence (Henley and Schott, 1999). The weight and quality of the information that the parent receives to support one side of an argument or the other is all too often eclipsed by the volume of alarming messages delivered. Research (Mishel, 1981, 1983; Horner, 1997) has shown how uncertainty over prognosis and management in childcare can inhibit a parent's reasoning and decision-making processes.

Reassurance, albeit on the back of evidence, is seldom sufficient by itself to secure informed consent, especially where the treatment in question has received unfavourable coverage at some point in the media. In such situations, it is vital that shared exploration of the basis for a patient's concerns and interpretations takes place (Hall, 1964). Choice is much less bewildering when one is able to weigh options for their implications. The practitioner uses this knowledge to present the client with choices that are informed by the benefits and risks as they are proportionate to each decision. This is patient-centred planning in prescribing practice.

CONCORDANCE

Concordance comes from an old French word meaning 'harmony' and the term describes an egalitarian relationship based on an agreement or contract between two individuals or groups. In the healthcare setting it has been described as 'a consultation process between a healthcare professional and a patient' (Weiss and Britten, 2003: 493). The concordance ideal is one in which the patient's knowledge of their illness experience together with the beliefs and judgements that accompany or even issue from that experience form part of shared decision making and care planning (Marinker, 1997; Department of Health, 2000). Patients also bring information about the social context of their health state – their housing conditions, geographical placement, employment and employment patterns, family and family dynamics and financial situation – which shape care planning and prescribing behaviour (Russell et al., 2003).

For the practitioner seeking concordance, the patient's dimension of expertise is a vital and highly valued source of information that assists them to frame the problem in hand, reach a diagnosis and draft a plan of care. Practitioners bring evidence-based biomedical, social and behavioural scientific expertise to the consultation. They have interpersonal skills and are aware of the socioeconomic variables at work in people's lives. They are pathophysiologically aware and select the appropriate clinical examination, test, procedure or referral to confirm their diagnosis based on current understanding. However, such professional skill and knowledge are incomplete without the contribution of the patient. It is not that one body of applied knowledge is superior to another, but rather that both are necessary to reach an accurate diagnosis and definitive care plan (Marinker, 1997; Hopkins et al., 2000).

AN ALTERED BALANCE OF POWER

This is a huge cultural shift from the traditional way in which healthcare practice in general and medical practice in particular have been conducted in the past. Until the latter part of the twentieth century, health professionals were viewed by society as 'knowing what was best' for their patients. Patients were seen as sensible if they followed the instructions of a health professional, even at the cost of their own beliefs and values. Patients who ignored, questioned or even attempted to negotiate in the face of expert health advice were seen as 'foolish' or 'difficult'. This is the 'compliance' model of treatment.

Compliance is a measure of patient cooperation with professional explanations and instructions. In the compliance model, the diagnosis, treatment and plan of care are strictly the domain of the practitioner. The patient's role is to inform the practitioner accurately of their health state (usually in the shape of a record of signs and symptoms) and then to listen, understand and 'comply' with the treatment plan. In contrast, the consultation process that promotes concordance is a phased interaction cycle (Figure 2.1), where the practitioner listens to the patient's story and sifts the resultant evidence with behavioural evidence from the interview and clinical evidence from an examination. The practitioner shares a provisional diagnosis with the patient, who then has the opportunity to provide further evidence to refute, confirm or refine this. This process in which partners in the consultation compare their respective 'pictures' continues through diagnosis, treatment options and personalised care plan formulation until a 'best fit' is agreed and concordance achieved.

The transition from compliance to concordance as the dominant mode of approach to practice means that the balance of power between prescriber and patient is altered in favour of the patient. For the prescriber, the patient is no longer the passive recipient of treatment but a partner with whom diagnosis and care planning are negotiated. The practitioner may work to persuade the patient of the way forward using research-based evidence and risk-assessment tools, but this is done from the perspective of informing choice instead of one of imposed authority.

The balance of responsibilities has also shifted. The prescriber retains responsibility for diagnosis and treatment. All healthcare professionals have a duty of care and this means that the prescriber's role in concordance is mandatory. The patient's role is voluntary in as much as they may disengage from treatment at any time, but whether or not they commit to a plan of care, they are responsible for their decisions and the consequences of those decisions (Marinker, 1997). They have the responsibility to be honest in their dealings with the practitioner. Shared decision making means that responsibility for the contract of care is also shared. Professional records need to reflect the details of this contract and these records are ideally in a format that can be shared with patients.

Madge and Harry are a couple in their early 60s whose children have left home. They enjoy travelling and are about to depart for a holiday in Spain. Harry has read that nurses are now allowed to prescribe antibiotics and he and Madge recall that when they were recently in California they both contracted chest infections and had to buy antibiotics at considerable cost at a drugstore.

Harry and Madge would like you to prescribe some antibiotics for both of them just in case the same thing happens in Spain.

What interpretations, past and present, do Madge and Harry place on antibiotics? How do those interpretations explain their concerns and how can these concerns be reconciled with issues of public health?

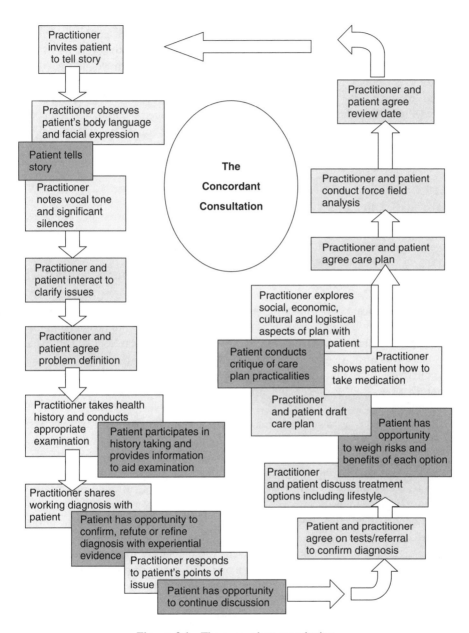

Figure 2.1   The concordant consultation

CONCEPTUAL ORIGINS OF CONCORDANCE

Concordance has evolved from a number of synergistic social, political, psychological and ethical themes. These warrant discussion for more than reasons of idle historical interest. Patient-centred values in care are very much in vogue and on the lips of every policy maker, but it does not necessarily follow that this will always be so. Realising and sustaining principles in practice requires advocacy built on knowledge of how concepts in care are related to each other. Understanding conceptual origins means that nurses and allied health professionals are able to make a more informed stand in favour of shared decision making should such values ever be challenged.

MESSAGES FROM PRACTICE

'Be alert to the faults of the patients which make them lie about the taking of the medicines prescribed and when things go wrong, refuse to confess that they have not been taking their medicine.'

Hippocrates, 200 BC

Widespread concern about the the chasm between prescribed medication directives and the medicine-taking behaviour patterns of patients led to the inauguration of a working party under the direction of the Royal Pharmaceutical Society (Marinker, 1997). A systematic review of the literature was conducted covering qualitative and quantitative research on the subject (McGavock et al., 1996). A disturbing picture emerged of wasted resources and life chances resulting from suboptimal use of medicines.

The composite message from practice was that up to one third of prescribed medication was never even dispensed and around half of medicines prescribed as part of chronic disease management were not taken properly. The breakdown of these figures to inform on clinical categories showed an 80 % default among asthma patients, 55 % among diabetics and 40 % among patients suffering epilepsy and patients with hypertension.

Researchers were also shocked to find that even in areas where medicine offered or performed a dramatic life-saving function, as in the case of the role of immunosuppressive drugs in post-operative organ transplantation management, 18 % of patients were not taking their medication as it had been prescribed. Mortality and organ failure were more than five times higher in this group than among patients who were adhering to prescribed medical directives.

These findings have profound implications for public health in terms of reduced life expectancy, morbidity and quality of life. While there is disagreement about the general extent of the health gain that improved regimen adherence would produce, it has been estimated that in the field of cardiovascular disease alone, cerebral vascular accidents and coronary heart disease could be reduced by one half and one fifth respectively.

There are implications too for the national economy in terms of days at work lost through sickness and health service expenditure. In 2001 prescription costs exceeded £6 billion, approximately 10 % of the NHS budget. In addition, the invalidity costs arising from increased morbidity are substantial.

Parallel and subsequent research (Haynes et al., 1996; Horne and Weinman, 1999; Dowell et al., 2002) has endeavoured to examine the patient psyche in the face of prescribed medicine. These studies, like the ones before them, produced a powerful consensual message. It seems that patient behaviours associated with prescribed medicine were based on very different values and beliefs from those of the prescriber, which had never been shared or elicited at the time of prescription.

There were indications that at least some of the failure to have medicine dispensed was also due to logistical and practical issues such as affordability and access to services.

Patients were found to harbour doubts about the efficacy of their medicine and would sometimes put this to the test by taking 'drug holidays'. This would sometimes become manifest in 'white coat adherence' (Marinker, 1997), a form of deceitful behaviour in which a return to appropriate adherence precedes an appointment with the prescriber. The fear that drug dependency would ensue with continued adherence, or conversely that the clinical condition in question would over time become immune to the therapeutic agent, was common. A tacit caution or even hostility towards prescribed medicines on moral grounds, which might have been more readily expected in connection with illegal drugs kept for a recreational purpose, has been noted among some patients. In contrast, patients seemed much less fearful of herbal and other alternative remedies. The patient's perception of the severity of a diagnosed illness and of the need for medication to treat that illness was often at variance with that of the physician.

The impact on patients' daily lives proved a highly influential factor in compliance with medical prescriptions. Prescribed drugs such as tranquillisers were often used to manage stress arising from the complexities of life, but equally the complexities of life such as work and eating patterns, child and family responsibilities interfered with sound management of medication timetables.

Addressing the intentional and unintentional issues of human, therapeutic and economic cost contained within these research findings requires practitioners to engage in a different level of discussion, an exploratory partnership that is not permitted by the compliance model of care. A new approach is required to address the gaps in diagnosis and care planning that only the patient contribution can fill.

Indeed, evidence exists within social science to question whether an effective therapeutic relationship could develop in any other way.

MESSAGES FROM PSYCHOLOGY

Compliance is not consistent with how we as humans act and behave (Figure 2.2). Learning and assimilating new behaviour is not simply the product of a unilateral transfer of information. As intentional beings, our behaviour indicates what motivates and matters to us much more than it reflects what we have been told to do

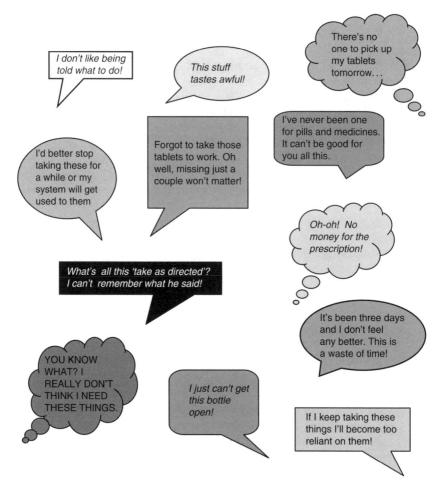

Figure 2.2 Why compliance fails

(Armitage and Conner, 2000). It would seem that much of this begins with how we perceive ourselves in relation to everything else.

In what has come to be known as his attribution theory, Rotter (1966) argued that each individual can be placed on a continuum of generalised expectancy between positions of attribution: two points of view regarding the source dictates of their decisions and behaviours. At one extreme a person can be said to have an internal locus of control, in which the individual attributes their decisions, efforts and degree of success or failure to their own abilities. At the other end of the continuum a person is said to have an external locus of control, in which they attribute the life events that affect them largely to external circumstances.

There are two different challenges here for the prescribing situation. The person with an internal locus of control will wish to take responsibility for their own health and their commitment to their share in the care plan will generally be good. However, they will by nature require and demand accurate and current information from the prescriber to assist them in making choices and they will not be easily turned from a particular opinion that they believe to be evidence based. The patient with an external locus of control will at least appear more compliant with the instructions of the prescriber, but may be just as easily swayed afterwards by other external influences. In areas of a care plan where commitment is required from such a patient, they will be less likely to take responsibility for their behaviour and may return to place this firmly with the prescriber. The 'sick role' in which a disease state excuses an individual from responsibility is closely allied to this positioning of the self.

Most crucially, neither of these patient positions can be addressed by a practitioner who expects habitual compliance.

The power of a patient's interpretations, beliefs and concerns as determinants of health behaviour is demonstrated well by Icek Ajzen (2002) in his theory of reasoned action. Ajzen exposed discrepancies between attitude and actual behaviour and argued that other factors exerting influence on intentions explain these discrepancies, namely subjective beliefs about the reactions of others to their intended behaviour and beliefs about their ability to perform the behaviour. There is some similarity between Ajzen's work and that of the health belief model (Maiman and Becker, 1974). The authors of this model argue that an individual's perception of the severity of a condition, their susceptibility to that condition and the benefits of changed behaviour all affect their motivation to challenge barriers to change. The same factors seem to influence ability to achieve and sustain that change.

Behaviourists such as Rotter, Ajzen and Becker present the prescriber with root areas of intention, which can be manipulated through compensatory interventions such as providing extra information, boosting self-confidence and offering support, reassurance and incentives.

Humanistic psychologists such as Carl Rogers (1994) take issue with such a pre-structured approach as inconsistent with the uniqueness and unpredictability of each human being. Rogers places emphasis instead on removing the perceived threat to someone's world as represented by new information or experience (e.g. a diagnosis or health lifestyle recommendation) and relating this information to their purposes, doing so in a carefully crafted atmosphere of mutual trust. This approach is closest to that adopted in the first section of this chapter.

Despite some philosophical differences, there is a clear consensus that compliance models have not kept pace with behavioural science and that a model is needed that recognises and interacts with the complexities of decision making and intentional behaviour.

CONCORDANCE AND SOCIAL CHANGE

For many the chief rationale for adopting concordance is one of human rights. The seminal work of the sociologist Ivan Illich (1977) has been deeply influential in reducing the power of the medical profession, making them more accountable to the public they serve. Placing health firmly in the broader social context, Illich portrayed doctors very differently from the traditional picture of society's chief benefactors. Drawing on public health research, he argued that twentieth-century populations owed the extent of their wellbeing to social provision, reform and the alleviation of poverty, rather than to medical science. A central point in Illich's critical appraisal of the medical profession was that their position of power had been gained through the medicalisation of social problems and the social construction of disease. This had in Illich's view led to the enforced reliance of communities on medical services. This radical perspective caused many within society to re-establish alternative health models through self-help initiatives and exploration of other therapeutic avenues. Most pertinent to issues of concordance are the challenge to the power of medicine and the championing of patients' rights that arose from this crucial change in public mood.

The 1986 World Health Organization Ottawa Convention on Human Rights (WHO, 1986) resolved that individuals had the right to participate in their own healthcare. Since that time, a series of high-profile cases of professional negligence, incompetence and even malevolence has driven public demands for still greater accountability and evidence of safe and effective practice from the medical profession. Concordance is therefore seen as a way of addressing this imbalance of power by enfranchising patients and their families.

Paternalism has been deeply ingrained in professional life and the discomfort with which some medical professionals contemplate a loss of power is evident from the alarm and confusion that have punctuated debate about concordance in health practitioner publications since the mid-1990s (Marinker and Shaw, 2003; Jones, 2003). The lack of awareness of concordance as a concept among prescribers and the lack of motivation to assimilate it within daily practice would seem to be similar to that found in connection with patient centredness (Hopkins et al., 2000; Rossi, 2003). More than a degree of self-deception would appear to be at work. According to a study conducted by Makoul et al. (1995), doctors grossly underestimate the unilateral nature of their consultations and overestimate the extent to which they conduct shared decision making with patients. The authors found that only 15 % of patients were asked their views about treatment or the care plan and 46 % were not informed of the benefits of the medication. Bond (2003) fears that just as in patient-centred planning, lip service is being paid to the notion of concordance while compliance models are what patients experience.

This superficial approach to a new culture of care in therapeutics is problematic for a number of reasons. First, to use concordance as a mere synonym for compliance is to place in jeopardy the goals of improved medicine taking set by the Royal Pharmaceutical Society's Working Party (Marinker, 1997), and with them the projected human and economic benefits.

Second, the patient experience will not improve, serving to further diminish confidence in healthcare professionals. The opportunity and ability to provide leadership at a critical time in public health history could be seriously compromised.

Third, in the case of antimicrobials, continued misuse by patients is likely to accelerate resistance and render whole groups of drugs therapeutically invalid.

Finally and perhaps most important of all, surreptitious adherence by a prescribing practitioner to a paternalistic model of treatment is illegal, as it denies the very self-determination in healthcare catalogued by the WHO Convention. Concordance is the outcome of consent. Government guidelines (Department of Health, 2001a) clearly state that consent is not valid if it can be argued that it was obtained under duress and that sensitivity was not shown as to time, place and patient perspective.

No matter how benign, in the absence of specific statutory conditions paternalistic approaches are incompatible with modern prescribing behaviour. There are three groups who may present special challenges in this regard.

CONCORDANCE AND CHILDREN

With the advent of the 1989 Children Act, children have equal rights in law with adults (Department of Health, 1989). This means that they too deserve to be consulted about treatment and to be allowed to share in decisions about their care. The law stipulates that while the extent of autonomy afforded to children should be commensurate with their development, their active involvement should be encouraged as early as possible.

Statutory specification is weighted to permit maximum possible child consultation. This is observable in the fact that parents may give consent in the face of child refusal (as in the case of childhood immunisation), but cannot override child consent (as in the case of an adolescent request for contraception; Department of Health, 2001a). While parents or other identified guardians and carers are seen as intermediaries through whom care plans may be negotiated and implemented, the health professional who engages in child healthcare is also an advocate for the child's rights (Doyle and Maslin-Prothero, 1999).

The subject of concordance and child healthcare practice calls for some honest, in-depth reflection on the part of practitioners. In Britain, child rights legislation has not been simultaneous with any supportive resources to invest in a child-friendly society or even to encourage a re-evaluation of how children are treated by individuals and communities (Leach, 2000). It is important, therefore, to be able to untangle the reality of what children are capable of understanding with appropriate assistance from our own assumptions and prejudices regarding how we expect them to behave. For example, Sanz (2003) notes that although traditionally paediatric consultations have confined communication with the child to pleasantries aimed at putting them at their ease, children have been known to eavesdrop and correct their parent's narrative. Many children between the ages of 7 and 11 are very conversant with their respective conditions and autonomous in the use of their medicines. Striving to understand a child's perception of health and illness, preventive and curative treatments opens up new possibilities in terms of concordance with the very young. The imaginative use of models, sketches and conversation skilfully pitched at the appropriate level has led to active involvement of children much younger than 7 years old (Sanz, 2003; Department of Health, 2004).

Children's rights require that medicines be palatable and with a formulation and appearance that are acceptable to a child. These issues have also been shown to boost adherence (Matsui, 1997). Children do not usually possess the coordination and dexterity of adults. Administration equipment that facilitates handling by small hands and consumption by small mouths promotes the practical aspects of drug efficacy. Oral syringes, breath-activated devices and masks are all examples of this.

A child-centred approach recognises that children are neither the property of their parents nor mini-adults. They are instead seen as individuals who want to know about their health state, their treatments and the effect that both will have on their lives (Webb, 2004). To meet these needs and achieve concordance with children, prescribers need to focus on the child. This must nevertheless be done in a way that does not alienate the parent. On the contrary, the practitioner works with the parent in a triangular partnership to fully exploit their skill as a mentor, observer, interpreter, teacher and exemplar (McklinDon and Schlucter, 2004).

The parent is a mentor in that they accompany and help the child negotiate unfamiliar situations such as the clinical setting, the new relationship with professionals and the therapeutic implications of a changing health status. This provides stability and security of emotional attachment. A child who would otherwise be uncomfortable in a clinical situation is often able to engage comfortably if sitting on their parent's knee. Listening to a child does not rule out use of the parent's observational skills. More often than not the parent's account will complement rather than conflict with that of the child. The role of interpreter is also best filled by the parent, in that whenever professional efforts at communication falter, the parent is best placed to compensate. They do this by drawing on their intimate personal knowledge of a child's personality and perception through spontaneous use of alternative language, which sometimes is known only to the parent and the child, to convey the clinician's meaning. The parent's teaching skills in reinforcement of good practice in a child's daily life and in encouraging appropriate drug administration routines and techniques are valuable assets. Finally, parents are exemplars. Children learn by watching and listening to their parents every day. This reflective observation within the family can be harnessed in the concordance partnership to help children achieve competence and responsibility in taking and safeguarding their medicines (Department of Health, 2005; Mason and Fattore, 2005).

Parent-held child records (PHCRs) consolidate the parent's role in securing concordance with children. They provide an ideal place in which to record clear, specific instructions for the administration of drugs in a way that accounts for the individual needs and understandings of both parent and children. Pre-printed information leaflets, while useful, are no substitute for this. Fully exploiting PHCR use means that parents may contribute to the individualised care of their children through planning implementation and evaluation. The content of such records often says much about the commitment of health professionals to their place in practice. Ideally, the PHCR should colourfully inform on the individuality of a child's world and personality far beyond that delivered by mere biographical detail. Contributions of the parent and child to care plans, whether sketched, written or indicated by

Table 2.1   Concordance and children

- Children are entitled to information about their health status and treatment pitched at their developmental level.
- Remember children are individuals. Don't make assumptions about their level of ability or interest.
- A child's power of consent grows with their understanding of their health status and treatment.
- Communicate directly with the child. Speak to them at eye level whenever possible. This may involve you sitting on the floor!
- Use models, pictures and drawings to improve the quality of your dialogue.
- Children are able to grasp the purpose of curative medicine more easily than that of preventative medicine.
- Negotiate the taste and formulation of prescribed medicine with the child.
- Encourage the child's interest in medicine safety.
- Recruit the support of the parent as mentor, observer, interpreter, teacher and exemplar for the child.
- Use the parent-held child record to record the prescription and care plan details. Encourage parent and child to use the record to evaluate the plan.

souvenirs about progress made and milestones achieved, mean that health concordats and the individually focused needs on which they were built are mobile and follow the child through life. This information can be used to help achieve best practice for a child served by professionals who will never meet.

Elizabeth is 14 years old and for about four months has had problems with what she calls 'her spots'. Her mother, who accompanies her to the consultation, says she arranged the appointment following a quarrel that ensued between them when Elizabeth began using her mother's facial scrub. Elizabeth's mother says she puts the problem down to her daughter's age and the fact that Elizabeth eats too much chocolate and wants you to reinforce this view. 'Everyone' at school reportedly calls Elizabeth 'pit face'.

On examination you find that Elizabeth's face, upper back and chest are covered in open and closed comedones along with some papules and pustules.

How do the different interpretations that Elizabeth and her mother place on Elizabeth's skin condition shape their concerns? How can these differences be reconciled?

How does your relationship with Elizabeth differ from your relationship with her mother and what legal issues exist in relation to Elizabeth's treatment?

What potential barriers are there to acheiving and sustaining concordance?

CONCORDANCE AND OLDER PEOPLE

In contemporary western society old age has largely been socially constructed as a time of deteriorating health and ability. Consequently, older people have often been stereotyped and marginalised, when in fact the majority are in good health and able to make sound decisions about their lives (Heath and Scofield, 1999). If these influences go unacknowledged by the prescriber, health gain will be adversely affected. Establishing a brand of concordance with the old that is real and effective requires that the practitioner be mindful of a number of special considerations.

In her critical review of the literature, Westbury (2003) found that many professional concerns about old people and medicine taking, while founded in fact, were exaggerated and that the main reasons for poor adherence in the old were very similar to the young. In some cases, adherence was actually better among the old than in younger groups.

Old people do want to be involved in decisions about their care. Cultivating the patient's knowledge of their disease process and treatment creates motivation and promotes concordance. Cultural expectations of health professionals associated with birth cohorts currently in old age have given the impression of a preference for a compliance model of care, but when concordant approaches are employed, old people have been found to respond positively (Department of Health, 2001b; Westbury, 2003).

Past research (Cornwell, 1984) has shown that many old people disguise or minimise their social and medical problems, believing these to be the unavoidable companions of old age and fearing that they will be perceived as a burden on resources and on their communities. These beliefs and fears require high levels of discretion and vigilance in history taking, on the part of the prescriber.

A number of studies (Department of Health, 2001b; Furniss, 2002) have shown that although multiple disease states in older people may necessitate a large therapeutic package, many of the drugs within medication profiles have no rationale or

Table 2.2 Concordance and older people

- Do not assume that older patients are easily confused and forgetful.
- Conduct an individual assessment to confirm level of neurological and cognitive function, sensory ability, vital organ function, mobility and level of dependence.
- Explore and encourage patient's knowledge of disease process and treatment.
- Explore lifestyle options in relation to prescription with patient.
- Explore social and physical practicalities of drug regimen with patient.
- Keep daily administration times to a minimum.
- Ensure appropriate dosage formulation.
- Ensure drug container suitability.
- Where appropriate, tailor use of aides-mémoires and dispensing kits to patient's needs.
- Where necessary, recruit support from family and friends, with the patient's agreement.
- Review medicine profile regularly.
- Cross-reference adverse reactions with new pathology states and new drug interventions.

---

are for conditions that have been reversed. It is interesting that many of these findings were in nursing homes, where on average patients were on four times as many prescribable items as their peers elsewhere and where the degree of consultation with the recipient of care may have been low.

In the older patient, individual assessment is necessary to separate stereotype from reality. The patient's mobility, level of independence, cognitive function, sensory and neurological status, as well as vital organ function all need to be profiled. The circumstances of administration are important. No matter how suitable the drug, a prescription will not be effective if the patient's arthritis prevents them from opening the container, they experience swallowing difficulties or muscle wasting makes some injection sites non-viable. Ingestion problems can be resolved by tailoring the medicine formulation and advising on technique (e.g. upright body positioning; taking tablets with water). Reducing the administration times to as few as possible may address issues of polypharmacy that cannot otherwise be resolved. Dispensing kits and the use of aides-mémoires such as calendars and diaries are usually all that is required to deal with forgetfulness. Support from family, friends and appointed carers can also be recruited (Heath and Scofield, 1999).

CONCORDANCE AND THE MENTAL HEALTH PATIENT

The nature of mental illness and the manner in which it may affect patient concentration, perception and judgement mean that there are times when the capacity to exercise autonomy with accountability is compromised in a way that could cause harm to the patient themselves or to others. This has special implications for prescribing, which are explored by Stuart Kennedy in Chapter 10.

THE RELATIONSHIP BETWEEN CONCORDANCE AND PATIENT-CENTRED PLANNING

When judging quality care, patients have been shown to ignore or forgive clumsily performed technical tasks when these are accompanied by caring behaviour that respects their individuality (Reiman, 1986). The pride of place allocated to patient-centred planning in the hierarchy of service user priorities is endorsed by Attree (2001), who noted that patients were more likely to engage and form a rapport with practitioners who anticipated their needs as individuals and built care around this. Research in medical practice also shows that the quality of the relationship between prescriber and patient is related to the calibre of health outcome (Little et al., 2001).

Concordance can therefore be seen to have a positive sequential link with patient-centred care planning. The type II diabetic, for example, will most likely concur with prescribed diet and medication when they perceive that these are tailored to interface best with their dietary preferences and essential daily routine (Crow, 2004). In fact, the work of Jacobson and colleagues (1997) has shown that failure to give attention to the psychological trauma of diabetes diagnosis can cause a lack of motivation towards self-care, further threatening concordance.

Concordance will also be more likely to be achieved with the adolescent asthmatic when they can see that their recreational needs and image in the eyes of their peers are accounted for (Anderson, 1997). Patient misgivings and doubts about prescribed treatment that in a compliance model may have led to costly and even harmful misuse of medicine are more likely to be shared in a consultation that takes its cues from the patient themselves. Pollock (2001) has demonstrated how lay explanatory models of care and diagnosis assist both concordance and health literacy. On the other hand, concordance can have no real meaning unless the patient's concerns contained within their frame of reference are heard, respected and addressed.

Methods that have previously been demonstrated to improve adherence to prescribed regimens, such as aides-mémoires, dispensing kits and the involvement of family members and carers, are best used as part of a comprehensive patient centredness. Even modest medication profiles often involve complex regimens in which more than one route is used, with some orally administered drugs requiring to be taken with food and others without, for example. Faithfully adhering to administration times may result in disturbed sleep or other disruptions in lifestyle routines. The effort, energy and sheer inconvenience affecting patients and their carers already heavily burdened with illness, discomfort and other life responsibilities would appear to occur all too infrequently to those of us broadly identified as healthcare professionals.

Concordance can never be just about taking prescribed medicines in isolation. It must involve the patient's whole world.

SUSTAINING CONCORDANCE

'The mornings are the worst. I lie in bed and curl up in a ball. My insides feel like they're shrivelling up. I'm too frightened to get up because of what may happen if I do, but the longer I lay there the worse I feel. I know you said these pills would take a while to kick in, but right now I don't think I'm ever going to get better.'

In recent years, theorists have recognised that patients not only uniquely interpret their world but reflect on their experience of receiving care, just as practitioners reflect on their experience of care giving (Perry, 2000; Edwards, 2003). In view of this, it is one matter to achieve concordance but quite another to sustain it. In mental healthcare perhaps more than in any other field, the concerns, interpretations and overall mood of the patient are crucial to sound diagnosis and care management. For instance, although it is one of the more popular selective serotonin reuptake inhibitors (SSRIs), fluoxetine is recognised as having an efficacy gap of 10 to 15 days between commencement of treatment and satisfactory therapeutic plasma levels being attained (Anderson and Edwards, 2001). While it is good practice to inform the patient of this in advance, the level of physical and psychological discomfort that must be endured during this interim period may still take the patient by surprise. Clinical judgement based on the timing of the patient's concern and sound pharmaceutical knowledge would have to be used to decide whether perseverance with current treatment should be recommended. Alternatively, if the patient is not responding to treatment within the expected time frame, the drug of choice might be changed to a selective noradrenaline reuptake inhibitor (SNRI) such as reboxetine (Fava et al., 2003).

The prescriber and patient need to exercise foresight by exploring potential hurdles: 'what if' scenarios in therapy that the patient in isolation may have to negotiate along with a range of proposed helpful responses. Such strategies are forms of forcefield analysis that provide support for anticipated problems. These are skills that have been transferred from specialist areas such as smoking cessation and drug and alcohol withdrawal, where they have proved useful in strengthening the patient's resolve (West, 2004).

However, the unpredictable nature of professional practice and the lives in which it intervenes mean that there are many areas that threaten sustained concordance about which no one can know in advance. A family crisis may undermine the ability to adhere to the prescribed regimen. Illness may disguise side effects or an adverse reaction; and indeed, as in the example captured in the scenario above, drug action or the progress of a condition for which the drug is prescribed may not match the patient's expectation.

The clinically measured recovery from a diagnosed condition and the patient's experience of illness as a result of that condition are two distinct trajectories that are not always parallel (Stewart and Roter, 1989). It is when the patient perceives that a beneficial clinical response is not being achieved that the carefully woven fabric of trust between them and the practitioner is tested and the integrity of concordance threatened.

Initial care planning that is sensitive and reciprocal to evidence gained through insight into the patient's perspective is the key to good prescribing practice. Sequential and interim care planning that is not only sensitive and reciprocal but also contingent on the changing face of the patient experience is the key to sustaining concordance. Of course, interim planning can only take place if the patient has been encouraged to take part in reviews. Such reviews are integral to the initial plan, but are ideally instigated by the patient when concordance is unexpectedly threatened. This reminds us that in this culture of partnership, the patient has responsibilities as well as rights. The part played by clinical management plans in this process is discussed further in Chapter 6.

Helen has influenza and has been diagnosed with a chest infection. She is considerably stressed as she is missing work and the annual production meeting is in four days' time. She is not eating and informs you that she is an insulin-dependent diabetic.

What are Helen's concerns and in what order of importance might she place these?

What are the barriers to her acheiving and sustaining concordance?

A FOUNDATION FOR ETHICAL PRACTICE

In Chapter 3 we will discuss how the use of ethical frameworks can help to clarify and resolve dilemmas in prescribing. It is clear, however, from issues considered in this chapter that while ethical knowledge can be applied to practice, it may also be extracted from it. The application of individualised patient care to prescribing behaviour means that ethical movement comes as an implicit prepackaged accessory (Redfern, 1996). For example, respect for autonomy is evident when a patient's religious, cultural and moral positioning is respected in relation to prescribable agents such as certain methods of contraception, blood or animal pharmaceutical constituents and the plan of care offers viable alternatives (Murphy and Tallis, 2003). Beneficence is exercised in the humanity and compassion extended while an exhausted mother tries to describe her idiopathic back pain. Patient-centred planning is the paramount principle in prescribing practice through which other principles, approaches and ways of knowing operate (Perry, 2000).

PRESERVING AN EPISTEMOLOGY OF CARING

The advent of non-medical prescribing means that pathophysiology and other technical knowledge are high on the agenda for discussion. Highlighting these glamorous but essentially contemporaneous skills achieves professional recognition within a time frame that is only as long as it is politically expedient. Moreover, such recognition potentially detracts from perennial core values in caring. Effective prescribing or non-prescribing behaviour cannot take place without the patient seeing the practitioner as an interpretative helper as well as a knower. Technical knowledge and skill, while important, must not concern the practitioner to the extent that caring loses its cultural identity.

Patient-centred practice helps preserve an epistemology of caring. Reflection on the perspective of the patient as an individual maintains the centrality of patient need and serves to prevent a loss of focus in favour of preoccupation with biomedical models of care.

REFERENCES

Ajzen, I (2002) Perceived behavioral control, self-efficacy, locus of control, and the theory of planned behavior. *Journal of Applied Social Psychology* **32**(4): 665–683.

Anderson, IA & Edwards, JG (2001) Guidelines for choice of selective serotonin reuptake inhibitor in depressive illness. *Advances in Psychiatric Treatment* **7**(3): 170–180.

Anderson, J (1997) Patient behaviour and attitudes to asthma. In *Asthma Adherence Workshop Report*. Melbourne (Victoria): National Asthma Campaign.

Armitage, CJ & Conner, M (2000) Social cognition models and health behaviour: A structured review. *Journal of Psychology and Health* **15**(2): 173–189.

Attree, M (2001) Patients' and relatives' experiences and perspectives of 'good' and 'not so good' quality care. *Journal of Advanced Nursing* **33**(4): 456–466.

Benner, P, Tanner, CA & Chesla, CA (1996) *Expertise in Nursing Practice, Caring, Clinical Judgement and Ethics.* New York: Springer.

Bond, C (2003) Concordance: Is it a synonym or a paradigm shift? *Pharmaceutical Journal* **271**(7270): 496–497.

Cornwell, J (1984) *Hard Earned Lives.* London: Tanstode.

Crow, J (2004) Consultation and diagnostic skills: Holistic care and concordance. *Prescribing Nurse* **1**(2): 22–26.

Department of Health (1989) *The Children Act: An Introduction for the NHS.* London: The Stationery Office.

Department of Health (1998) *The New NHS, Modern and Dependable.* London: The Stationery Office.

Department of Health (2000) *Pharmacy in the Future: Implementing the NHS Plan.* London: The Stationery Office.

Department of Health (2001a) *Good Practice in Consent.* London: The Stationery Office.

Department of Health (2001b) *National Service Framework for Older People.* London: The Stationery Office.

Department of Health (2003) *Supplementary Prescribing by Nurses and Pharmacists with the NHS in England: A Guide for Implementation.* London: The Stationery Office.

Department of Health (2004) *National Service Framework for Children: Children's Version.* London: The Stationery Office.

Department of Health (2005) *National Service Framework for Children, Young People and Maternity Services: Core Standards* (2nd edition). London: The Stationery Office.

Dowell, J, Jones, A & Snadden, D (2002) Exploring medication use to seek concordance with non-adherent patients: A qualitative study. *British Journal of General Practice* **52**(474): 24–32.

Doyle, KA & Maslin-Prothero, S (1999) Promoting children's rights: The role of the children's nurse. *Paediatric Nursing* **11**(8): 23–25.

Edwards, C (2003) The reflective patient: Intrapersonal care. *Nursing Standard* **17**(38): 33–36.

Epstein, O, Perkin, GD, de Bono, DP & Cookson, J (2000) *Clinical Examination* (2nd edition). London: Mosby.

Fava, M, McGrath, PJ & Sheu, WP (2003) Switching to reboxetine: An efficacy and safety study in patients with major depressive disorder unresponsive to fluoxetine. *Journal of Clinical Psychopharmacology* **23**(4): 365–369.

Furniss, l (2002) Use of medicines in nursing homes for older people. *Advances in Psychiatric Treatment* **8**(3): 198–204.

Hall, L (1964) Nursing: What is it? *The Canadian Nurse* **60**(2): 150–154.

Haynes, RB, McKibbon, A & Kanani, R (1996) Systematic review of randomised trials of interventions to assist patients to follow prescriptions for medications. *Lancet* **388**(9024): 383–386.

Heath, H & Scofield, I (1999) *Healthy Ageing: Nursing Older People.* London: Mosby Harcourt.

Henley, A & Schott, J (1999) *Culture, Religion and Patient Care in a Multi-ethnic Society.* London: Age Concern UK.

Hopkins, H, Wade, T & Weir, D (2000) 'Take as directed', whatever that means. *Australian Prescriber* **23**(5): 103–104.

Horne, R & Weinman, J (1999) Patients' beliefs about prescribed medicines and their role in adherence to treatment in chronic illness. *Journal of Psychosomatic Research* **47**(6): 555–567.

Horner, SD (1997) Uncertainty in mothers' care for their ill children. *Journal of Advanced Nursing* **26**(4): 658–663.

Illich, I. (1977) *Limits to Medicine: Medical Nemesis: The Expropriation of Health.* New York: Penguin.

Jackson, T (2002) Both sides now (editorial). *British Medical Journal* **325**(7364): 603.

Jacobson, AM, Hauser, ST, Willett, JB, Wolfsdorf, JI, Dvorak, R, Herman, L & de Groot, M (1997) Psychological adjustment to IDDM: 10 year followup of an onset cohort of child and adolescent patients. *Diabetes Care* **20**(5): 811–818.

Jones, G (2003) Prescribing and taking medicines (editorial). *British Medical Journal* **327**(7419): 819.

Leach, P. (2000) *Children First: What We Are Not Doing and Should Be Doing for Children Today* (2nd edition). London: Michael Joseph.

Little, P, Everett, H, Williamson, I, Warner, G, Moore, M, Gould, C, Ferrier, K & Payne, S (2001) Observational study of patient centredness and positive approach on outcomes of general practice consultations. *British Medical Journal* **323**(7318): 908–911.

Maiman, LA & Becker, MH (1974) The health belief model: Origins and correlates in psychological theory. *Health Education Monographs* **2**(4): 336–353.

Makoul, G, Arnston, P & Scofield, T (1995) Health promotion in primary care: Physician–patient communication and decision making about prescription medications. *Social Science Medicine* **41**(9): 1241–1254.

Marinker, M (1997) *From Compliance to Concordance: Achieving Shared Goals in Medicine Taking.* London: Royal Pharmaceutical Society of Great Britain.

Marinker, M & Shaw, J (2003) Not to be taken as directed. *British Medical Journal* **326**(7394): 348–349.

Mason, J & Fattore, T (2005) *Children Taken Seriously: In Theory, Policy and Practice.* London: Jessica Kingsley.

Matsui, DM (1997) Drug compliance in pediatrics: Clinical and research issues. *Pediatric Clinician of North America* **44**(1): 1–14.

McGavock, H, Britten, N & Weinmann, J (1996) *A Review of the Literature on Drug Adherence.* London: Royal Pharmaceutical Society of Great Britain.

McklinDon, DD & Schlucter, J (2004) Parent and nurse partnership model for therapeutic relationships. *Pediatric Nursing* **30**(5): 418–20.

Miller, E (2003) Measles-mumps-rubella vaccine and the development of autism. *Seminars in Pediatric Infectious Diseases* **14**(3): 199–206.

Mishel, MH (1981) The measurement of uncertainty in illness. *Nursing Research* **30**(5): 258–263.

Mishel, MH (1983) Parents' perception of uncertainty concerning their hospitalized child: Reliability and validity of a scale. *Nursing Research* **32**(6): 324–330.

Murch, SH, Anthony, A, Casson, DH, Malik, M, Berelowitz, M, Dhillon, AP, Thomson, MA, Valentine, A, Davies, SE & Walker-Smith, JA (2004) Retraction of an interpretation. *The Lancet* **363**(9411): 750.

Murphy, A & Tallis, R (2003) How to achieve concordance through ethnic sensitivity and lateral thinking. *Pharmaceutical Journal* **271**(7270): 511–512.

National Prescribing Centre (1999). *Signposts for Good Nurse Prescribing.* http://www.npc. co.uk/nurse_prescribing/bulletins/signposts1.1.htm [accessed 26 September 2006].

Perry, MA (2000) Reflections on intuition and expertise. *Journal of Clinical Nursing* **9**(1): 137–145.

Pollock, K (2001) 'I've not asked you see and he's not said': Understanding lay explanatory models of illness is a prerequisite for concordant consultations. *International Journal of Pharmacy Practice* **9**(2): 105–117.

Redfern, S (1996) Individualised patient care: A framework for guidelines. *Nursing Times* **92**(5): 33–36.

Reiman, D (1986) Non caring and caring in the clinical setting. *Topics in Clinical Nursing* **8**(1): 30–36.

Rogers, C (1994) *Freedom to Learn* (3rd edition). London: Macmillan.

Rossi, S (2003) Compliance or concordance? (editorial). *Australian Prescriber* **23**(5): 105.

Rotter, J (1966) Generalized expectancies for internal versus external control of reinforcements. *Psychological Monographs* **80**(609): 1–28.

Rubin, J (1996) Impediments to the development of clinical knowledge and ethical judgement in critical care nursing. In P. Benner, CA Tanner & CA Chesla (1996) *Expertise in Nursing Practice: Caring, Clinical Judgement and Ethics*. New York: Springer.

Russell, S, Daly, J, Hughes, E & Hoog, C (2003) Nurses and 'difficult' patients: Negotiating non-compliance. *Journal of Advanced Nursing* **43**(3): 281–287.

Sanz, E (2003) Concordance and children's use of medicines. *British Medical Journal* **327**(7419): 858–860.

Schwartz, J (2000) Have we forgotten the patient? *American Journal of Nursing* **100**(2): 61–63.

Seagroatt, V & Goldacre, MJ (2003) Crohn's disease, ulcerative colitis, and measles vaccine in an English population, 1979–1998. *Journal of Epidemiology and Community Health* **57**(11): 883–887.

Stewart, MA & Roter, D (eds) (1989) (eds) *Communicating with Medical Patients*. Newbury Park, CA: Sage.

Webb, E (2004) Discrimination against children. *Archives of Disease in Childhood* **89**(9): 804–808.

Weiss, M & Britten, N (2003) What is concordance? *Pharmaceutical Journal* **271**(7270): 493.

West, J (2004) ABC of smoking cessation: Assessment of dependence and motivation to stop smoking. *British Medical Journal* **328**(7435): 338–339.

Westbury, J (2003) Why do older people not always take their medicines? *Pharmaceutical Journal* **271**(7270): 503–504.

World Health Organization (1986) *Resolution of the Convention of Human Rights*. Ottawa, Canada: World Health Organization.

3 The Application of Ethical Frameworks to Prescribing

JOHN McKINNON

The aim of this chapter is to acquaint the reader with the better-known ethical frameworks and their application to prescribing. Prescribing practice does not take place in a morally neutral environment. As part of modern healthcare it involves complex decision making and an infinite number of moral quandaries that may confront the practitioner.

Ethics (originating from the Greek word *ethos* meaning character, conduct or custom) and a closely allied word, morals (from the Latin word *mores* meaning custom or habit), form a branch of philosophy concerned with measuring and determining right and wrong.

In order to apply ethics to prescribing practice, it is necessary to have an understanding of the range of ethical frameworks. To this end, a number of ethical frameworks will be critically discussed, focusing on the major tenets of deontology and utilitarianism. As part of this process, we will be helped to apply these frameworks through use of fictitious scenarios. Related legal obligations will form part of a parallel discussion and the concept of accountability will receive special attention. We will begin with an examination of the rationale for such frameworks in healthcare.

RATIONALE FOR ETHICAL FRAMEWORKS IN HEALTHCARE

It is true that most of us operate satisfactorily in our own private lives using our own value and belief systems. However, as practising healthcare professionals, our involvement with large numbers of people negotiating crises brought about by health problems means that we are confronted by large numbers of complex moral predicaments, many of which we have never previously encountered. Frameworks

Towards Prescribing Practice. Edited by J. McKinnon.
© 2007 John Wiley & Sons, Ltd.

that draw on more diverse philosophical ground than the system that we may personally use are necessary to guide our actions in such situations.

Furthermore, patients and their families also use their own moral frameworks as guides for living, but on being confronted by mental or physical trauma, coping mechanisms become paralysed or fragmented. Such individuals rely on healthcare professionals to provide support in their decision making. It is important that practitioners do not permit their own values and beliefs to bias the support they provide. To remain impartial as an ethical helper requires the use of a theoretical model to maintain objectivity.

Contained within our own personal codes of moral reasoning, many of us harbour ideas about right and wrong that we consider to be absolute in certain situations. Theft, fidelity to one's partner and the sanctity of life are only three examples in which many take an absolutist stance. In the role of healthcare practitioner, however, we provide care for many individuals and groups who do not share our views or who may take an absolutist stance on issues we consider to be relative to the context of the situation. Diverse moral codes issue from diverse sources, ranging from the teachings of a holy book to a self-constructed framework based on lived experience. Not infrequently, individuals allow what is aesthetically pleasing, what intuitively feels right or what seems most practical to guide their actions. Prostitutes, criminals, drug addicts and people with resolute religious or political beliefs will all own frameworks of moral reasoning from which we may wish to distance ourselves or which we may find potentially provocative. Ethical models assist us in acknowledging the right of such patients to receive our care and participate in their own healthcare plans in a way that fits with their own value system, placing moral relativism as a prerequisite to good practice.

The continuing advancement of medical technology presents us with new situations that can blur previously perceived clear borderlines between right and wrong. For example, neonatal intensive care facilities make viable the lives of babies born weeks before term who would not have survived in previous times. For some, this does not rest easily with decisions to terminate a pregnancy involving a fetus of similar gestation. Ethical frameworks supplying principles applicable in fluid situations are essential here too.

Ethics are very much related to the notion of human beings as separated from other life forms in the universe, as rational beings deserving of individual rights and also bound by certain duties and responsibilities. Ethical frameworks form the basis for expected standards of behaviour, but they are not static phenomena. They constitute a continual process by which society has a discussion with itself. An individual or group rarely thinks that their ideas are initially bad. It is only after ideas are shared and subjected to wider consultation that objections may be raised and/or amendments made to produce a standard that is acceptable to the majority if not to all. In time this standard may be revisited as society evolves and new or previously unnoticed factors come to light.

DEONTOLOGY

The term deontology comes from the Greek word *deon* meaning duty. Deontology is not the only ethical philosophy employed in healthcare, but with its emphasis on duties of care, it is perhaps the one with which practitioners in healthcare most often identify themselves. Certainly, professional codes of conduct derive from deontological themes.

We will see in our consideration of the deontological perspective that duties issue from the existence of rights. Rights are just claims or entitlements that are owed to an individual or a community on a moral, ethical or legal basis. Duties are the corresponding obligations of others. So it follows that the right to free speech gives rise to a duty to be tolerant, the right to peace and security gives rise to a duty to be peaceable and the right to healthcare gives rise to the duty to care. Both rights and duties are seen by philosophers as being related to moral convictions. In a deontological framework emphasis is placed on the morality of actions.

The most widely published theory of deontology rests on the ideas of the eighteenth century Prussian philosopher Immanuel Kant (Kant, 1996). Dr Sam Brock of Georgetown University conceived a framework of key concepts that facilitate the application of deontological principles in practice. This framework has come to be known as the Georgetown mantra (Beauchamp and Childress, 2001). The mantra consists of four principal concepts: autonomy, non-maleficence, beneficence and justice. These principal concepts are closely related to others that also form a founding part of ethical healthcare practice.

AUTONOMY

Autonomy, the first core concept of the Georgetown mantra, is self-regulation, the notion that an individual may decide for themselves the correct course of action and behave accordingly. The concept is closely related to ideas of free choice on the basis of a person's ability to reason on factual evidence. Kant made the distinction between *heteronomous* will, in which an individual submits to externally imposed rules and regulations, and *autonomous* will, in which an individual is guided by their own sense of right and wrong. In Kant's view, people act with autonomy when they move towards aims and objectives of which they themselves have ownership.

Dworkin (1988: 20) defined autonomy as 'a second order capacity to reflect critically upon first order preferences, desires and wishes and so forth and the capacity to accept or attempt to change them in the light of higher order preferences and values'.

Professional practitioners act autonomously when they apply their own knowledge and judgement in unique situations, executing practice in order to frame and resolve problems or to meet desirable outcomes. To the extent that such behaviour is independent of protocols and decision-making trees, with the practitioner exercising the freedom to choose the way forward at each juncture, this is autonomous practice. In the prescribing situation, the patient exercises autonomy when they decide to refuse or consent to immunisation, decline the offer of a prescription in the belief that self-care will resolve their condition more effectively, or question the judgement of the prescriber as to the accuracy of their diagnosis. In each case, decisions are made on the basis of the evidence the individual believes is available to them. The place of autonomy as the first deontological concept in the Georgetown mantra reminds us of the importance of the rights of service users to individuality and self-determination in modern healthcare.

Critique of Autonomy

The concept of autonomy assumes a vision of human beings as willingly reflecting openly, honestly and scrupulously on their actions, making adjustments as they deem appropriate. This is a highly questionable perspective. Human beings do not always reflect on their actions, and when they do it is not always in a well-structured, well-reasoned, consistent and honest way (Daly, 1998; De Bono, 2000; Cuypers, 2004). On the contrary, the propensity for self-justification is strong (Mezirow, 1981). The 'second-order capacity' to ethically monitor one's own decisions and behaviour described by Dworkin is often far from evident. The absence of a ubiquitous and perpetual selfless reflective mode in human deportment *is* evident in problems of bullying and discrimination in the workplace, road rage and political corruption, to name but a few examples.

People often hold beliefs and make decisions that are not soundly based on evidence. Failing to make a search of all or any of the facts, they may act on the basis of others' influence or their own prejudices. They may even act out of belief in the face of evidence to the contrary (Harris, 1995).

Autonomy is the companion of power. Clearly, the vision of anyone with complete personal or professional autonomy, able to make choices and act in whatever manner they please, leaves others vulnerable. Furthermore, people whose powers of reason are compromised, either because of a disease process, learning difficulty or post-traumatic state, are potentially disadvantaged in a world where the expressed wishes of the individual are key to healthcare provision. Some patients may wish to surrender their autonomy because they believe that the choices in a specific situation are too complex and therefore beyond their grasp. Such patients may wish to leave decisions to the judgement of professionals, trusting that they will do what is in their best interests.

Autonomy has also arguably become rather overrated in contemporary western society, where consumer power and the creation of personal wealth and individual security are often portrayed as paramount and synonymous with success. Many non-western cultures do not reason in this way. For them, the wellbeing of a collective and the strength and ability of a community to support its members are paramount. In this type of society, decisions that in a western culture are left to personal choice are considered best taken in consultation with a centrally appointed hierarchy or body of elders.

Autonomy must therefore be bounded by a number of related concepts, which are explored below.

Autonomy and Accountability

For healthcare practitioners, levels of autonomy must be commensurate with levels of accountability. Accountability is the obligation to render an account or to be answerable to identified authorities for one's professional conduct and it relates directly to the duty of care binding on a practitioner. The importance of power being matched by a corresponding degree of accountability was borne out by the infamous case of cardiac surgeons at Bristol Royal Infirmary performing operative procedures on children that were neither viable nor within their field of competence, at the cost of many of those children's lives. The fact that such a situation continued unchecked for a substantial length of time was the result of lines of accountability that were either dysfunctional or completely absent. The inquiry that followed found that such was the level of power of the consultants involved that allied professional staff did not feel able to address the matter effectively (Klein, 1998).

The four areas of accountability are:

- the patient through civil law
- the employer through contractual law
- the public through criminal law, and
- the practitioner's professional body through a ratified ethical code of conduct.

The practitioner's duty of care to the patient means that this relationship usually comes first in the hierarchy of accountability, the exceptions being where the greater public good is placed at risk, such as cases of child abuse or intended criminal activity (Dimond, 2000).

Prescribing practitioners are accountable for assessment, diagnosis and any prescribing or non-prescribing behaviour that issues from these. Non-prescribing behaviour refers not simply to the decision not to prescribe but also to any health action agreed with the patient, including directives to purchase over-the-counter items, general sales list or pharmacy-only medicines.

A prescription is one of several possible outcomes arising from an assessment and diagnosis. As the prescribing act cannot be disembodied from the roles of assessment and diagnosis, prescribers cannot prescribe at the request of non-prescribing practitioners. Where a repeat prescription is being written by a prescriber who is not the practitioner who issued the first prescription, the repeat prescription and the review assessment that accompany it are the responsibility of the second prescriber (McHale, 2003; Nursing and Midwifery Council, 2006).

Prescribing, like any other aspect of professional practice, cannot be performed merely by rote. The prescriber must be able to conduct a critical evaluation of their behaviour, evidencing the rationale on which the plan of care was based. Delegation of any role must be appropriate to the scope of practice of the one who is in receipt of the delegation. If this is not the case, then both parties in the delegation process are liable. This shows the importance of acting strictly within one's own area of competence and how accountability demands a progressive, dynamic education and practice base that sustains a prescriber practising with a current theoretical understanding (National Prescribing Centre, 2001).

Competence is the desirable measure of skilled knowledge in practice. The breadth of competency in prescribing is different from the breadth of the licence to prescribe. A prescriber may be legally permitted to prescribe from the greater part of a drug formulary, but in reality only be competent to prescribe from the parts of that formulary that relate to practice in which they are proficient. Depending on the situation, awareness of the limits of competence may mean deferring to a prescriber who is more experienced or specialised, or consulting another source of authority such as a pharmacy adviser prior to a prescribing decision. Failure to work within these parameters courts negligence of the duty of care (Nursing and Midwifery Council, 2006).

Employers are also legally obligated to have procedures and policies in place that guide good practice, maximise use of limited resources and protect the public. Prescribing practitioners have a duty to their employers by virtue of their contract of employment to practise within these guidelines. In situations such as a severe adverse drug reaction, in which the prescriber is found to have met the criteria of duty of care and acted within employer guidelines, the employer will usually meet and manage any litigation that arises. This is vicarious liability. However, if the prescriber is found either to have acted negligently or to have strayed outside their employer's policies and procedures or the boundaries of their contract, they will be held personally responsible for any related untoward incident involving the patient's wellbeing (McHale, 2003; Dimond, 2004).

In Chapter 8, Jo West discusses the specifics of prescribing legally in greater depth.

Accountability and Conflicting Interests

The prescriber's duty of care for the patient also carries meanings of guardianship and advocacy, in that they must at all times act to protect and defend the best interests of the patient. There are grounds for potential conflict here between the duty of care to the patient and loyalty to employer-imposed rules. In such cases, the duty of care to the patient is paramount. One example of this is where the evidence base exists to show that a particular treatment not available for prescription from the local budgeted formulary is the superior one of choice in a particular patient's case. The practitioner is ethically obligated to present a case to their employer arguing for the patient to receive the said treatment. Deontological conflicts that result in confrontational situations are not pleasant. However, failing to represent the patient's interests or retreating from a position of patient advocacy breaches the professional code of conduct laid down by the practitioner's regulatory body (Nursing and Midwifery Council, 2006).

In exceptional cases, the practitioner may feel placed in a 'catch 22' situation in which the ethical course places their job in jeopardy, but it is better to lose a job and retain a licence to practise and prescribe than to lose both through loss of that licence by deregistration (Glover, 1999). An ethical philosophy of personal integrity in life as well as in professional practice, while temporarily traumatic, often proves ultimately fulfilling in the way one is respected and remembered by others.

Accountability and Commercial Interests

It has always been important for healthcare practitioners to be seen to be impartial in their recommendations of treatment and undivided in their loyalties to their service user groups. Practitioners are not permitted to sacrifice or compromise clinical judgement and patient protection in favour of personal gain. The role of prescribing, however, introduces a powerful but often subtle variable to this equation: the pharmaceutical industry.

Pharmaceutical companies invest heavily in clinical research and therapeutic development. The combined cost of this is estimated to be approximately $6 billion in the United States alone. In Britain the figure is closer to £3.3 billion, six times that of the British government's investment. Such vast expenditure and the competition that exists in the global marketplace mean that companies are pressed to promote their products as superior to those of their rivals in an effort to reclaim their costs and achieve a sizeable profit margin. In addition to advertising, hospitality, gifts and sponsorship of research, education and conference programmes are included in what can be broadly defined as promotion and marketing. Given that a reputed 25 % of a drug company's annual budget is spent on promotional activities, the claims of some prescribers that they are able to accept the benefits of such promotion and simultaneously resist influence on their prescribing behaviour would appear self-deceiving and naïve (Hartley, 2004; House of Commons Health Committee, 2005). Komesaroff and Kerridge (2002) cite seven major pieces of research all showing that physicians, most of whom claimed to be uninfluenced by advertising and patronage, were in fact more likely to prescribe those products that were promoted in this way. There is no evidence to support the suggestion that non-medical prescribers are automatically immune to such influence (Shaw, 2003).

Prescribers need to be mindful of their accountability to their patients and professional regulatory bodies. Guidelines for prescribers working with the pharmaceutical industry, such as those published by the Royal Pharmaceutical Society of Great Britain (2003), reflect principles accepted across all prescribing healthcare professions (Komesaroff and Kerridge, 2002).

Features of ethical practice in this area should include:

- Dual interest, such as sponsorship from a pharmaceutical company, should always be declared, particularly in published work.
- Entertainment/hospitality should be modest, appropriate, secondary to the occasion and no more extravagant than if the practitioner were paying for themselves.
- Gifts should not be accepted by prescribers unless they are both modest and relevant to practice, e.g. diaries, pens etc.

- Meetings with the pharmaceutical industry should be organised by independent bodies and prearranged with an appropriate agenda and equal time given to all representatives.
- Critical appraisal of claims made by pharmaceutical companies should be shared with all interested prescribers and pharmacy advisers.
- Sponsorship should not blatantly promote the sponsor and should be limited to non-product-specific events such as local education programmes and funding partnerships with other organisations.

The pharmaceutical industry in Britain must abide by the code of practice set out by its own association (Association of the British Pharmaceutical Industry, 2001). This code is regularly reviewed in consultation with the major health professional bodies and the Medicines and Healthcare Products Regulatory Agency (MHRA).

Paul is a nurse consultant in pain assessment. He is contacted by the representative for Gottya Pharmaceuticals plc, which is promoting its new product, Deflamaton 5. Paul agrees to meet for lunch, which is paid for by the representative. At face value there appears to be no difference between Deflamaton 5 and three other similar products in the *BNF* except that Deflamaton 5 is slightly more expensive. The representative insists that his company's drug has faster absorption and distribution rates and provides a more effective level of pain relief. The representative produces a paper published in an American journal that appears to support these claims. After lunch, Paul leaves saying that he will think over their discussion. Two days later Paul receives an offer of part sponsorship of his PhD studies from Gottya.

What steps is Paul obligated to take before agreeing to prescribe Deflamaton 5? Describe the potential issues of conflicting interest for Paul.

Accountability, Informed Choice and Concordance

The concept of informed choice is important to the practitioner required to honour the patient's autonomy but also to fulfil their duty of care. The end-stage decisions of the patient to accept or reject a prescription or opt for a particular healthcare package must be based on their conscious knowledge of the potential harm and benefits, advantages and disadvantages of each choice open to them. Patients may come to a consultation with a firm set of values and beliefs about health and illness, and some may also bring a measure of knowledge of research findings relating to therapeutic substances and lifestyle choices. Especially where there is controversy surrounding treatment, the prescriber must ensure that the patient is given an accurate picture of the reliability of research findings, balanced against misconception born of sensationalism, together with a record of current established practice.

The values of informed choice, concordance and autonomy all relate to the practitioner having earned the patient's trust by evidencing both their expertise and their ability to grasp the patient's frame of reference and establish shared goals (Emmanuel and Emmanuel, 1992).

There are a number of situations where the patient is not able to express a preference or may exercise their autonomy with difficulty. A patient with cerebral palsy, while in full possession of their mental faculties, may experience problems making themselves understood, and a patient with severe multiple learning difficulties may not be able to communicate verbally. Successfully ascertaining the wishes of patients who are mentally ill, unconscious or have died may seem completely beyond reach.

When patients cannot communicate verbally, forms of non-verbal communication can be used. The involvement of close family members and carers who can help represent the wishes of the patient, at least in part, play a positive role in this area. Because of knowledge and experience born of close association with a patient with a disability, relatives are often able to interpret agitation and anxiety, approval and preference in behaviour that would be otherwise meaningless to the practitioner. In Chapter 10, Stuart Kennedy discusses how windows of improved insight and recovery can, in addition to family partnerships, be used by the practitioner to negotiate concordance with patients in mental health. Living wills and advanced medical directives, when detailed and well maintained, help healthcare professionals be aware of a patient's wishes when unconscious or posthumously. No matter how valuable the contribution of related others in preserving the autonomy of a patient, this is a 'second best' option. No one can give consent on behalf of another. Rather, the information supplied by literary evidence and personal testimony is used to build a picture that resembles as closely as possible the autonomous views of the patient had they been able to express them (Department of Health, 2001).

Where a patient elects to surrender their autonomy, it is good practice to have this recorded, signed, dated and witnessed by another member of the professional team and a relative or friend of the patient. The record should reflect that such a decision does not presume to cover all decision making associated with this patient's care, but relates specifically to the area in which the patient experienced difficulty (Dimond, 2000).

Alan is a healthy 19-year-old man who still lives with his mother. He does not carry an organ donor card but, while watching a television documentary on transplant surgery, he casually tells his mother that he likes the idea of his organs benefiting someone else when he dies. The following week, Alan is involved in a motorcycle accident, sustains a serious head injury and several weeks later is declared 'brain dead'. His mother is approached by the medical staff of the intensive care unit and asked if Alan's organs may be donated for transplant.

(Continued)

What part might the recent conversation between Alan and his mother play in her decision? How does this relate to respect for Alan's autonomy after his death?

The Nature of Consent

The relationship between consent and concordance has been discussed in Chapter 2 as well as above. However, there is a need to consider the nature of consent and the forms it may take. Consent is the autonomous expression of agreement by an individual or group to an act or procedure. It may be given verbally, non-verbally or in writing. Consent may also be implicit (for example when the patient presents on invitation for specific treatment) or explicit, when the patient responds positively to consent having been sought. Consent can be withdrawn by the patient at any time and for this reason there are very few occasions when written consent is of value. The exceptions to this rule are when the patient is receiving a general anaesthetic and is not in a position to reverse their decision once treatment has commenced (Hendrick, 2000).

Kathy visits the nurse practitioner following the onset of the menopause to discuss her symptoms. The possibility of prescribing hormone replacement therapy (HRT) is discussed. Kathy is reluctant to agree to HRT because she read in a tabloid newspaper some years ago that the chances of developing cancer are increased for women who opt for this treament.
   What do the concepts of duty of care, informed choice and patient autonomy require of the nurse practitioner?

Accountability and Record Keeping

Contemporaneous professional records are central to ethical practice, in that they show how accountability in practice has been behaviourally demonstrated. Patient-centred assessment, diagnosis and treatment are evidenced in a plan of care. As such, records include a rationale for care and this structure means that they can be used as an effective teaching tool. Patient records are also a contract that documents the concordat between patient and practitioner. In this way, records constitute a legal document that may be used as evidence (Hendrick, 2000).

NON-MALEFICENCE

Non-maleficence is the second concept of the deontological framework. Non-maleficence means doing no harm and in healthcare relates to the prevention of iatrogenesis. Iatrogenesis is illness, disease, injury or trauma that arises from health-care intervention. Practitioners acting on the ethical principle of non-maleficence ensure that the patient leaves professional care in a condition that is at least no worse as a result of that care. Non-maleficent prescribing practice is concerned with the prevention of iatrogenesis by means of the measures discussed in Chapter 6.

Iatrogenesis is often the result of negligence. Negligence can broadly be defined as failure to perform a task to the standard that might be reasonably expected of another individual with the same level of skill. This may be characterised by acts of omission; failure to perform a task or element of a task essential to good care or commission; performing a task that could potentially prove harmful to a patient. For negligence to be proven in the litigation process, it must be established that a duty of care existed, that this duty was breached and that any harm that occurred was related to the said breach of duty. It therefore behoves practitioners to consider any harmful effects of prescribed medication in advance of administration and report any hazard or hazardous practice that may cause harm (Griffith and Tengnah, 2004).

Critique of Non-Maleficence

A sociological perspective on healthcare points to many sources of iatrogenesis that are not traditionally associated with acknowledged suboptimum practice. Nosocomial infections, side effects of therapeutic agents and post-operative complications all number among harmful factors resulting from practices with which healthcare professionals identify the doing of good.

Determining non-maleficence is made all the more difficult in situations that may appear paradoxical, for example the prescribing of syringes and needles for drug addicts. Such a practice, while helping to prevent the spread of hepatitis C and human immunodeficiency virus (HIV), might also be viewed as condoning and perpetrating the consumption of illegal drugs and the health and social problems that such consumption creates. Conversely, to withhold such a service would be to neglect a major public health issue. Thus, both options appear fraught with elements of harm (Lazarini, 2001).

Rumbold (1999) has argued that harmful consequences resulting from morally good actions are acceptable when their cumulative effect is less than that of the resultant good. Furthermore, choice of action is conditional on harm being merely a side effect rather than a descriptor of the action itself. Judging on the basis of Rumbold's criteria, the prescribing of syringes and needles to drug addicts is ethically acceptable as the prevention of incurable disease is the central moral act. This would seem to be confirmed by the findings of the Joseph Rowntree Foundation (2006), which cites the provision of drug-consumption rooms in a number of European countries as a positive factor in reducing not only infection but also illegal drug taking by bringing addicts into contact with support services.

BENEFICENCE

Beneficence, the third deontological concept, is the doing of good. Good has been defined as that which is 'characterised by desirable qualities, virtuous' (*The Concise*

Oxford Dictionary, 1998). Doing good can be expected to produce favourable results. The philosophical roots of beneficence are closely linked to virtue theory, which argues that for the concept to prove functional, certain qualities must be actively present in the benefactor. Plato (Cooper, 1997) listed 'courage, wisdom, restraint, generosity and fortitude' among the virtues that are prerequisites to beneficence. For the virtue ethical theorist, good in doing results from good in being. Beneficent deeds and practices explain the nature of the benefactor. The classic case of this is the 'Good Samaritan'.

Much of this reasoning has survived to retain a place in modern writing (MacIntyre, 1984). The American Philosophical Association (1990) identified personal qualities such as tolerance, flexibility, prudence, honesty, humility, diligence and reasonableness as predisposing someone to sound discriminating clinical judgement. The idea that ethical practice inculcates virtues in the practitioner and that, conversely, virtuous practitioners will produce beneficial practice is an integral part of twenty-first-century philosophy. Nursing theorists such as Patricia Benner (2000) often speak of the 'wisdom and goodness' in nursing, while other healthcare professionals speak of the desire to do good as the main driving force in their practice.

Critique of Beneficence

Beneficence is a subjective concept. There is no cross-cultural consensus as to what constitutes doing good. In fact, so diverse and divisive is the interpretation of beneficence that it can be said that one person's sin really is another's virtue! This causes problems for the practitioner intent on doing good as it may be understood in the world of health science. Beneficence carries potential links with paternalism: the idea that one knows what is best for another by virtue of one's expertise. Paternalism serves to steal or at least limit the autonomy of a person or a community. As such, it has no place in modern healthcare except to prevent the majority from harm.

Nineteenth-century philosopher and economist John Stuart Mill (1859: Chapter 1, p. 6) expressed the proper relationship between personal autonomy and paternalism in the following way:

> The only purpose for which power can be rightfully exercised over any member of a
> civilized community, against his will, is to prevent harm to others. His own good, either
> physical or moral, is not sufficient warrant.

A libertarian perspective on beneficent healthcare practice facilitates good as the patient perceives this to be, with the proviso that this does not affect others adversely. Patients' lifestyles or lifestyle choices often work in opposition to the treatment prescribed for a disease state. While public health advice and referrals are appropriate, healthcare practice exists to fit the needs of patients and not the reverse. To try to coerce or blackmail a patient by threatening to discontinue their prescribed medication unless they comply with advice is an illegitimate use of paternalism, an assault on the patient's autonomy.

The relationship between beneficence and accountability is clear in terms of what beneficence requires of the practitioner. The concepts of veracity and confidentiality are essential to doing good.

David is a 42-year-old manager of a local supermarket. His wife has recently left him for another man. He is also under pressure at work to meet targets that he believes are unrealistic. He is currently working 52 hours a week and is is having trouble sleeping. In the course of the consultation he occasionally becomes tearful, although he states when asked that he has never contemplated harming himself in any way. He is adamant that he will not accept medication, but would accept a referral for counselling. He adds that he is not happy about going on sick leave, although he would consider this.

It is the prescriber's judgement that David is on the verge of a depressive illness and that counselling and sick leave are by themselves an inadequate response to this. A prescription for an antidepressant is judged to be essential.

What does the relationship between beneficence, paternalism and autonomy mean for the prescriber seeking to care for David?

Veracity

Truth telling is a foundation for any relationship of trust. The practitioner cannot presume to know what the patient would and would not rather know. Neither can the wish to be kind justify the withholding of information that relates directly to the patient's health; this would be paternalism. The term 'therapeutic privilege' describes the decision temporarily to withhold information until a time when the patient is better disposed to absorb and reflect on it. However, such occasions are comparatively rare and the burden of proof rests with the practitioner in evidencing that the patient's best interests were served by this action (Edge and Groves, 1999).

Privacy

The concepts of dignity and personhood discussed in Chapter 2 are closely associated with the right of the patient to privacy: to be permitted periods of solitude free from intrusion. Patients who are acutely or chronically ill may by the very nature of the high levels of observation, care and treatment they require enjoy very little privacy. There is a profound need to build episodes of intensive care and therapy around observation, leaving time gaps where the patient may enjoy privacy and the peace of mind that this supplies.

In prescribing practice, the named preparation box abbreviated as 'NP' on the prescription sheet is used in many parts of Britain. Deletion of this box by the prescriber signals to the pharmacist that the name of the prescribed medicine should not appear on the container. This is useful in safeguarding the patient's privacy in cases such as human immune deficiency virus, when the name of their medication might inform others of their condition. In this way the patient's privacy is respected.

Confidentiality

Confidentiality is also a core value in the beneficent patient–practitioner relationship. Therapeutic partnerships move forward positively when there is a clear understanding that information shared by the patient is not divulged to anyone else outside the immediate care team without their explicit consent. Furthermore, the law requires that within the relevant team of professionals, confidential information should only be shared and recorded on a 'need to know' basis. Professional practitioners must be able to establish that the information shared was necessary to facilitate care.

Even in cases where confidentiality is breached in the interests of the greater public good, the patient should be informed unless such an act increases the risk of harm to the public (Edge and Groves, 1999).

Fidelity

Fidelity is faithfulness and is a prerequisite to personal integrity. If ethics are the principles by which good practice is guided, then the practitioner is obliged to be faithful to these principles. For example, prescribers who profess to practise by a code of ethics and set of standards cannot pay lip service to concordance, act dishonestly or waive those responsibilities that may cause them discomfort. The course of fidelity is not always the populist one. For example, a prescriber who refuses to prescribe antibiotics inappropriately or who acts as advocate for a vulnerable patient should not expect their fidelity and integrity to be rewarded or even acknowledged.

JUSTICE

Justice is the fourth deontological concept. It describes fairness, the idea that an individual's rights and entitlements should be equitable. Justice is arrived at through impartial judgement of different layers of evidence and measured examination of many 'truths' as individuals and groups perceive truth to be. Judgement rests on the extent to which these different truths can or cannot be reconciled and judicial decisions are executed accordingly (Memon et al., 2003). Natural justice is not always the same as legal justice. Legal justice is sometimes attained when the conclusion of a dispute between parties is reached that is merely within the rules. Natural justice is attained when the human rights of all parties are respected, sometimes at the expense of rules.

Critique of Justice in Healthcare

Attempting to achieve justice is often a slow, laborious task that involves the gathering and sifting of relevant data. Not all data may be accessible and even the most judicious person or body can only make a judgement on the evidence available at the time. The process may be subject to all manner of political and economic pressures. The National Institute of Clinical Excellence (NICE) has been criticised for the length of time taken to assess the cost effectiveness and clinical value of drugs. However, the decisions of that organisation are not the end of the justice process, as it does not provide a critical comparison of the clinical value of the drugs that it licenses. This is often left to individual NHS provider groups or even prescribers themselves.

In healthcare, distributive justice has been administered on the basis of a number of criteria such as need, contribution and merit of the patient case. This is closely allied with explicit healthcare-rationing approaches and is highly controversial, not least because it is fraught with inconsistency. For example, if a patient of advanced age is to be assessed for treatment on the grounds of contribution or merit, on what grounds are the neonate and the patient who is HIV positive to be assessed (Baumrin, 1991)?

Healthcare rationing is based on the dubious assumptions that demand will always outstrip supply and that healthcare spending is out of control. Neither is an absolute truth. Public-sector healthcare funding in Britain has only recently matched the percentage of gross domestic product of major European neighbours. Each generation of medical and biotechnology costs less in real terms than it did at its inception. There are only a finite number of people who can demand a given treatment and the size of the budget available for 'rationing' can be reduced or increased at the will of government (Hogg, 1999).

It has been argued that implicit rationing such as queue management of resources is fairer than the explicit forms that use criteria that are open to ethical questioning. Moreover, rationing approaches do not remove the right of an individual to a particular available treatment (Haydock, 1992). The legal battle won in 2006 by Ann Marie Rogers to be treated with the drug Herceptin for a stage of breast cancer for which it had not yet been licensed is evidence of this.

Healthcare rationing is often justified by providers as a means of ensuring fairness, but often the criteria for treatment relate more to the objectives and values of healthcare politics than to justice. Bennett and Chanfreau (2005) describe the different rationing criteria for treatment of HIV with antiretroviral drugs used in Mexico, Senegal, Uganda and Thailand. In Mexico, the government made a commitment to facilitating treatment for all AIDS patients, managing distribution by clinical criteria and waiting lists. However, 'distinct patterns of access' (p. 544) were observed between insured and uninsured groups. A lack of funding was also reported to threaten supply of drug treatment. In Senegal, the ability to pay is viewed as qualification for priority treatment over those who are poor. In Uganda, the prioritisation of infected children on the grounds of their 'innocence' suggests the apportioning of blame to other infected parties. In Thailand criteria are in place, but implementation was left to individual practitioners. Such international variance in distribution criteria further perpetrates a lack of justice in healthcare.

Nevertheless, the controversy illustrates that in attempting to resolve dilemmas of distributive justice, practitioners are subject to external forces over which they have no control.

ETHICAL SYNERGY

From the foregoing discussion, we can evaluate the Georgetown mantra as a theoretical framework that is greater than the sum of its parts. Zealously pursuing any one of the concepts alone means that individuals and society suffer as a result of a lack of attention being paid to one of the others. Excessive autonomy means that justice is not always served. Beneficence without due attention to non-maleficence may be fundamentally flawed. Beneficence when possessed of paternalism robs individuals of their autonomy. The framework displays a synergy that helps maintain a balanced ethical assessment that is valuable in prescribing practice. However, deontology is not the only ethical framework warranting attention.

UTILITARIANISM

Utilitarianism, literally 'the doctrine of usefulness', is an ethical standpoint that emphasises the morality of aims or projected outcomes rather than the means by which those aims and outcomes are met. Utilitarian values extend back to the Epicurean philosophers of Ancient Greece, who believed that anything resulting in the shared pleasure of the majority was good. These values were developed for modern times in the writings of John Stuart Mill (1869) and Jeremy Bentham (1996; orginally published in the nineteenth century). Once again, the greatest happiness and least pain and suffering of the greater number form the moral basis for reasoning. Actions are measured on the basis of experience as to the favourable or unfavourable outcomes that are thought likely to result. The actions of choice are those that have been estimated to have the greater number of favourable outcomes. Not surprisingly, many writers correctly refer to utilitarianism as a form of consequentialist theory, in that good and bad actions are judged on the basis of the estimated consequences for the majority (Beauchamp and Childress, 2001).

Although deontology may appear to be the natural ethical approach of healthcare practice, utilitarian approaches are used frequently by healthcare professionals and managers and punctuate prescribing policy and practice. Healthcare-rationing approaches described by Bennett and Chanfreau (2005) and discussed above contain strong utilitarian themes. Prescribers assist informed choice and negotiate concordance by helping patients to estimate the harm and benefits of each option for treatment. Care pathways are built on what has been found to be best practice, and the concept of risk management functions by calculating the positive and negative outcomes of a way forward. Immunisation programmes are endorsed when the benefits are shown through clinical trials and pilots to dwarf any risk in the shape of adverse reactions for a minority. All these ways of working have a flavour of utilitarianism, although they may not solely be governed by such.

CRITIQUE OF UTILITARIANISM

Both Mill and Bentham lived in a time of great optimism and radical change, when philosophers struggled to define the principles by which a new utopian society of the future should be governed. They viewed lists of duties as cumbersome and unnecessarily time consuming. The world has changed a great deal since the nineteenth century and we are able to reflect on the worth of utilitarian approaches with hindsight. Utilitarianism is not necessarily deployed nowadays in the way in which it was intended.

Utilitarian philosophy is related to the present time frame, in that decisions are made on the basis of what is known and predicted at that time. However, much of the future is unpredictable and there are circumstances and therefore consequences that cannot be known in advance.

Happiness is not necessarily a measure of goodness. Some actions may seem to provide happiness but cannot sustain it. On evaluation, such actions may be seen as having provided a false sense of security or fuelling only short-term gain. Policies that generate the greatest happiness of the greatest number in any area of ethnic or religious conflict would not mean an end to the violence and hatred that often characterise such conflict. This shows how a utilitarian ethos, by favouring the majority, may often devalue the interests of minority groups and so ignore justice and equity (Seedhouse, 1998).

FEMINIST ETHICS AND EMOTIVE APPROACHES

From a feminist perspective, much moral philosophy is dominated by reasoning that is male oriented, originating in a culture of political power manoeuvres. An alternative ethical philosophy has evolved from the concept of female morality as distinct from male ethics, one that views justice and logic as an insufficient basis on which to judge right and wrong. To the extent that feelings and spontaneous creative caring responses to the uniqueness of each situation are valued, this is an emotive brand of ethical reasoning (Noddings, 1984). Subsequently, radical feminists such as Patricia Spallone (1992) and Lesley Doyal (1995) used this approach to considerable effect in forcing professional recognition of the rights of women to define their own health states for themselves.

Prescribers allow such reasoning to guide their practice when patients' emotions and the link between these emotions and their health state are acknowledged and allowed to play their part in shaping a care plan. For example, a patient may speak of her fear of radical invasive surgery in spite of her awareness of the need for such surgery. Anxiety and embarrassment may cause a man to be reticent at an appointment he has made to discuss a testicular lump.

CRITIQUE OF EMOTIVE APPROACHES

While tempered emotion can assist sound reasoning, excessive emotion can warp it (Damassio, 2000). Forging practice on the basis of what is emotionally comforting at a critical time such as the determination of a poor prognosis may risk breaching other principles of autonomy and justice. Emotions inform on what matters to an individual, but as in the case of respect for autonomy this must be balanced against what matters to everyone else.

PHILOSOPHICAL CONFLICT

In modern healthcare, there is a demand for more innovative, cost-effective and clinically effective ways of planning and working. Practitioners possessed of duty principles may find themselves working within utilitarian approaches. The different value systems underpinning the ethical frameworks and approaches inevitably mean that conflict will punctuate any or all policy and practice discussions.

For example, a utilitarian will value the aims of the private finance initiative in providing new healthcare facilities with a delayed fiscal impact. Deontologists, on the other hand, will be concerned that the involvement of the private sector in provision and management of any public service threatens to compromise the principles of universalist provision of care that is free at the point of delivery.

In an effort to use the best features of different ethical models, some theorists have devised frameworks that combine features of several perspectives. Newdick (2005) outlines the Berkshire Priorities Committee (BPC) Ethical Framework designed to fairly resolve ethical conflict in healthcare rationing. The framework rests on five pillars:

1. Evidence of clinical effectiveness.
2. The cost of healthcare.
3. The need for treatment.
4. The needs of the community.
5. National standards.

While the aims of this framework may be laudable, in practice it is likely that the five criteria will compete much more than they will complement one another, creating more conflict than they resolve. Seedhouse (1998) has designed a framework for comprehensive use in healthcare that combines utilitarian and deontological dimensions with a dimension taking account of external pressures such as the law, professional codes and the quality of evidence available.

However, it is interesting that when Amoroso and Otway (2006) applied Seed-house's framework to three very different prescribing case studies, a consensual conclusion was reached in only one. In the latter case, while the framework helped resolve the dilemma that was central to the discussion, the authors were left feeling that somehow natural justice had eluded them and that beneficence could have been executed more satisfactorily had they not been restrained by issues of legal accountability.

CONCLUSION

Ethical frameworks help guide professional judgement in prescribing. Deontology or duty-based ethics help the prescriber balance respect for the patient's autonomy with the virtue-driven desire to do good and prevent harm. Accountability to employer, public and professional body is facilitated by reflection on justice. Accountability to the patient holds primacy in the majority of cases, regulating the provision of informed choice and obliging the prescriber to maintain competence built on a current evidence base in practice. Accountability to the patient also means that the practitioner must critically reflect on relationships that carry the potential of conflicting commercial interests.

However, the different value systems on which these frameworks are built mean that new conflicts may replace the ones that the frameworks are used to resolve. The use of ethical models does not mean that decision making will be without stress, but the moral integrity of the patient–practitioner relationship and that of the practitioner and other authorities is best protected by their implementation.

REFERENCES

Amoroso, J & Otway, C (2006) Ethics in prescribing practice: A review of topical issues. *Nurse Prescribing* **4**(1): 38–42.

American Philosophical Association (1990) *Critical Thinking, as Statement of Expert Consensus for the Purposes of Educational Assessment and Instruction*. Millbrae, California: California Academic Press.

Association of the British Pharmaceutical Industry (2001) *Code of Practice for the Pharmaceutical Industry*. London: Association of the British Pharmaceutical Industry.

Baumrin, B (1991) Putting them out on ice, curtailing care of the elderly. *Journal of Applied Philosophy* **8**(2): 145–154.

Beauchamp, TL & Childress, JF (2001) *Principles of Biomedical Ethics* (5th edition). New York: Oxford University Press.

Benner, P (2000) The wisdom of caring practice. *Nursing Management* **6**(10): 32–37.

Bennett, S & Chanfreau, C (2005) Approaches to rationing antiretroviral treatment: Ethical and equity implications. *Bulletin of the World Health Organization* **83**(7): 541–547.

Bentham, J (1996) *The Collected Works of Jeremy Bentham: An Introduction to the Principles and Morals of Legislation*, Hart, HLA & Rosen, F (eds). Oxford: Clarendon Press.

Cooper, JM (ed.) (1997) *The Complete Works of Plato*. Indianapolis: Hackett Publishing.

Cuypers, SE (2004) Critical thinking, autonomy and practical reason. *Journal of Philosophy of Education* **38**(1): 75–90.

Daly, W (1998) Critical thinking as an outcome of nurse education. What is it? Why is it important to nursing practice? *Journal of Advanced Nursing* **28**(2): 323–331.

Damassio, A (2000) *The Feeling of What Happens: Body and Emotion in the Making of Consciousness*. New York: Vintage.
De Bono, E (2000) *New Thinking for a New Millennium*. London: Penguin.
Department of Health (2001) *Good Practice in Consent*. London: The Stationery Office.
Dimond, B (2000) *Legal Aspects of Nursing*. London: Prentice Hall.
Dimond, B (2004) Accountability and medicinal products 3: Employment. *British Journal of Nursing* 13(5): 276–279.
Doyal, L (1995) *What Makes Women Sick*. London: Macmillan Press.
Dworkin, G (1988) *The Theory and Practice of Autonomy*. Cambridge: Cambridge University Press.
Edge, RS & Groves, JR (1999) *Ethics of Health Care: A Guide for Clinical Practice*. Albany, NY: Delmar Publishing.
Emmanuel, E & Emmanuel, L (1992) Four models of patient–physician relationship. *Journal of the American Medical Association* 267(16): 2212–2226.
Glover, D (1999) *Accountability*. London: NT Books.
Griffith, R & Tengnah, C (2004) A question of negligence: The law and the standard of prescribing. *Nurse Prescribing Journal* 2(2): 90–92.
Harris, J (1995) *The Value of Life*. London: Routledge.
Hartley, J (2004) Lifting the lid on the drug industry. *Nursing Times* 100(47): 21–22.
Haydock, A (1992) QALYs – A threat to our quality of life. *Journal of Applied Philosophy* 9(2): 183–188.
Hendrick, J (2000) *Law and Ethics in Nursing and Healthcare*. Cheltenham: Nelson Thornes.
Hogg, C (1999) *Patients, Power and Politics: From Patients to Citizens*. London: Sage.
House of Commons Health Commitee (2005) *The Influence of the Pharmaceutical Industry*. London: The Stationery Office.
Joseph Rowntree Foundation (2006) *Drug Consumption Rooms*. London: Joseph Rowntree Foundation.
Kant, I (1996) Foundations of Metaphysics of Morals, Gregor, MJ (ed.). Cambridge: Cambridge University Press.
Klein, R (1998) Competence, professional self regulation and the public interest. *British Medical Journal* 316(7146): 1740–1742.
Komesaroff, PA & Kerridge, IH (2002) Ethical issues concerning the relationships between medical practitioners and the pharmaceutical industry. *Medical Journal of Australia* 176(3): 118–121.
Lazarini, Z (2001) An analysis of ethical issues in prescribing and dispensing syringes to injection drug users. *Health Matrix Cleveland* 11(1): 85–128.
MacIntyre, AC (1984) *After Virtue: A Study in Moral Theory* (2nd edition). London: Duckworth.
McHale, J (2003) A review of the legal framework for accountable nurse prescribing. *Nurse Prescribing Journal* 1(3): 107–112.
Memon, A, Vrig, A & Bull, R (2003) *Psychology and Law: Truthfulness, Accuracy and Credibility*. Chichester: John Wiley and Sons Ltd.
Mezirow, J (1981) A critical theory of adult learning and education. *Adult Education* 32(1): 3–24.
Mill, JS (1859) *On Liberty*. London: Longmans, Roberts and Green.
Mill, JS (1869) *Utilitarianism*. London: Longmans, Green, Reader and Dyer.
National Prescribing Centre (2001) *Maintaining Competency in Prescribing*. Liverpool: National Prescribing Centre.

Newdick, C (2005) Accountability for rationing – theory into practice. *Journal of Law, Medicine and Ethics* **33**(4): 660–668.

Noddings, N (1984) *Caring, a Feminine Approach to Ethics and Moral Education*. Berkeley, CA: University of California Press.

Nursing and Midwifery Council (2006) *Standards of Proficiency for Nurse and Midwife Prescribers*. London: Nursing and Midwifery Council.

Royal Pharmaceutical Society of Great Britain (2003) *Guidance for Pharmacists on Working with the Pharmaceutical Industry*. London: Royal Pharmaceutical Society of Great Britain.

Rumbold, G (1999) *Ethics and Nursing Practice* (3rd edition). London: Baillière Tindall.

Seedhouse, D (1998) *Ethics: The Heart of Health Care*. Chichester: John Wiley & Sons Ltd.

Shaw, M (2003) Freebies, favours and the seven deadly sins: Keeping on the straight and narrow. *Nurse Prescribing* **1**(3): 134–136.

Spallone, P (1992) *Generation Games: Genetic Engineering and the Future of our Lives*. Philadelphia: Temple University Press.

Thompson, D (ed.) (1998) *The Concise Oxford Dictionary*. Oxford: Clarendon Press.

4 The Public Health Context

JOHN McKINNON

'Health is not bought with a chemist's pills, nor saved by the surgeon's knife.
Health is not only the absence of ills, but the fight for the fullness of life.'
Piet Hien, World Health Organization 40th Anniversary
Conference, October 27th 1988.

In this chapter, the meaning of public health and the public health dimension of
prescribing will be discussed. Three areas – antimicrobial resistance, use and misuse
of drugs and iatrogenesis – have been given special attention because of their
relevance to prescribing practice. Consideration will be given to the values of the
modern public health era and their pertinence in the twenty-first century. Health
statistics will be sifted and the health states they represent will be understood in the
light of the lived experience of communities. Lifestyle choice will be placed in the
context of health inequality.

None of this is a digression from the core purposes of this book. Rather, we
will see that a public health philosophy in prescribing helps to maintain a focus on
the true determinants of health, serves justice in healthcare and promotes a holistic
approach to practice.

PUBLIC HEALTH PRINCIPLES

Public health is concerned with the ability of the many to live healthily and any
intervention aimed at sustaining or improving this. Such a concept, although vast,
is governed by universal principles of community collaboration, empowerment and
health as a human right.

Public health has been the concern of civilisation since ancient times, but the
huge shifts in population that accompanied the industrialisation and urbanisation of
Victorian Britain and the resultant increase in squalor, poverty and disease created
a backdrop for major humanitarian campaigns in favour of prison reform, sanitary
regulation, effective systems for sewage and waste disposal, the provision of basic
clean housing, and education regarding hygiene and nutrition. It was also during
this time that limits began to be set on working hours and conditions, not least
those pertaining to children (Baggott, 2000; Naidoo and Wills, 2005b).

Towards Prescribing Practice. Edited by J. McKinnon.
© 2007 John Wiley & Sons, Ltd.

The worth of public health provision lies in its long-term epidemiological and economic benefits when measured against its cost to the public purse. Social reforms of the past have arisen out of the realisation that to do nothing would ultimately be more costly. The preventive health principle at the heart of such measures was captured by Florence Nightingale when, following her return from the Crimea, she conducted a study of deprivation in provincial communities. Nightingale said,

> We seem to be watching . . . murder going on, and to be waiting for the rates of mortality to go up before we interfere; . . . And then, when enough have died, we think it time to spend some money and some trouble to stop the murders going further, and we enter the results of our masterly inactivity neatly in tables. (Ridgely Seymer, 1954: 382)

The near-apocalyptic proportions of the death rates in the mid to late nineteenth century from infectious diseases such as typhus, smallpox, measles, scarlet fever, whooping cough, tuberculosis and cholera raised fears that disease would spread to higher social groups, threatening recruitment to the armed forces and socioeconomic meltdown. These fears, rather than any sudden sense of altruism among the upper classes, provided the impetus for the reforms that followed (Naidoo and Wills, 2005a).

The view that public health legislation and practice infringe civil liberties, allied to fears of a 'nanny state', was common in the nineteenth century and survives today. However, in reality societies prosper on the back of how individuals relate to one another rather than what they achieve in isolation. Absolute individual autonomy is neither attainable nor desirable. It is not truly attainable in that each member of society at one time or another relies on the integrity of others to inform and support their decisions and judgements. It is undesirable because the rights of the individual are best preserved when consideration is given to how the acquittal of those rights affects others and the general wellbeing of the population at large. Legislation on compulsory use of car seatbelts, water fluoridation and prohibition of smoking in public places are examples of state enforcement of this principle. Moreover, where there is voluntary acknowledgement of these 'relational' values of shared welfare – where childless adult citizens willingly pay taxes to support those raising young families in the knowledge that such future generations will support them as tomorrow's aged; or where the privileged and prosperous in society support the underprivileged, chronically ill and impoverished in the confidence that they too would receive support were they to fall on unanticipated hardship and poor health – we might contend that our nation is a better, more stable place (Wanless, 2002).

NEW CHALLENGES FOR OLD

The public health reforms of the nineteenth and twentieth centuries, together with better healthcare, have led to an improved level of health for all, which is observable in average life expectancy increases from 45.5 years in men and 49 years in women in 1901 to 76 years for men and 81 years for women in 2000 (Amaranayake et al., 2000). However, the infectious disease epidemics linked to former prevailing social conditions have been replaced by a new breed of conditions – cardiovascular disease, cancer, diabetes, acquired immune deficiency syndrome (AIDS) and mental illness – which are also linked to the prevailing social conditions of our era (Colgrove, 2002). All these conditions have the potential to outstrip the capacity to treat them (Department of Health, 2004).

The increase in mobility of populations across western continents, whether for reasons of economic migration, trade and commerce or political asylum, has led to a greater multicultural mix in most nations and with it a more complex variety of health needs. The economic world recession of the latter part of the twentieth century left many communities in need of investment and regeneration. Relative poverty and social exclusion have bred low social morale and fragmented neighbourhood networks. The advent of the 24-hour or '24/7' society has brought with it changing patterns of working and living, which do not sit well with an inflexible primary healthcare provision confined to office hours.

Increasingly sedentary routines, widespread use of labour-saving technology and the reduction of time and space reserved for sport as part of school curricula mean that physical exercise no longer assumes a natural place at the heart of individual lifestyles. Dietary habits have changed so that a greater proportion is occupied by foods with a high glycaemic index as well as saturated and hydrogenated fats (Ebelling et al., 2002). 'Fast' and 'convenience' foods, in company with potentially misleading information about their content, have exacerbated this trend. These factors have been blamed for increased levels of obesity and cardiovascular disease (Baltas, 2001; Dietz, 2001). Type II diabetes mellitus, once a condition of middle and old age, is increasingly found among younger people (Zimmet et al., 1997; Ludwig and Ebelling, 2001).

Prolonged life expectancy has brought with it an increase in chronic illnesses and greater caring responsibilities for a shrinking younger population. A larger ageing population and the unprecedented number of immunosuppressed patients recovering from organ transplant surgery or receiving treatment for an immune disease who would not have survived in previous times mean that the population is more rather than less vulnerable to disease. A new generation of infectious disease is feared. Tuberculosis, once thought to be wholly containable if not a disease of the past, is re-emerging as a potent threat to health (Minten et al., 2004). The ability of viruses to mutate means that the influenza pandemic of 1918 is thought certain to be repeated at some point in the future (Department of Health, 2002a).

THE DETERMINANTS OF HEALTH

The definition of health given at the beginning of the chapter was coined by the late Danish philosopher, poet and scientist Piet Hien on the 40th anniversary of the inauguration of the World Health Organization (WHO). Among many such definitions, this one stands out as superior by virtue of its comprehensiveness.

THE PLACE OF BIOMEDICAL INTERVENTIONS

Hien's reference to 'chemist's pills and the surgeon's knife' highlights the limitations of biomedical science. While it is true that modern medical care has had a positive impact on the lives of many, it is, at best, one dimensional and episodic in nature. Biomedical interventions are not root factors in health; they may palliate or remove illness and disease, but they do not of themselves create health. Health is not one dimensional. It is a state that is born from the security, hope and optimism brought about by an individual's ability to shape their surroundings (Freund et al., 2003). Public health is not synonymous with public health medicine. The provision of comprehensive advanced healthcare in a community with no leisure facilities, lacking access to affordable fresh food and fragmented by crime and violence illustrates the tertiary and one-dimensional contribution of biomedical science to health.

INEQUALITIES IN HEALTH

The utopian idealism implicit in the WHO's 1946 definition of health is conspicuously absent from Hien's definition. His mention of the need to 'fight' implies the existence of injustice. Successive studies (Townsend et al., 1992; Acheson, 1998) have shown that health status has much less to do with what an individual does in isolation than the geographic and socioeconomic circumstances into which they are born and the behaviours that these circumstances engender.

The statistics alone expose the social polarisation of health in terms of class, gender, ethnicity and place of residence. Seven years separate the life expectancy of a man born in the lowest socioeconomic group from a man born in the highest. An infant born in poverty is 2.2 times more likely to die before one year old than a baby born into affluence. The incidence of chronic illness among members of the lowest socioeconomic group is double that of those born into the most prosperous levels of society. Women live on average six years longer than men, yet they record higher morbidity rates in both acute and chronic illness. Poverty is over 60 % more common in Britain among Black Caribbean and Indian families and twice as common among Black non-Caribbean families than in those of Caucasian peoples. Among Bangladeshi and Pakistani families poverty is more than three times as common as in white families. This affluence gap between ethnic groups is matched by a corresponding chasm in wellbeing. For example, higher rates of cardiovascular disease, schizophrenia and suicidal behaviour are found among black men (Department for Work and Pensions, 2003; Nazroo, 1998).

Health would also appear to be dictated by the places in which people live out their lives. A health divide exists not just between rich and poor but also between the north and south of the UK, with morbidity and mortality rates higher in the north.

Much of the political rhetoric of our time is concerned with lifestyle choice and its relationship to health. In particular, consumerist approaches to health promotion such as those enshrined in the 1992 *Health of the Nation Report* (Department of

Health, 1992) imply that good health is attained as a commodity in a marketplace. In this vision of public health the emphasis is on effective giving and receiving of advice and information that service users are required to apply (Baggott, 2000; Naidoo and Wills, 2005a). However, health inequality speaks of a plethora of factors influencing wellbeing over which an individual has little or no control, such as gender, genetics, ethnicity and socioeconomic status. The four constructs of power – standard of education, economic status, mental health and physical ability – are all compromised among lower socioeconomic groups. Individuals who lack one or more of these are less able to exercise choice. Choice equates with power and is therefore constrained by poverty (Marmot and Wilkinson, 2006). Graham (2000) confirmed this when she found that lifestyle choice was responsible for only 20–30 % of the socioeconomic health gradient. The remainder is the result of the cumulative effect of adverse circumstances (Moore, 2002).

Strong, intertwined threads of social and epidemiological evidence running from the antenatal period through childhood and deep into adulthood have recently been exposed that show the lamentable plight of the poor in our time: developmentally and nutritionally disadvantaged *in utero* and in infancy, burdened with anxiety, suffering from poor concentration and low self-esteem in childhood, which threatens failure at school and promotes adolescent and teenage crime and disorderly behaviour. This early disadvantage is said to 'cast long shadows forward over future health' in terms of high morbidity and mortality (Graham and Power, 2004: 16). Those affected find their own child-bearing and parenting capacities compromised, as did their parents before them, and a well-trodden cycle of deprivation continues.

Arguments formed in a culture of blame that seek to dismiss the health inequalities are discharged by these findings, opening up new understandings of why and how the poor remain relatively ill and the rich remain relatively well.

THE ROLE OF PERSONAL AND CULTURAL FRAMEWORKS

The term 'fight' also permits a role for empowerment of the individual and their right to define and measure their health as it has meaning for them. While it is true that there are universal evidence-based determinants of good health, these are fluid rather than inflexible when they interface with an individual or group frame of reference. A rigid, standardised interpretation of what constitutes health can work to exclude groups who are merely at odds with some preset societal norm.

People who have physical or mental impairments, for example, do not require 'treatment' as if they were ill. People with impairments require a change in society's values expressed in an environment that they may access on equal terms with others. This should take the shape of change in the physical situation, such as facilitating wheelchair access, and change in the political process to include the voices of the socially excluded (Hales, 1996; Laverack, 2005). Hien's definition therefore values a personal state where health may exist in the presence of impairment and even chronic illness, because of the ability to realise dreams and ambitions.

A postmodernist perspective on health does not simply require an understanding of statistical patterns or a striving for healthcare targets, but a grasp of the daily practical, structural and legislative obstacles that people must negotiate in any attempt to improve their own health (Marmot and Wilkinson, 2006). Promoting health among the public at large means listening to how cultural and personal frameworks shape perception and expression of need and, by extension, receipt of information.

Familiar surroundings, social networks and peer support are essential to facilitating good public health. A man's willingness to accompany his wife to weekly dancing lessons at a local village hall may increase when he learns that a number of his male friends already attend with their partners. Teenagers will find sexual health services less embarrassing and more palatable within the walls of a youth club than those of a clinic or doctor's surgery (Ellis and Grey, 2004). At other times the pressure of caring responsibilities, such as the demands of childcare or the needs of infirm relatives, may cause a woman to postpone decisions about smoking cessation, recreation or holidays (Naidoo and Wills, 2005a).

The salience of social networking to wellbeing is borne out by the findings of a long-term study in which North American single-parent families in receipt of a nurse home-visitation programme experienced positive health outcomes in the face of otherwise worsening social conditions (Olds et al., 1998).

The role of religious belief and moral positioning in health is also observable among many groups. The fasting requirements of the Islamic festival of Ramadan may make evening classes less appealing to Muslims. Vegetarians will require reassurance about the non-animal sources and constituents of many drugs. For these groups and others like them, practices aimed at improving health must sit well with a moral and spiritual basis for living. To compromise on such issues occasionally is to devalue their sense of self-worth and purpose, negating any apparent temporary health gain in another area.

Public health is not merely a combination of tasks designed to achieve healthy living. Health-enhancing activities may not be viewed as such if better health as a commodity is the only visible end. A daily five-mile bike ride will almost certainly be more appealing when it also serves as transport to and from work.

The breadth, depth and nature of exposure to healthy living are sometimes predictors of the confidence with which people will approach and engage with health advice. It is not reasonable to expect children or adults who have never experienced properly cooked vegetables or had access to a wide variety of fresh fruit to act eagerly on advice to include them in their daily diet. The cost alone may prove prohibitive. Parents in lower socioeconomic groups often perceive as wasteful the purchase of foodstuffs that they fear their children will not eat. The health gain inherent in evidence-based life practices is real to someone only when it is able to function within personal and cultural frameworks woven within the fabric of their life. Experienced healthcare professionals work to promote health within these frameworks rather than opposing or ignoring them. Personal and cultural frameworks hold the key to the design of strategies for health improvement that are tailored to individuals, communities and groups (Naidoo and Wills, 2005b).

THE ROLE OF ENVIRONMENT AND INFRASTRUCTURE

Hien speaks of health and the 'fullness of life'. Fullness of life is concerned with access to diverse experience that permits individual growth and development and a sense of self-worth and purpose. Denial of fullness of life, conversely, results in suppressed development, low life expectation, low self-esteem and lack of purpose. Life fullness is closely linked with principles of lifelong learning that embrace formal education, travel, social interaction and community participation. Unemployment has negative impacts on health through disenfranchisement and social exclusion. Moreover, lack of worker control over a situation in the workplace is linked to ill health (Mausner-Dorsch and Eaton, 2000). Opportunities for social interaction and community participation are related to longevity (Sugarman, 2005). Populations living in the shadow of excessive toxic chemical efflux or with no clean water supply often suffer from a range of illnesses.

The demographic composition of a community and the level of facilities for employment and education, trade and consumption, transport and safety, crime and law enforcement, healthcare, housing, sanitation and clean air, nutrition, food production and storage standards, recreation and leisure, religion and culture all contribute to the grand narrative of public health analysis. This grand narrative is a map of health need that is the community health profile (see Table 4.1). This profile includes short- and long-term plans and strategies for how these needs might be met (see Table 4.2). Many such strategies are the result of alliances between a range of disciplines across the public and private sectors. The provision of a public swimming pool is one example of how many health needs can be met within one community project. It functions as a meeting place, a centre for exercise and recreation and a tool for ill-health prevention that is acceptable and affordable to all races, classes

Table 4.1 Community profiling

Describe the district in which you practise and how it has changed in the last 100 years.
What is the size and composition of the population? Include an assessment of mobility, birth and death rates.
What are the main areas of employment and the proportion of unemployment?
Profile the proportion of low income households and their distribution across race and gender.
Analyse the effectiveness of local environmental health services.
Critically assess facilities for preschool, school, further and higher education and lifelong learning.
Detail the primary, secondary and tertiary care services, assessing the ease of public access and relevance to local epidemiology.
Measure the universality and appropriateness of local sports and leisure facilities.
Detail the local mix of housing and the proximity of other services and facilities.
Critically appraise the accessibility of public transport infrastructure, its alignment with commuter routes, health, education, trade and leisure facilities.

Table 4.2   Public health professional action plan

Do my clinical priorities match the needs of the community in which I work?
What are the implications of my community profile shape for my practice in relation to

- Health needs of specific client groups, e.g. migrant workers, ethnic minorities, travelling people, homeless, mentally ill, geographically isolated, children, women, men, older people
- Antimicrobial resistance
- Free prescriptions and dispensing services
- Drug abuse and misuse
- Immunisation programmes
- Health promotion and screening
- Non-attendance and uptake of services?

What developments are necessary to make my practice more accessible, effective, appropriate and equitable?
What professional and lay partnerships do I need to build?

---

and cultures, and has repeatedly been shown to be a positive infrastructural health determinant within disadvantaged communities (Laverack, 2005).

The perpetually expanding role of therapeutics in the prevention and management of disease has brought its own specific problems to the modern public health picture. Effective prescribing in the public health context requires practitioners to be aware of these issues and the implications they have for practice.

ANTIMICROBIAL RESISTANCE

Antimicrobial resistance is a collective term referring to the changes that take place in microbes that serve to protect them by reducing or negating the effectiveness of therapeutic agents designed to fight infection.

Antimicrobials have stood at the helm of medical treatment and biomedical scientific advancement for almost three-quarters of a century. Yet a place for discussion has been reserved here not because of the problems this has addressed, but for those that have been created. Resistance to penicillin was observed (Abraham and Chain, 1940) as early as 1940. Now the ability of microbes to develop a variety of mechanisms that sustain them in the face of the most powerful antimicrobial agents poses one of the biggest threats to public health in the twenty-first century. The trend is observable in every group of antimicrobials: the resistance of *Staphylococcus aureus* to methicillin, *Escherichia coli* to gentamicin, *Enterococcus faecalis and Enterococcus faecium* to vancomycin, and *Streptococcus pneumoniae* to penicillin and erythromycin have all increased, most dramatically since 1990. Consequently, major infectious diseases have become more difficult to treat. The scale and immi-nence of the presenting danger should not be underestimated. Our generation will be the one to succeed or fail in stemming this trend and we may also be the ones to reap the rewards of success or pay the price of failure (Department of Health, 1999, 2000; Health Protection Agency, 2005a, 2005b).

ROUTES OF RESISTANCE

Microbes exist in a world where resistant strains of organisms survive the sensitive organisms and sensitive organisms become resistant. Pharmacodynamic variety in antimicrobials means that bacteria have the capacity to develop and retain multiple resistances.

Resistance has been spread by spontaneous mutation, by transposons and by exchange of DNA material via plasmids. In spontaneous mutation, a mutant gene imparts resistance to a microbe, which then thrives and divides (Figure 4.1). Trans-posons are sections of DNA that can replicate themselves and code for resistance. Each section has end segments at either end that, aided by the enzyme transposase, migrate to other parts of the microbe's genome and insert themselves there, rather like a 'cut and paste' editing tool in a computer program (Figure 4.2). This migration property has led to transposons being informally labelled 'jumping genes'. Plasmids are circular 'pockets' of genetic material that often exist close to the bacterial cell wall and that code for replication of resistance, which can be unilaterally transferred during conjugation with other bacteria (Figure 4.3). Transposons use plasmids as stepping-stones. Resistant DNA can also be absorbed by the bacterium from the external environment. Recombinant DNA technology used in controlled laboratory manipulation is in fact an artificial simulation of this natural process.

ANTIMICROBIAL ACTION AND THE MECHANISMS OF RESISTANCE

Antimicrobials have been traditionally divided into those agents that are directly bactericidal (they kill the bacteria) and those that are bacteriostatic (they inhibit cell growth). However, in modern therapeutics these boundaries have become blurred.

Antimicrobial action takes place in a number of ways (Figure 4.4) and patterns of resistance have developed that are aligned with these routes.

Inhibition of Cell Wall Synthesis

Human cells and bacterial cells are first of all distinguishable from one another by the fact that bacterial cells have a wall and human cells do not. Gram-negative and Gram-positive bacteria can be identified by 'Gram staining' of any body fluid that is normally sterile.

The cell wall is assembled in a series of 'steps' beginning with the cytoplasm and ending outside the cytoplasmic membrane. The outer cellular coverings of Gram-negative and Gram-positive bacteria differ. In Gram-negative bacteria the outer

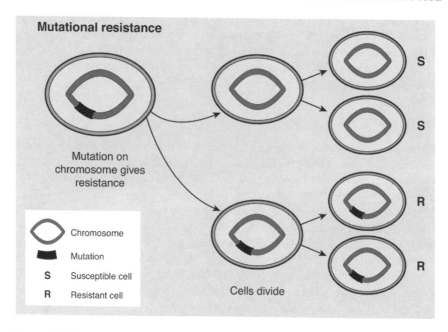

Figure 4.1 Spontaneous mutation. Reproduced by permission of MA Healthcare. (See also colour plate 16).

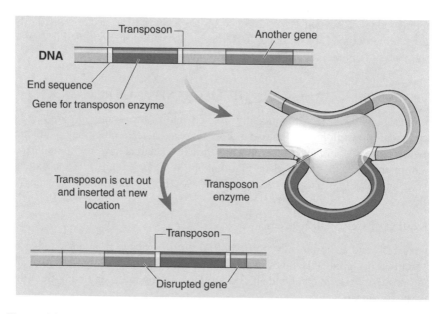

Figure 4.2 Transposons or 'jumping genes'. Reproduced by permission of MA Healthcare. (See also colour plate 17).

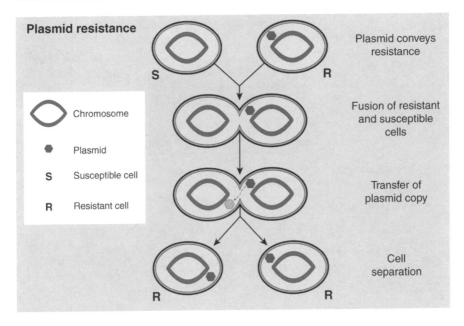

Figure 4.3 Exchange of DNA material via plasmids. Reproduced by permission of MA Healthcare. (See also colour plate 18).

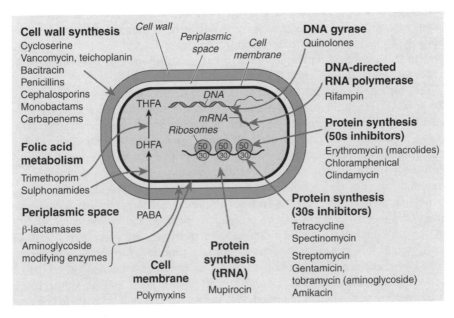

Figure 4.4 Diversity of antimicrobial action. Reproduced by permission of MA Healthcare. (See also colour plate 19).

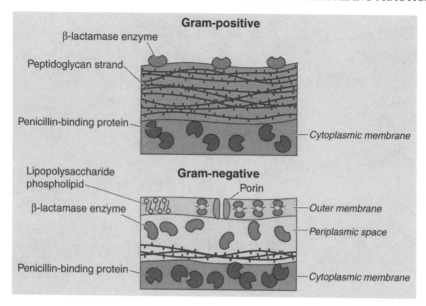

Figure 4.5 Gram-positive and Gram-negative bacteria. Reproduced by permission of MA Healthcare. (See also colour plate 20).

membrane of lipopolysaccharide is located exterior to a few layers of interwoven peptidoglycan, with a periplasmic space in between. In Gram-positive bacteria the lipopolysaccharide layer is missing and many more layers of peptidoglycan are present (Figure 4.5). It is the peptidoglycan chains that are vital to wall integrity, as they maintain rigidity (Seeley et al., 2000).

Beta-lactams (penicillins, carbapenems, cephalosporins and monobactams) inhibit the cross-linking of the peptidoglycan chains by inhibiting transpeptidase, the relevant catalyst, and by activating autolytic enzymes. Osmotic pressure in the cytoplasm is high and a break in the wall results in rapid cell death. Vancomycin and bacitracin are two antimicrobials whose inhibitive actions take place particularly early in the peptidoglycan biosynthetic process, interfering with lipid carrier transport from the cytoplasmic membrane to the developing peptidoglycan matrix.

Beta-lactamases, degradative bacterial enzymes that thrive in the periplasmic space and outer membrane of Gram-negative microbes and on the outer surface of the peptidoglycan wall of Gram-positive microbes, are the chief agents of resistance in this area. Beta-lactamases inactivate the beta-lactams by hydrolysis. Beta-lactamases are also responsible for altering penicillin-binding sites, rendering beta-lactams ineffective (Patterson, 2003; Rupp and Fey, 2003). Although the cephalosporin generation of antimicrobials has served to counter this, there is recent evidence to show that it too is proving ineffective against new extended-spectrum beta-lactamases (ESBL), which have adapted through exchange of genetic material (Carbonne et al., 2005).

Disruption of Cell Membrane

The cytoplasmic membrane of Gram-negative bacteria acts as a diffusion barrier for water, ions, nutrients and transport systems. A number of antibacterial agents can cause disorganisation of the outer membrane. These agents can be divided into cationic, anionic and neutral agents. The best-known compounds are polymyxin B and colistemethate (polymyxin E), and these are commonly used. They are nephrotoxic and can only be used for non-systemic infection. Polymyxins are bactericidal cationic detergents with both lipophilic and lipophobic parts that interact with phospholipids and disrupt bacterial cell membranes. The divalent cationic sites on the lipopolysaccharide component of the outer membrane of Gram-negative organisms interact with the amino groups of polymyxins. The lipophilic tail portion of the drug molecule penetrates the hydrophobic areas of the outer layer to produce holes in the membrane through which cellular constituents can leak (Figure 4.6).

Resistance has been observed taking place as a result of modification of the transmembrane proteins or porins. These cell surface changes reduce the affinity of the polymyxin drug molecule (Gunn et al., 1998). Drug efflux pathways have also been shown to be instrumental in the resistance of some microbes to polymyxin (Bengoechea and Skurnik, 2000). Antimicrobial agents can be ejected through these pathways by altering the gradient of diffusion across the bilayer.

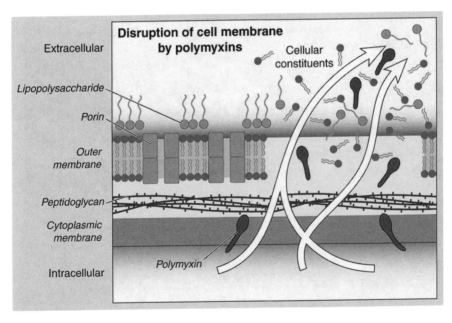

Figure 4.6 Disruption of the cell membrane by polymyxins. Reproduced by permission of MA Healthcare. (See also colour plate 21).

Inhibition of DNA Replication

Quinolones and metronidazole inhibit DNA synthesis by blocking DNA gyrase enzymes which catalyse the direction and extent of DNA supercoiling.

Resistance takes place when mutative changes occur in the target enzymes or in the permeability of the organism (Engberg et al., 2001).

Inhibition of Protein Synthesis

Protein synthesis takes place in the cytoplasm of the microbe. Therapeutic agents bind with the 30S ribosomal subunit (in the case of gentamicin, tobramycin, amikacin, streptomycin, neomycin and tetracycline) and with the 50S ribosomal subunits (in the case of erythromycin, clindamycin and chloramphenicol) to inhibit the process. Rifampin acts on enzyme RNA polymerase, which is responsible for constructing the RNA that reads the microbe's genetic code and for giving instructions to the ribosomes on protein synthesis. The topical antibiotic mupirocin acts to inhibit the latter process.

Resistance has developed through chromosomal mutation, resulting in reduced binding capacity, and also through the development of the efflux pumps illustrated in Figure 4.7 (Engberg et al., 2001).

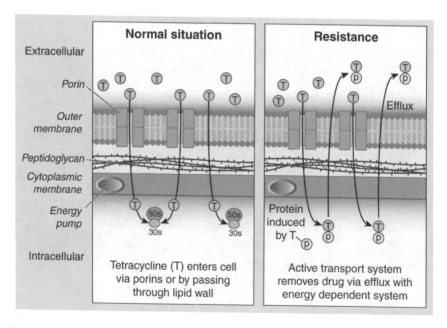

Figure 4.7 Development of efflux pumps. Reproduced by permission of MA Healthcare. (See also colour plate 22).

Folate Antagonists

Here there is competitive inhibition of the folate metabolic pathway. In turn, RNA and DNA replication are compromised. Sulphonamides such as co-trimoxazole block the conversion of P-amino benzoic acid (PABA) to dihydrofolic acid (DHFA). Trimethoprim blocks the conversion of dihydrofolic acid to tetrahydrofolic acid (THFA).

Resistance to this group of antimicrobials has been observed for many years and can occur in a number of ways. The microbe may simply produce excessive amounts of PABA or, because of plasmid-mediated DNA changes, the therapeutic agents may not bind so well to PABA, DHFA or THFA. Microbial permeability may also be reduced (Enne et al., 2001; Grape et al., 2003).

A UNIQUE SITUATION IN THERAPEUTICS

Resistance is a unique entity because antimicrobial use is widespread. Apart from analgesia, no other form of medication is so commonly prescribed or taken. The communal consequences of this are also unique. The capacity for resistance to spread means that the efficacy of treatment prescribed for one individual is related to the dexterity of prescribing by other practitioners for other patients in other situations in the past, present or future. Conversely, the extent to which those patients adhere to the prescribed regimen will also influence the efficacy of that agent elsewhere. This cannot be said of any other drug group.

The use of antimicrobials is not limited to the world of human pathogens. Antimicrobials are also used in veterinary practice and prophylactically in animal husbandry to promote growth. These practices have implications for the control of antimicrobial resistance in the wider population, in that they may compromise the potency of agents used in human biomedical intervention (Teale, 2005). There is also a risk that these undermine those new antimicrobial groups still in development. Spontaneous resistance and cross-resistance in a shared environment may cause pathogens to acquire a cellular defence against such new groups before they are ever prescribed.

CONTRIBUTORY FACTORS

There is no one solitary causative factor at the root of this situation. Many features of our modern world that at a glance may appear unrelated have contributed to the rise in resistant microbes. It is likely, however, that these factors fall within one or more of the following categories:

- mobility among individuals, communities and groups
- herded populations
- suboptimum prescribing practice
- poor adherence to prescribed regimens

- suboptimum standards of infection control
- other misuse of antimicrobials.

In the world of domestic hygiene antibacterial agents have become popular, performing functions where disinfectants or soap and water would suffice. Conversely, complacency relating to basic hygiene and infection control such as hand washing among both the public and health professionals has encouraged plasmid transfer (Wise, 2004).

Hospitals present a special challenge in that, although in the UK only one tenth of antimicrobial prescribing takes place there, prescribing patterns are more concentrated and the target group more vulnerable to infection. This increased 'selective pressure' makes hospital settings ideal breeding grounds for resistance and 'opportunistic pathogens' that in another situation may have proved harmless. The increased throughput of patients in acute hospital settings further accelerates resistance spread. The growing prevalence of nursing and residential homes for older people and pre-school care provision for children constitutes further 'herding' of members of the population who have less robust immune systems.

The propensity among patients towards discontinuing antimicrobials when illness subsides rather than at the end of the prescribed course encourages the development of resistance in microbes that may not yet have been penetrated. The propensity among healthcare professionals to prescribe non-specifically in advance of or without culture of organism sensitivity or inappropriately for viruses or other self-limiting conditions leads to unnecessary exposure of bacteria to therapeutic agents, nurturing resistance still further. These practices, together with the suboptimum infection control discussed above, are what have led to infections such as methicillin-resistant *Staphylococcus aureus* (MRSA) reaching endemic proportions in many hospital and community settings (Department of Health, 2000; Scottish Infection Standards and Strategy Group, 2006).

Resistance in the UK remains lower than in many of its European neighbours, including France, Spain or Italy, but there is a feature of our modern life that may pose a threat to this. Although international travel and trade are far from recent phenomena, the contemporary availability of cheap airfares and consumer demand for imported, out-of-season produce have resulted in aircraft, shipping and juggernauts trailing 'corridors' of resistance transfer back and forth across continents (Department of Health, 1999).

PUBLIC PERCEPTION

Public perception and expectation constitute a major challenge to any initiative aimed at changing prescribing practices in this area. Despite the evidence that better public health has arisen because of better living standards and improved living conditions, biomedical interventions appear to receive the majority of the credit for delivering better health in the eyes and minds of the public. A number of studies (Milandri, 2004; Bozoni et al., 2006) carried out among primary school children in

Italy and Greece have shown that many youngsters view health as inextricably tied up with doctors and medicine. This suggests that the 'pill for every ill' culture may be deeply embedded in our minds from an early age. Milandri's work is of particular concern because of the way her young subjects saw antimicrobials as a blanket response to viruses and bacteria, with no distinction being made between cleansing and disinfecting. These are the very misconceptions that have led to complacency and negligence in everyday basic hygiene and overuse of antimicrobials.

The findings of research seeking to measure the success of public knowledge and expectation of antimicrobial therapy are less than heartening. In one study in north-east Scotland (Emslie and Bond, 2003), 351 patients with a variety of respiratory tract complaints responded to a postal questionnnaire enquiring into their attitudes, knowledge and behaviour towards antimicrobial use. Less than half of the respondents were concerned about antimicrobial resistance and although only a very small minority expected antimicrobial treatment for a cold, half said they would expect such treatment for influenza or a sore throat. In a much larger international study involving 3000 patients in Spain, France, Germany and Italy, Pechere (2004) found that the majority of sample members expected influenza to be treated with antibiotics.

A climate of consumerist values in which patients are encouraged to demand the treatment of their choice may mean that a change of prescribing or non-prescribing behaviour is met with opposition or even hostility. There is no ethical conflict here. Patients need help to understand the futility and danger of inappropriate antimicrobial prescribing for themselves and the communities in which they live. Concordance and public health are both served when there is sound communication of shared care plans that are clinically robust and evidence based. Practice that shrinks back from evidence-based behaviour for fear that the relationship with the patient will suffer serves no one.

THE WAY FORWARD

Antimicrobial resistance is inevitable. Conservation of the existing bank of anti-microbial drugs for as long as possible is essential. If resistance continues to outflank the development of new agents, antimicrobials will eventually become useless. This would in turn render most modern major surgery impossible. Entire groups of patients who currently rely on prophylactic antimicrobial therapy would not survive. Vital time currently bought by antimicrobials for the critically ill would be lost. Recovery times, morbidity and mortality rates would all rise.

The overall picture, although disturbing, is not a totally pessimistic one. The Health Protection Agency (HPA), incorporating the function of the decommissioned Public Health Laboratory Service, requires all microbiology centres to monitor and report resistance trends. In turn, the HPA collates these statistics to produce a national picture and make recommendations as to good proactive prescribing practice and infection control through evidence-based guidelines.

Evidence-based prescribing of antimicrobials includes short, three-day courses matched with penetration times for conditions such as uncomplicated cystitis or otitis media. Non-prescribing behaviour, refraining from unnecessary treatment with antimicrobials, is equally important Computerised decision-making systems and swifter microbiological diagnosis are also playing a part. Infection control involves not only the maintenence of high standards in personal and domestic hygiene, but also the control of the movement of air within clinical areas. This requires limiting the number of patients cared for in a bay and an increase in the quota of single rooms. The trend towards open visiting times in hospitals that has grown in recent years now, with hindsight, seems clinically inappropriate and is being curtailed and reversed (Department of Health, 2000).

The relevance to resistance of antimicrobial use in animal husbandry and veterinary practice has been recognised and collaborative working is taking place between the Department of Health, the Food Standards Agency and veterinary bodies.

Antimicrobial prescribing rates in the UK are being reduced. It is also encouraging that in Scandinavia, programmes to reduce the pace of resistance have met with some success (Wise, 2004) although some of the studies purporting to evidence this have been criticised for their lack of vigour.

Pharmaceutical companies are working towards developing a new generation of antimicrobials through genomics. This involves a number of techniques, including manipulation of genome sequencing to produce more powerful but specific antimicrobial therapy and comparative analysis of identified genes within bacteria to ascertain more precisely the spectrum and specificity of a precise target such as an efflux pump (Mills, 2003).

The *Haemophilus influenzae* type B vaccine protects against what hitherto has been the most common cause of bacterial meningitis in children under 5 years old and is offered routinely to all young children. The vaccine is an example of how immunisation is playing a growing part in the fight against bacterial infection.

One of the most potentially exciting developments in this field is still in its infancy. Britton et al. (2002) have observed that crocodiles thrive in highly infectious environments. While bacterial pathogens may survive in human blood for long periods of time, they are killed almost instantaneously when they enter crocodile blood. Britton and his colleagues have argued that crocodile immunology holds promise for the discovery and development of a new generation of potent antimicrobials.

DRUG MISUSE AND ABUSE

Substance abuse, or the use of drugs for non-therapeutic and recreational purposes, has been present in developed and underdeveloped societies for millennia. In our modern age, however, substance misuse has reached epidemic proportions and lies at the root of many of the dysfunctional features of society. In many cities around the world, drug barons have invaded legitimate businesses and drug crime has become part of the permanent economic infrastructure (Jansen and Bruinsma, 1997). It is estimated that in England and Wales alone, 11 million people between 16 and 59 years old have at some time taken illicit drugs (Home Office, 2005). Crime is perpetrated indirectly to feed the habit and directly to perpetuate trafficking (Jarvis and Parker, 1989; Hough, 1996). Depending on the substance of choice, addictive behaviour may result and lead to unemployment and family problems. The abuse of major toxic substances has been linked to cardiocascular disease (Mittleman et al., 1999), hepatitis C (Patrick et al., 2001), the induction of mental illness (Fergusson et al., 2005; Weaver et al., 2003), HIV/AIDS and premature death (Edlin et al., 1994).

ALCOHOL

The term 'substance abuse' is most commonly associated with illegal drugs such as cannabis, dextro lysergic acid diethylamide tartrate (LSD), cocaine and amphetamines, but in reality the most commonly abused substances are also those that are most freely available. Alcohol is the most commonly abused drug. Sold legally in a wide range of outlets, it has long assumed a fashionable image together with implied mythical properties of enhanced sophistication, maturity and even sexual prowess for the consumer. It is easily the most socially tolerated substance widely used as an integral part of relaxation and celebration alike, with often little conscious thought as to the effects of immoderate or excessive use. It is nonetheless estimated as being directly or indirectly responsible for over 40 % of admissions to accident and emergency units in the UK (Rainer et al., 1996; Charalambous, 2002).

TOBACCO

Smoking tobacco is the biggest single cause of preventable disease and premature death, responsible every year for 120,000 deaths in Britain alone at an annual cost of £1.7 billion to the health service (Department of Health, 2002b). The average cigarette contains a number of substances that are both toxic and carcinogenic, including nicotine, carbon monoxide, formaldehyde and hydrogen cyanide. The 30-minute half life of the stimulant nicotine explains why most smokers smoke an average of between 15 and 20 cigarettes per day. Temporary paralysis of the bronchial cilia is reversed during sleep and other periods of abstinence and is responsible for the 'smoker's cough' experienced on wakening. Withdrawal from tobacco can be very unpleasant and is characterised by anxiety and irritability, lethargy and exhaustion, increased thirst and hunger, dizziness and a sensation of 'pins and needles' at the extremities caused by peripheral vasodilation (Mera, 1997).

The numbers of people smoking tobacco have been falling for three decades, so that approximately 25 % of the population now engage in the habit. However, these statistics may give a misleading impression of the real trend, in that more young people are now smoking. This may be disguised in the general statistics by a reduction in the proportion of the population under the age of 25. A coordinated approach – including the availability of nicotine-replacement therapy on prescription, peer and professional support and anti-smoking campaigns, together with the prohibition of cigarette advertising and smoking in public places – appears currently to be having a positive impact on the prevalence of smoking (Naidoo et al., 2004).

The epidemiology of illnesses linked to non-therapeutic legalised drugs such as tobacco and alcohol remains a potent argument in opposition to further legalisation of other commonly abused substances, although this continues to be a highly contested issue.

DRUGS AND ABUSE POTENTIAL

Most drugs have a legitimate therapeutic use and, alternatively, an abuse potential. Arguments for the use of cannabis in the treatment of multiple sclerosis are merely a contemporary example of this. According to Longo and Johnson (2000: 2126), a drug can be said to have a high abuse potential if it has 'a rapid onset of action, a high potency, a brief duration of action, high purity and water solubility (for intravenous use) or high volatility (ability to vaporize if smoked)' among its profile characteristics. Commonly abused substances reflect this, as well as ease of access by the illicit drug user. Readily prescribable agents therefore number highly among such substances.

OPIATE DERIVATIVES

Although opiates prescribed for pain relief are not commonly abused and addiction as a result of legitimate therapeutic use is rare, opiate derivatives such as kaolin–morphine mixtures, Gee's linctus and codeine linctus have a long history of widespread abuse (Anderson and Berridge, 2000).

METHYLPHENIDATE (RITALIN)

Methylphenidate or Ritalin is a central nervous system stimulant after the fashion of an amphetamine. It is used in the treatment of patients with attention deficit hyperactivity disorder (ADHD), although how it achieves its mood-moderating effect is not strictly understood. Methylphenidate's pharmacodynamics are similar to cocaine, but methylphenidate has a slower clearance rate from the brain. When taken orally, its peak plasma concentration occurs after two hours in children, with a half life of 2.4 hours. However, when crushed and injected or inhaled, plasma concentration is achieved much more swiftly. When dissolved in water and injected there is an additional danger that insoluble excipients may act as emboli (Volkow et al., 1995). Methylphenidate is an appetite suppressant and can be abused by individuals trying to lose weight or simply for the euphoric effects it can supply. It has a street value and is otherwise known as Vitamin R or kiddie coke. It may increase the likelihood of seizures in people who have a previous history of this and should not be taken in pregnancy. Effects typical of sympathetic stimulation will result from overdosage: vomiting, agitation, tremors, muscle twitching, euphoria, confusion, hallucinations, delirium, sweating, flushing, headache, raised body temperature, tachycardia, palpitations, cardiac arrhythmias, hypertension, mydriasis and dryness of mucous membranes.

DRUG COCKTAILS

The use of cocktails in which one drug is used to reinforce the effects of another is common. The antihistamine chlorpheniramine or piriton enhances the effects of alcohol absorption and distribution and is misused by drug addicts and alcoholics.

Benzodiazepines, anxiolytics used in the treatment of anxiety and depression, while not usually sole drugs of abuse, are often primary drugs of recreation in combination with other agents, including alcohol. As with methylphenidate, abusers sometimes resort to alternative routes and methods of administration to achieve the desired altered mood. It seems that the highly lipophilic benzodiazepines such as diazepam are often favoured by polydrug abusers because of their ability to cross the blood–brain barrier more rapidly. Others associated with abuse are lorazepam and temazepam (street name 'wobbly eggs'), because of their short half life and high potency. These properties make drugs effective reinforcers of other agents (Longo and Johnson, 2000).

ANABOLIC STEROIDS

Anabolic steroids, synthetic derivatives of the male sex hormone testosterone, are used in moderate quantities to treat a range of inflammatory conditions, blood disorders and cancers. This drug group is abused by body builders seeking to enhance skeletal tissue growth and by athletes seeking to increase erythropoiesis, which in turn facilitates faster performance during any aerobic exercise through increased oxygen-carrying capacity. Common street names include 'roids', 'sauce' and 'slop'. These drugs can be taken orally (e.g. methandienone, oxymetholone and oxandrolone) or by intra-muscular injection (e.g. testosterone enanthate, nandrolene and sustanon). They can also be taken in conjunction with a range of products, including caffeine, to reinforce the effect. Side effects include growth of facial hair, irregular menstruation or amenorrhoea and deepening of the voice in women, and gynaecomastia, baldness and testicular atrophy in men. Hypertension, hyperlipidaemia, sequential heart disease and mood swings have been observed in abusers of anabolic steroids of both sexes (Kutscher et al., 2002; Payne et al., 2004).

LAXATIVES

Laxatives are commonly abused in the pursuit of weight loss by patients suffering from anorexia nervosa. Such weight loss is of course shortlived, as it is mainly as a result of water and electrolyte loss rather than loss of nutrients, which are absorbed at a higher location in the alimentary tract. Chronic laxative abuse/misuse will eventually present with one or more of a range of adverse reactions, including abdominal cramping and pain, diarrhoea and vomiting, which can lead to dehydration, electrolyte, fluid and mineral imbalances, weak muscles, metabolic acidosis, tetany and, in extreme cases, heart failure (Downie et al., 2000). Traces of stimulant laxatives such as Bisocodyl can be found in the urine of such consumers.

UNINTENTIONAL MISUSE

Often drug misuse is the product of poor consultation or a lack of education. For example, people who seek to procure laxatives suffer from constipation often because they have insufficient levels of fibre and fluid in their diet and/or because they do not take enough exercise. Such patients may not consider their practices as a misuse but as a logical step in self-medication.

'WEEKEND' DRUG ABUSE

The party and clubbing culture of recent years has created a new market for synthetic stimulants that produce fast, euphoric effects (McCambridge et al., 2005). They are all class A drugs and as such are illegal substances.

Liquid Ecstasy

Gammahydroxybutyrate, better known by its street names 'liquid ecstasy', GBH and GHB, is an anaesthetic and a class A drug with narrow distribution margins between energetic euphoria, sedation and coma. Used therapeutically in North America in the early 1990s, it was quickly withdrawn following a series of adverse reactions and dosage problems. GHB has been used illicitly alone, but can be reinforced using benzodiazepines or alcohol. Once ingested it has an average absorption time of ten minutes and a half life of two hours. Headache, nausea, vomiting, hallucinations, loss of peripheral vision, hypoventilation, cardiac arrhythmias, seizures, short-term coma and on rare occasions death are all documented side effects (Timby et al., 2000).

Ecstasy

The street name 'ecstasy' is shared with other substances: 3,4-methylene-dioxy-methamphetamine (MDMA), also known as 'Adam', 3,4-methylenedioxy-ethylamphetamine (MDEA), also known as 'Eve', and N-methyl-1-(3,4-methylene-dioxyphenyl)-2-butanamine (MBDB), also known as 'Methyl-J' or 'Eden'. There are also many unregulated variations. Drugs in this group are believed to be the illegal substances most commonly taken in Britain after cannabis and cocaine (Home Office, 2005). These 'designer' drugs stimulate the dopamine and serotonin receptors to produce an accelerated euphoric feeling. Memory problems, depression, restlessness and confusion are common experiences for days after consumption (Smith et al., 2002).

Ketamine

Ketamine hydrochloride (street names include 'angel dust', 'special K', 'Kit Kat' and 'Ket') is an anaesthetic used in humans and animals. It has also been a recreational drug since the 1960s and is taken intramuscularly, intravenously, orally, nasally and rectally, with a half life of 2.5 hours. Given parenterally it has an onset of five minutes, ten to twenty minutes when taken orally, depending on the last time food was consumed, and five to ten minutes when administered rectally or nasally. Its powerful anaesthetic properties mean that users have suffered serious injury without being immediately aware. Side effects include loss of motor control, temporary memory loss, numbness, drowsiness and nausea, along with 'out-of-body' and 'near-death experiences' (Dotson et al., 1995; Curran and Morgan, 2000).

Anaesthetic properties and the generated feelings of intimacy and enhanced libido also make both GHB and ketamine commonly used 'date rape' drugs.

'Weekend' Drugs and Public Health

Individuals who are known to take recreational drugs as part of the clubbing culture should be warned to refrain from driving, to remain among trusted others, not to dance incessantly but to rest intermittently in a well-ventilated area, to wear light clothing and to refrain from wearing head gear in order to avoid overheating. They should also avoid alcohol and drink approximately 500ml of water per hour when dancing. In addition, it is best to rest the following day. To facilitate this reputable clubs supply 'chill-out' rooms and water dispensers (Smith et al., 2002).

CRACK COCAINE

Cocaine is a derivative of the South American coca plant, which was used by the ancient Inca peoples in a variety of religious and hedonistic rituals. When inhaled or injected, cocaine blocks the uptake of dopamine in the midbrain, creating a state of euphoria (Mash and Staley, 1999). It presents as a white, bitter-tasting powder, but since the 1990s it has become popular to concentrate cocaine by heating the drug in a solution of ammonia or baking soda until the water evaporates. The end product of this is crack cocaine, so called because of the cracking sound produced by the heating process. Crack has the appearance of small crystal rocks and can be snorted. The effects are virtually instantaneous but last for about ten minutes. The substance has a wide variety of street names, including badrock, devil drug, french fries, grit, hotcakes, nuggets, prime time, rocks, scrabble, snow coke and sleet, to name only a few.

Crack use has been linked to pulmonary, cardiovascular and circulatory disease in addition to mood swings, anxiety, paranoia and aggression, together with cognitive difficulties (Hatsukami and Fischman, 1996; Constable, 2002). The British Crime Survey (Home Office, 2005) indicated that trends in the illicit use of cocaine showed a marked increase between 1998 and 2000. It remains the most commonly abused class A drug in Britain.

THE LAW AND DRUG ABUSE/MISUSE

Legislation is in place to regulate the import, production and supply of drugs, making them available for therapeutic use through prescription, but restricting their distribution where there is concern about the impact of abuse on individual and public health. There is currently grave concern that inappropriate sale and purchase of drugs over the Internet is bypassing this legislation.

Table 4.3 outlines drug classification under the 1971 Misuse of Drugs Act.

The Advisory Council on the Misuse of Drugs (ACMD), established under the 1971 Act, has a membership appointed by the Secretary of State for Health and representatives of the main prescribing professions, the pharmaceutical industry and other persons from a variety of backgrounds deemed to be able to advise on the social problems connected with drug abuse.

The Council has a duty to report to the Home Secretary, the Secretary of State for Health and the Secretary of State for Education and has a wide range of responsibilities as an adviser. These include measures to prevent the misuse of drugs and health promotion relating to the dangers of substance abuse, levels of restriction on the supply and availability of drugs and the supervision of arrangements for supply. The recent reclassification of cannabis was an example of this (Home Office, 2002). The ACMD also promotes collaboration between professional and community services to enable anyone affected by the misuse of drugs to access treatment and support. It also plays a part in promoting research into misuse prevention.

A person is regarded as being addicted to a drug if they have as a result of repeated administration become chemically dependent and harbour a singular desire

Table 4.3   Misuse of Drugs Act 1971 classification

Class A
  Cocaine
  Diamorphine (Heroin)
  Opium
  Dextro lysergic acid diethylamide tartrate (LSD)
  Class B compounds formulated for injection
Class B
  Oral amphetamines
  Barbiturates
  Codeine
  Ethylmorphine
  Phenmetrazine
  Pentacozine
Class C
  Cannabis (originally class B)
  Anabolic steroids
  Benzodiazepines
  Gonadotrophin

for administration to continue. Downie et al. (2000: 243) suggest that there are six chief ways in which addictive drug-seeking behaviour may present:

- Implying that the only possible solution to a medical problem is a prescription for a controlled (addictive) medication.
- Describing symptoms that markedly deviate from objective evidence or the physical examination findings.
- Claiming that non-addictive medications 'don't work' or cannot be taken because of an allergy to them, that the person has a high tolerance to drugs, that they have lost a prescription or that they have run out early.
- Manipulating the situation by pitting the opinion of one doctor on treatment against that of another. For example, threatening to get the requested drug from a 'smarter' or 'more caring' doctor.
- Resisting non-pharmacological treatment recommendations, such as behavioural training or psychotherapy.
- Offering bribes or sex, or even making threats of harm to person or property. Patients may often sell or forge prescriptions.

The Home Office maintains an index of addicts that doctors may consult in confidence. Practitioners are required to notify the Home Office annually of patients' attendance for treatment.

Professional diligence is important to prevent addicts from abusing a prescribing facility; but equally, expert help should be made available to help them overcome their addiction. The work of the Maudsley Hospital Group (Marsden, 1994; Marsden et al., 1998) has been influential in shaping the treatment and rehabilitation of substance addicts by identifying the multifactorial nature of the causal roots of substance abuse and the key support factors, such as personal support, housing and employment, that build resilience and sustain recovery. Here, as in many other areas of healthcare, positive outcomes have been more common when peer support is involved, particularly when young people have been the recipients of care (Black et al., 1998).

Stuart Kennedy discusses therapeutic approaches to substance abuse in Chapter 10.

PREVENTING IATROGENESIS

Iatrogenesis as it relates to adverse drug events is a negative impact on a patient's health status as a result of prescribing, preparation, dispensing and administration of medicines. It has been estimated that drug errors constitute the single largest source of iatrogenic incidents, at 11% (Leape et al., 1995). There is a well-established evidence base (Reason, 1990; Kohn et al., 1999) to show that in the absence of proven malicious intent, a punitive approach to drug errors is ineffective and at times counter-productive to risk management in therapeutics. Modern responses to reducing drug errors recognise the complex, fast-paced world in which practitioners and patients interact. Optimum competence in numeracy alone is insufficient protection against errors in such an environment, in which healthcare professionals are frequently required to multitask. Drugs that are pre-packaged in pharmacies for administration are becoming commonplace, as is the use of the patient's own drugs in formal care settings and drug dispensers that can be used in patients' own homes. These measures help ensure that the volume and rate of patient care required of care givers is less likely to be related to the amount of drug errors (National Prescribing Centre and National Primary Care Research and Development Centre, 2002).

GOOD HISTORY TAKING

Good history taking is the primary weapon of prevention against adverse drug events. It helps assemble a patient portfolio of past allergies and reactions and present medication, to include over-the-counter, general sales list, alternative treatments and non-therapeutic as well as prescribed drugs. The more detailed the history, the better the assessment of risk that is facilitated (National Prescribing Centre, 1999). Vulnerable groups such as the elderly, children and those who have multiple disease states or are immunosuppressed deserve special attention (National Prescribing Centre, 1999; Walker and Edwards, 2003; Curtis et al., 2004).

SHARING BEST PRACTICE

Responsibility for continuous professional development, which is shared by healthcare practitioners and employers, also contributes to drug administration safety (Nursing and Midwifery Council, 2002). The use of significant event audit is now part of established good practice and serves to produce a common team learning process out of an individual error, rather than to apportion blame. Learning that arises out of good practice is also shared. Clinical care pathways and information systems such as PRODIGY help ensure that evidence-based practice guides and informs prescribing behaviour and provides maps for planning therapeutic intervention (National Prescribing Centre and National Primary Care Research and Development Centre, 2002).

REPORTING UNANTICIPATED DEVIATIONS FROM THE NORM

Most pre-marketing drug trials are carried out on sample populations with single-pathology illness states and therefore are unlikely to detect many potential adverse reactions. The role of post-marketing prospective and retrospective research studies in predicting adverse drug event potential cannot therefore be understated. The association identified between Reye's syndrome and the use of aspirin in adolescents and children (McGovern et al., 2001; Committee for Safe Medicines, 2002) is an example of this.

In 2002, in what many believe to be a long-overdue legislative amendment, nurses joined doctors, pharmacists and dentists as an identified group authorised to use the yellow card system to report adverse reactions to the Committee for Safe Medicines (CSM) and the Medicines and Healthcare Products Regulatory Agency (MHRA) (Callaghan, 2003). The yellow card reporting system is the point at which proactive and reactive medicines management meet. The reporting practitioner reacts in response to an undesirable clinical response to a prescribed treatment, but collation of such reports by the CSM and MHRA means that awareness and pharmacovigilance are increased among other prescribers and patient safety benefits accordingly. Case reports such as the one by Schatz et al. (1989) also inform other prescribers of dangers that may hitherto have been unknown in the prescribing community.

OPTIMUM TEAM WORKING

Electronic patient-centred records help enhance shared record systems, in that any singular update simultaneously informs a whole team of professionals who may be delivering care and prescribing treatment for the same patient. The consequent reduction in delay of shared knowledge within a team means that the potential for adverse drug events is also reduced (National Prescribing Centre and National Primary Care Research and Development Centre, 2002).

The role of the pharmacist in relation to the prevention of adverse drug events is a multifaceted one: an expert therapeutic consultant for all prescribers, a patient and practitioner educator, a prescriber, dispenser and supplier. The time period that lies between the acts of prescribing and dispensing may prove to be a period of reflection for the patient (McKinnon, 2004). The dispensing episode provides an opportunity for pharmacists to reinforce prescribing advice and clarify any misunderstandings. The same applies to the supply of general sales list medicines (Walker and Edwards, 2003). Supplementary prescribing affords an opportunity for a higher standard of patient medication portfolio review and safer controls on repeat prescribing (National Prescribing Centre and National Primary Care Research and Development Centre, 2002).

PATIENT INVOLVEMENT, EDUCATION AND CONCORDANCE

Research suggests that it is not merely the lack of patient education about prescribed treatment but the lack of sensitivity as to the timeliness of such education, along with failure to genuinely engage the patient's concerns, that results in a breakdown in concordance and consequent adverse drug events (Jacobs, 2002). Educating patients about their medication and treatment, therefore, cannot be merely the depersonalised transfer of information, but like all good teaching is couched in an awareness of the link between meeting learner needs and assimilation of new knowledge. However, in our efforts to secure safer medicines management, there may still be an even better way forward.

Public health initiatives are always more effective when appropriated by the public and when strengths of leadership and support grounded in the community are harnessed (Laverack, 2005). Practitioners have long recognised that many patients who suffer from chronic disease have through experience developed expertise and skill relating to their condition that can be shared with others. Formalising this concept of the expert patient (Department of Health, 2001), through the development of support and education programmes that are led by service users, has been linked to improved concordance. Such measures do more than confirm patients as partners in treatment. By nurturing patient leadership in therapeutics, we develop patient responsibility to new levels and take another step towards minimising adverse drug events.

THE PUBLIC HEALTH DIMENSION OF PRESCRIBING

GETTING PRESCRIBING IN CONTEXT

A public health model of prescribing practice does not conform to the traditional biomedical model of care that has until recent times dominated the prescribing franchise. Preventive public health medicine is an expanding science. Therapeutic management of cholesterol and obesity in the absence of specific disease states has joined immunisation in the area of primary public health medicine and produced beneficial results, but this is not primary prevention within a social model of care.

To prescribe in a context of public health is to own a public health philosophy in practice, appreciating the broader health consequences for the individual and the community of treatment options and care packages. The practitioner minded by a public health philosophy recognises the contribution made by therapeutics to health to be small in comparison to that of social, practical and environmental measures.

Both prescribing and non-prescribing behaviour should afford an opportunity for patients to explore ways in which they might be enabled to change their lifestyle for the better. Practical self-help, physical exercise (Hillsdon et al., 2004), a change of diet, recreation or social behaviour (Mulvihill and Quigley, 2003) and personal support to stop smoking (Naidoo at al., 2004) all provide solutions that are alternative or complementary to a prescription.

ENHANCING CARE THROUGH COLLABORATION

Health advice falls within a wider area of health promotion that can best be accomplished through collaborative working with a wide range of health and social care professionals, voluntary groups, community leaders and service users. The realisation that one cannot do everything oneself and the awareness of informed others who can play a valuable part in helping communities to help themselves are the beginnings of effective public health practice (Gillies, 1997). Service user partnerships result in initiatives such as food cooperatives established in food deserts[1] and after-school clubs, which embody health needs as they are expressed by the grass-roots community.

Prescribing in the public health context therefore means that while practitioners in primary and secondary care may not play a part in every health-promotion activity in the community, they are aware of all of them and are able to refer patients appropriately.

ALLOWING NEED TO SHAPE PRACTICE

The importance of healthcare practice located at times and places where people require it rather than the other way around has been recognised by a number of studies commissioned by government (Acheson, 1998; Department of Health, 2004). Public health prescribers profile the community in which they practise. Doing so means that they are able to tailor and target resources that are as accessible as they are effective. For example, clinics, surgeries and medical centres with flexible evening, early-morning and weekend opening times, walk-in centres, telephone and Internet services all help address the opportunistic access needs of people with complex life and work patterns. Outreach projects in schools, and mobile units for travelling families and geographically isolated groups, are advanced versions of the same approach. Ideally, the shape such services take will be as diverse as the populations they serve.

Systems need to be in place that facilitate audit of public health practice. This means more than monitoring prescribing patterns, but conducting an analysis of how these patterns sit with other aspects of care and treatment and whether they are meeting the most pressing health needs.

In particular, service-user-friendly explanations of the dangers for a community without herd immunity and the threat to health of inappropriate antimicrobial prescribing should be included in respective consultations about vaccines and antimicrobials in order to aid concordance and promote public health (Department of Health, 2000).

The prescriber who is also socially and politically aware will help promote justice in healthcare by practice that is non-discriminatory. Awareness of the inequalities in health means that prescribing practitioners realise the lack of room for manoeuvre endured by lower socioeconomic groups. Prescribing and non-prescribing behaviour for these groups includes provision of free prescriptions and, where this is not possible, negotiation with the patient over the use of products they may already have in the home or may obtain cheaply over the counter. Any attempt to guide the patient towards life-style change must be characterised by empathic engagement rather than paternalistic judgement, offering a range of options and support.

Equal access to healthcare by ethnic groups is promoted by the employment of practitioners who are members of these groups, along with interpreters and signers

---

[1] A food desert is the sociological term for a residential area where fresh produce outlets are either non-existent, or so expensive as to be beyond the means of the residents for the purposes of regular use.

and by literature that is multilingual as well as 'service user friendly' (Department of Health, 2004). Healthcare practitioners are also well placed to enable disadvantaged groups through advice and advocacy.

CONCLUSION

In the twenty-first century, as in the past, a public health approach is required to respond effectively to the challenges to health arising from the patterns of disease associated with our time. Wherever prescribing takes place, a public health philosophy serves to broaden care beyond the limited boundaries of therapeutics and promotes holistic practice. These approaches, while person centred, are mindful of the frames of reference through which wider communities perceive health and health need. Justice is also served through practice that serves the common good, balanced against the rights of the individual to whatever care is available.

REFERENCES

Abraham, EP & Chain, E (1940) An enzyme form bacteria able to destroy penicillin. Nature **146** (4136): 837–9.

Acheson, D (1998) *Independent Inquiry into the Inequalities in Health*. London: The Stationery Office.

Amaranayake, N, Church, J, Hill, C, Jackson, J, Jackson, JV, Myers, C, Saeed, Z, Shipsey, C & Symmonds, T (2000) *Social Trends, 30*. London: The Stationery Office.

Anderson, S & Berridge, V (2000) Opium in 20th-century Britain: Pharmacists, regulation and the people. *Addiction* **95**(1): 23–36.

Baggott, R (2000) *Public Health, Policy and Politics* (2nd edition). Basingstoke: Palgrave Macmillan.

Baltas, G (2001) Nutrition labelling: Issues and policies. *European Journal of Marketing* **35**(5/6): 708–721.

Bengoechea, JA & Skurnik, M (2000) Temperature-regulated efflux pump/potassium antiporter system mediates resistance to cationic antimicrobial peptides in Yersinia. *Molecular Microbiology* **37**(1): 67–80.

Black, DR, Tobler, NS & Sciacca, JP (1998) Peer helping/involvement: An efficacious way to meet the challenge of reducing alcohol, tobacco and other drug use among youth. *Journal of School Health* **68**(3): 87–93.

Bozoni, K, Kalmanti M & Koukouli, S (2006) Perception and knowledge of medicines of primary schoolchildren: The influence of age and socioeconomic status. *European Journal of Pediatrics* **165**(1): 42–9.

Britton, ARC, Diamond, G, Laube, D & Kaiser, V (2002) Antimicrobial activity in the blood of the saltwater crocodile (*Crocodylus porosus*) [abstract presented by G Diamond at the 16th Working Meeting of the IUCN/SSC Crocodile Specialist Group, Florida, USA, October 2002].

Callaghan, E (2003) Submit a Yellow Card to report adverse drug reactions. *Nurse Prescribing Journal* **1**(3): 138–139.

Carbonne, A, Naas, T, Blanckaert, K, Couzigou, C, Cattoen, C, Chagnon, JL, Nordmann, P & Astagneau, P (2005) Investigation of nosocomial outbreak of extended-spectrum Beta-lactamase VEB-1-producing isolates of Acinetobacter baumanni in a hospital setting. *Journal of Hospital Infection* **60**: 14–18.

Charalambous, MP (2002) Alcohol and the accident and emergency department: A current review. *Alcohol and Alcoholism* **37**(4): 307–312.

Colgrove, J (2002) 'The Mckeowan Thesis': A historical controversy and its enduring influence. *American Journal of Public Health* **92**(5): 725–730.

Committee for Safe Medicines (2002) Aspirin and Reye's syndrome in children up to and including 15 years of age. *Current Problems in Pharmacovigilance* **28**(4): 4.

Constable, N (2002) *This is Cocaine*. London: Sanctuary.

Curran, HV & Morgan, CA (2000) Cognitive, dissociative and psychotogenic effects of ketamine in recreational users on the night of drug use and 3 days later. *Addiction* **95**(4): 575–90.

Curtis, LH, Ostbye, T, Sendersky, V, Hutchison, S, Dans, PE, Wright A & Woosely, RL (2004) Inappropriate prescribing for elderly Americans in a large outpatient population. *Archives of Internal Medicine* **164**(15): 1621–1625.

Department for Work and Pensions (2003) *Households Below Average Income 1994/5–2001/2*. London: The Stationery Office.

Department of Health (1992) *The Health of the Nation*. London: The Stationery Office.

Department of Health (1999) *The Path of Least Resistance: Report by the Standing Advisory Committee on Antimicrobial Resistance*. London: The Stationery Office.

Department of Health (2000) *UK Antimicrobial Resistance Strategy and Action Plan*. London: The Stationery Office.

Department of Health (2001) *The Expert Patient: A New Approach to Chronic Disease Management for the 21st Century*. London: The Stationery Office.

Department of Health (2002a) *Getting Ahead of the Curve, a Strategy for Infectious Disease*. London: The Stationery Office.

Department of Health (2002b) *Smoking Kills, a White Paper on Tobacco*. London: The Stationery Office.

Department of Health (2004) *Choosing Health: Making Healthier Choices Easier*. London: The Stationery Office.

Dietz, WH (2001) The obesity epidemic in young children: Reduce television viewing and promote playing. *British Medical Journal* **322**(7282): 313–314.

Dotson, JW, Ackerman, DL & West, LJ (1995) Ketamine abuse. *Journal of Drug Issues* **25**(4): 751–757.

Downie, G, Hind, C & Kettle, J (2000) The abuse and misuse of prescribed and over the counter medicines. *Hospital Pharmacist* **7**(9): 242–250.

Ebelling, CB, Pawlak, DB & Ludwig, DS (2002) Childhood obesity: Public health crisis, common sense cure. *The Lancet* **360**(9331): 473–482.

Edlin, BR, Irwin, KL, Farugue, S, McCoy, CB, Word, C, Serrano, Y, Inciardi, JA, Bowser, BP, Schilling, RF & Holmbert, SD (1994) Intersection epidemics – crack cocaine use and HIV infection among inner-city young adults. *The New England Journal of Medicine* **331**(21): 1422–1427.

Ellis, S & Grey, A (2004) Prevention of sexually transmitted infections (STIs): A review of reviews into the effectiveness of non-clinical intervention. London: Health Development Agency.

Emslie, MJ & Bond, CM (2003) Public knowledge, attitudes and behaviour regarding anti-biotics – A survey of patients in general practice. *European Journal of General Practice* **9**(3): 84–90.

Engberg, J, Aarestrup, FM, Taylor, DE, Gerner-Smidt, P & Nachamkin, I (2001) Quinolone and macrolide resistance in Campylobacter jejuni and C. coli: Resistance mechanisms and trends in human isolates. *Emerging Infectious Diseases* **7**(1): 24–34.

Enne, VI, Livermore, DM, Stephens, P & Hall, LM (2001) Persistence of sulphonamide resistance in Escherichia coli in the UK despite national prescribing restriction. *The Lancet* **357**(9265): 1325–1328.

Fergusson, DM, Horwood, LJ & Ridder, EM (2005) Tests of causal linkages between cannabis use and psychotic symptoms. *Addiction* **100**(3): 354–366.

Freund, PES, McGuire, MB & Podhurst, LS (2003) *Health, Illness and the Social Body: A Critical Sociology* (2nd edition). New Jersey: Prentice Hall.

Gillies, P (1997) Effectiveness of alliances and partnerships for health promotion. *Health Promotion International* **13**(2): 99–120.

Graham, H (2000) *Understanding Health Inequalities*. Maidenhead: Open University Press.

Graham, H & Power, C (2004) *Childhood Disadvantage and Adult Health: A Lifecourse Framework*. London: Health Development Agency.

Grape, M, Sundstrom, L & Kronvall, G (2003) Sulphonamide resistance gene sul3 found in Escherichia coli isolates from human sources. *Journal of Antimicrobial Chemotherapy*. **52**(6): 1022–1024.

Gunn, JS, Lim, KB, Krueger, J, Kim, K, Guo, L, Hackett, M & Miller, SI (1998) PmrA-PmrB-regulated genes necessary for 4-aminoarabinose lipid A modification and polymyxin resistance. *Molecular Microbiology* **27**(6): 1171–1182.

Hales, G (ed.) (1996) *Beyond Disability Towards an Enabling Society*. London: Sage.

Hatsukami, DK & Fischman, MW (1996) Crack cocaine and cocaine hydrochloride. Are the differences myth or reality? *Journal of the American Medical Association* **276**(19): 1580–1588.

Health Protection Agency (2005a) *Antimicrobial Resistance – Inevitable but not Unmanageable*. London: Health Protection Agency.

Health Protection Agency (2005b) *Trends in Antimicrobial Resistance in England and Wales*. London: Health Protection Agency.

Hillsdon, M, Foster, C, Naidoo, B & Crombie, H (2004) *The Effectiveness of Public Health Interventions for Increasing Physical Activity among Adults: A Review of Reviews*. London: Health Development Agency.

The Home Office (2002) *The Classification of Cannabis under the Misuse of Drugs Act 1971*. London: The Stationery Office.

The Home Office (2005) *Drug Misuse Declared: Findings from the 2004/5 British Crime Survey*. London: The Stationery Office.

Hough, M (1996) *Drug Misuse and the Criminal Justice System: A Review of the Literature*. Home Office Drugs Prevention Initiative. London: The Stationery Office.

Jacobs, L (2002) Are your patients taking what you prescribe? *Permanente Journal* **6**(3): 59–61.

Jansen, E & Bruinsma, J (1997) Policing organised crime. *European Journal on Criminal Policy and Research* **5**(4): 85–98.

Jarvis, G & Parker, H (1989) Young heroin users and crime. *British Journal of Criminology* **29**(2): 175–185.

Kohn, LT, Corrigan, J & Donaldson, MS (eds) (1999) *To Err Is Human: Building a Safer Health System*. Washington: National Academy Press.

Kutscher, EC, Lund, BC & Perry, PJ (2002) Anabolic steroids. A review for the clinician. *Sports Medicine* **32**(5): 285–296.

Laverack, G (2005) *Public Health: Power, Empowerment and Professional Practice.* Basingstoke: Palgrave Macmillan.

Leape, LL, Bates, DW, Cullen, DJ, Cooper, J, DeMonaco, H, Gallivan, T, Hallisey, R, Ives, J, Laird, N, Laffell, G, Nemeskal, R, Peterson, LA, Porter, K, Servi, D, Shea, BF, Small, S, Sweitzer, B, Thompson, T & VanderVliet, M (1995) Systems analysis of adverse drug events. *Journal of the American Medical Association* **274**(1): 35–43.

Longo, LP & Johnson, B (2000) Addiction: Part I. Benzodiazepines – Side effects, abuse risk and alternatives. *American Family Physician* **61**(7): 2121–2128.

Ludwig, DS and Ebelling, CB (2001) Type 2 diabetes mellitus in children: Primary care and public health considerations. *Journal of the American Medical Association* **286**(12): 1427–1430.

Marmot, M & Wilkinson, RG (eds) (2006) *Social Determinants of Health* (2nd edition). Oxford: Oxford University Press.

Marsden, J (1994) *Treating Alcohol and Drug Problems: A Review of Assessment Domains, Outcome Measures and Instruments.* London: The Stationery Office.

Marsden, J, Gossop, G, Stewart, D, Best, D, Farrell, M, Lehmann, P, Edwards, C & Strang, J (1998) The Maudsley Addiction Profile (MAP): A brief instrument for assessing treatment outcome. *Addiction* **93**(12): 1857–1867.

Mash, DC & Staley, JK (1999) D_3 Dopamine and kappa opioid receptor alterations in human brain of cocaine-overdose victims. *Annals of the New York Academy of Sciences* **877**(1): 507–522.

Mausner-Dorsch, H & Eaton, WW (2000) Psychosocial work environment and depression: Epidemiologic assessment of the demand-control model. *American Journal of Public Health* **90**(11): 1765–1770.

McCambridge, J, Mitcheson, L, Winstock, A & Hunt, N (2005) Five-year trends in patterns of drug use among people who use stimulants in dance contexts in the United Kingdom. *Addiction* **100**(8): 1140–1149.

McGovern, MC, Glasgow, JF & Stewart, MC (2001) Reye's syndrome and aspirin: Lest we forget. *British Medical Journal* **322**(3702): 1591–1592.

McKinnon, J (2004) The importance of patient centred planning in prescribing practice. *Nurse Prescribing Journal* **2**(4): 163–166.

Mera, SL (1997) *Understanding Disease Pathology and Prevention.* Cheltenham: Stanley Thomas.

Milandri, M (2004) Children's views of microbes: Current beliefs about bacteria in Italian grade school children. *Pediatric Infectious Disease* **23**(12): 1077–1080.

Mills, S (2003) The role of genomics in antimicrobial discovery. *Journal of Antimicrobial Chemotherapy* **51**(4): 749–752.

Minten, J, Jani, Y & Grosso, A (2004) Treating drug resistant TB. *Pharmaceutical Journal* **273**(7318): 422–424.

Mittleman, MA, Mintzer, D, Maclure, M, Tofler, GH, Sherwood, JB & Muller, JE (1999) Triggering of myocardial infarction by cocaine. *Circulation* **99**(21): 2737–2741.

Moore, S (2002) *Social Welfare Alive* (3rd edition). Cheltenham: Nelson Thornes.

Mulvihill, C & Quigley, R (2003). *The Management of Obesity and Overweight: An Analysis of Reviews of Diet, Physical Activity and Behavioural Approaches.* London: Health Development Agency.

Naidoo, J & Wills, J (2005a) *Health Promotion, Foundations for Practice* (2nd edition). London: Baillière Tindall.

Naidoo, J & Wills J (2005b) *Public Health and Health Promotion, Developing Practice.* (2nd edition). London: Baillière Tindall.

Naidoo, B, Quigley, R, Taylor, L & Warm, D (2004) *Smoking and Public Health: A Review of Reviews of Interventions to Increase Smoking Cessation, Reduce Smoking Initiation and Prevent Further Uptake of Smoking.* London: Health Development Agency.

National Prescribing Centre (1999) Signposts for prescribing nurses – general principles of good prescribing. *Prescribing Nurse Bulletin* **1**(1): 1–4.

National Prescribing Centre & National Primary Care Research and Development Centre (2002) *Modernising Medicines Management, A guide to Achieving Benefits for Patients, Professionals and the NHS.* London: National Prescribing Centre.

Nazroo, J (1998) *The Health of Britain's Ethnic Minorities.* London: Policy Studies Unit.

Nursing and Midwifery Council (2002) *Supporting Nurses and Midwives through Lifelong Learning.* London: Nursing and Midwifery Council.

Olds, D, Henderson, CR Jr, Cole, R, Eckenrode, J, Kitzman, H, Luckey, D, Pettitt, L, Sidora, K, Morris, P & Powers, J (1998) Long-term effects of nurse home visitation on children's criminal and antisocial behavior: 15-year follow-up of a randomized controlled trial. *Journal of the American Medical Association* **280**(14): 1238–1244.

Patrick, DM, Tyndall, MW, Cornelisse, PG, Li, K, Sherlock, CH, Rekart, ML, Strathdee, SA, Currie, SL, Schechter, MT & O'Shaughnessy, MV (2001) Incidence of hepatitis C virus infection among injection drug users during an outbreak of HIV infection. *Canadian Medical Association Journal* **165**(7): 889–895.

Patterson, JE (2003) Extended-spectrum beta-lactamases. *Seminars in Respiratory Critical Care Medicine* **24**(1): 79–87.

Payne, JR, Kotwinski, PJ & Montgomery, HE (2004) Cardiac effects of anabolic steroids. *Heart* **90**(5): 473–475.

Pechere, JC (2004) The physician, patient and antibiotics. *Bulletin of the Academy of National Medicine* **188**(8): 1257–1267.

Rainer, TH, Swann, IJ & Crawford, R (1996) Critical analysis of an accident and emergency ward. *Journal of Accident and Emergency Medicine* **13**(5): 325–329.

Reason, J (1990) *Human Error.* Cambridge: Cambridge University Press.

Ridgely Seymer, L (ed.) (1954) *Selected Writings of Florence Nightingale.* New York: Macmillan.

Rupp, ME & Fey, PD (2003) Extended spectrum beta-lactamase (ESBL)-producing Enterobacteriaceae. Considerations for diagnosis, prevention and drug treatment. *Drugs* **63**(4): 353–365.

Schatz, PL, Mesologites, D, Hyun, J, Smith, GJ & Lahiri, B (1989) Captopril-induced hypersensitivity lung disease. An immune-complex-mediated phenomenon. *Chest* **95**(3): 685–687.

Scottish Infection Standards and Strategy Group (2006) *Guidance for the Hospital Management of Methicillin Resistant Staphylococcus Aureus.* Edinburgh: The Royal College of Physicians of Edinburgh.

Seeley, RR, Stephens, TD & Tate, P (2000) *Anatomy and Physiology.* Boston: McGraw Hill.

Smith, KM, Larive, LL & Romanelli, F (2002) Club drugs: Methylenedioxymethamphetamine, flunitrazepam, ketamine hydrochloride, and gamma-hydroxybutyrate. *American Journal of Health System Pharmacy* **59**(11): 1067–1076.

Sugarman, L (2005) *Life Span Development: Frameworks, Accounts and Strategies* (2nd edition). Hove: Hove Psychology Press.

Teale, CJ (2005) *Detection and Characterisation of Beta Lactamase Resistance in Gram Negative Bacteria of Veterinary Significance*. London: The Veterinary and Public Health Test Standardisation Group.

Timby, N, Eriksson, A & Bostrom, K (2000) Gamma-hydroxybutyrate associated deaths. *American Journal of Medicine* **108**(6): 518–519.

Townsend, P, Davidson, N & Whitehead, M (1992) *Inequalities in Health* (2nd edition). Harmondsworth: Penguin.

Volkow, ND, Ding, YS, Fowler, JS, Wang, GJ, Logan, J, Gatley, JS, Dewey, S, Ashby, C, Liebermann, J & Hitzemann, R (1995) Is methylphenidate like cocaine? Studies on their pharmacokinetics and distribution in the human brain. *Archives of General Psychiatry* **52**(6): 456–463.

Walker, R & Edwards, C (2003) *Clinical Pharmacy and Therapeutics* (3rd edition). Edinburgh: Churchill Livingstone.

Wanless, D (2002) *Securing Our Future Health: Taking a Long-Term View*. London: The Stationery Office.

Weaver, T, Madden, P, Charles, V, Stimson, G, Renton, A, Tyrer, P, Barnes, T, Bench, C, Middleton, H, Wright, N, Paterson, S, Shanahan, W, Seivewright, N & Ford, C (2003) Co morbidity of substance misuse and mental illness in community mental health and substance misuse services. *British Journal of Psychiatry* **183**(4): 304–313.

Wise, R (2004) The relentless rise of resistance? *Journal of Antimicrobial Chemotherapy* **54**(2): 306–310.

Zimmet, PZ, McCarty, DJ & de Courten, MP (1997) The global epidemiology of non-insulin-dependent diabetes mellitus and the metabolic syndrome. *Journal of Diabetes and its Complications* **11**(2): 60–68.

UNDERSTANDING BASIC PHARMACOLOGY

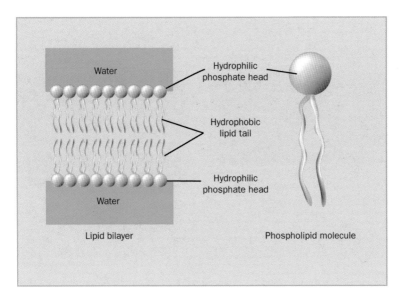

Plate 1 Structure of a cell membrane. Reproduced by permission of MA Healthcare.

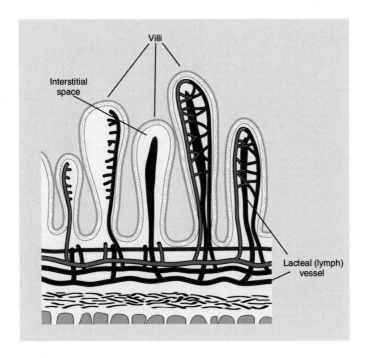

Plate 2 Structure of small intestinal wall, showing large surface area. Reproduced by permission of MA Healthcare.

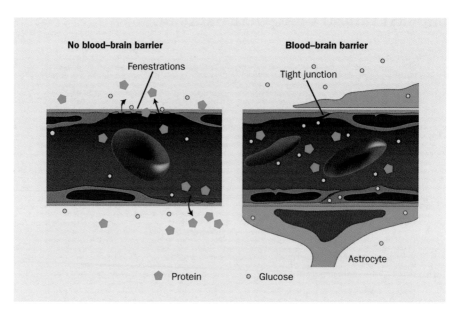

Plate 3 Blood–brain barrier. Reproduced by permission of MA Healthcare.

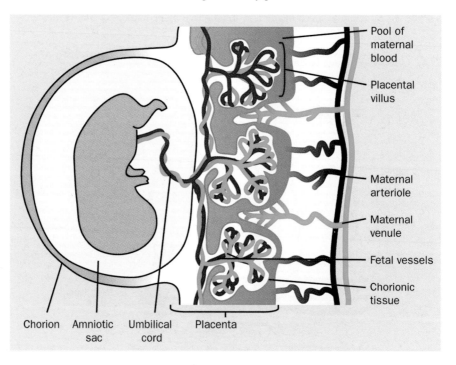

Plate 4 The placental barrier. Reproduced by permission of MA Healthcare.

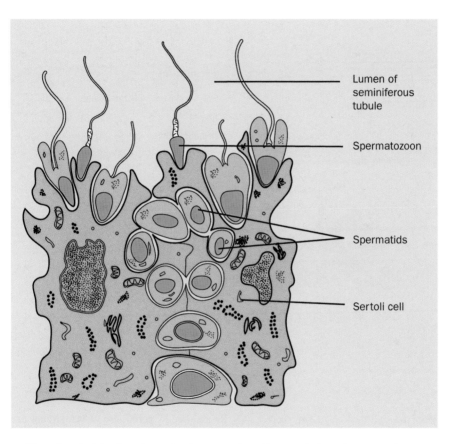

Lumen of
seminiferous
tubule

Spermatozoon

Spermatids

Sertoli cell

Plate 5 The blood–testicular barrier. Reproduced by permission of MA Healthcare.

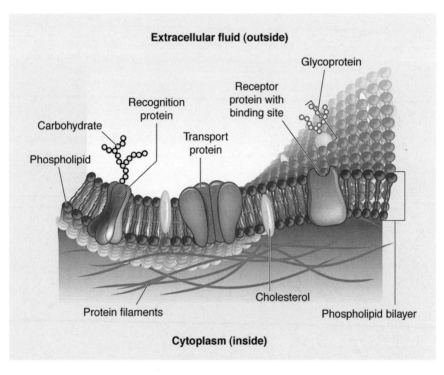

Plate 6 Cell membrane and receptor sites. Reproduced by permission of MA Healthcare.

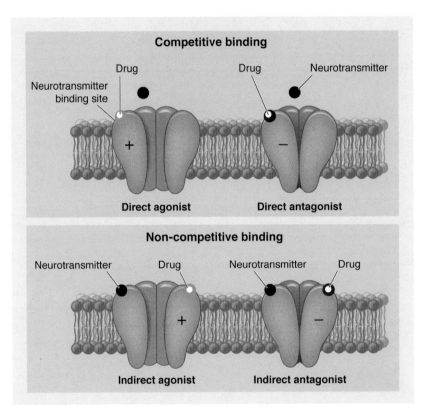

Plate 7 Competitive and non-competitive inhibition. Reproduced by permission of MA Healthcare.

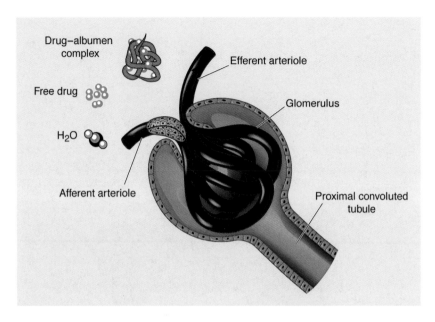

Plate 8 Glomerular filtration of drugs of low molecular weight. Reproduced by permission of MA Healthcare.

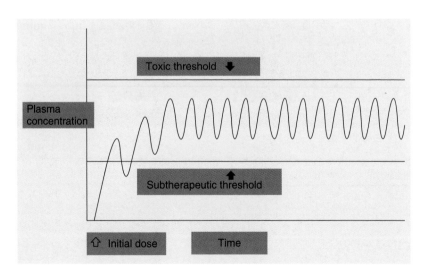

Plate 9 The therapeutic index

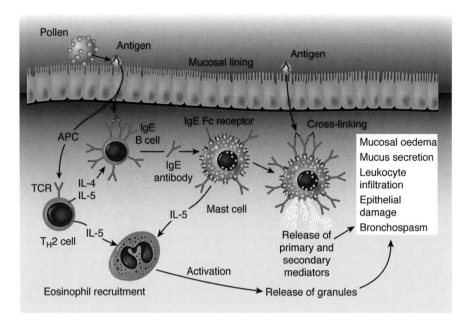

Plate 10 Type I hypersensitivity: excess antibodies bind to mast cells in the tissues. Reproduced by permission of MA Healthcare.

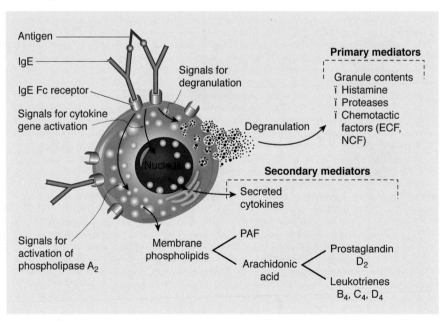

Plate 11 Type I hypersensitivity: antigens initiate a sense of intracellular messages. Reproduced by permission of MA Healthcare.

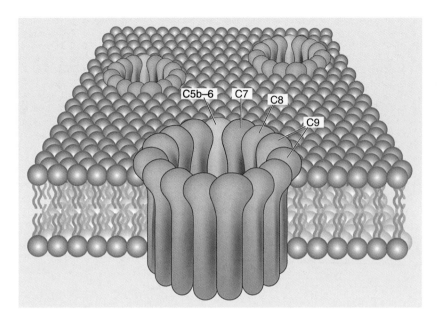

Plate 12 Type II hypersensitivity: the membrane attack complex. Reproduced by permission of MA Healthcare.

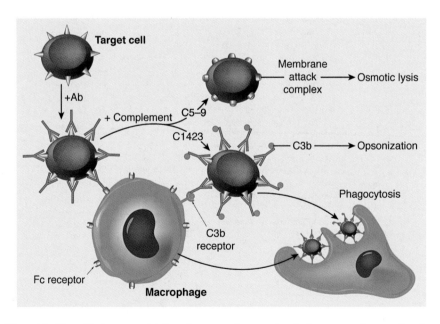

Plate 13 Type II: hypersensitivity: drug protein complex induces complement fixation. Reproduced by permission of MA Healthcare.

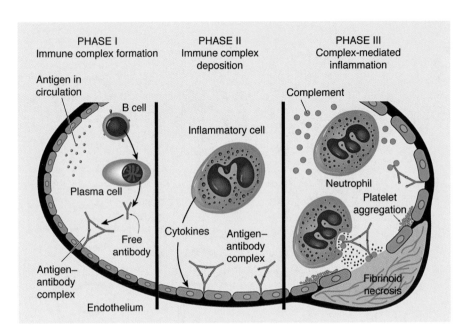

Plate 14 Type III hypersensitivity. Reproduced by permission of MA Healthcare.

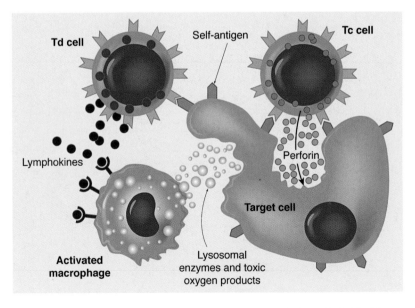

Plate 15 Type IV hypersensitivity. Reproduced by permission of MA Healthcare.

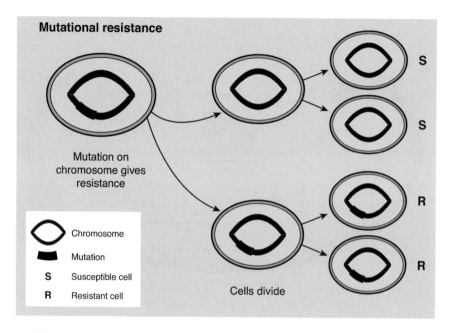

Plate 16 Spontaneous mutation. Reproduced by permission of MA Healthcare.

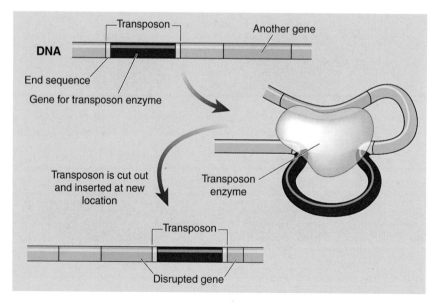

Plate 17 Transposons or 'jumping genes'. Reproduced by permission of MA Healthcare.

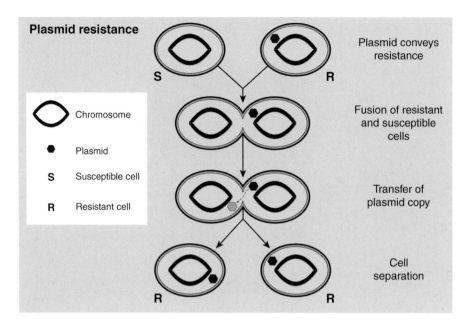

Plate 18 Exchange of DNA material via plasmids. Reproduced by permission of MA Healthcare.

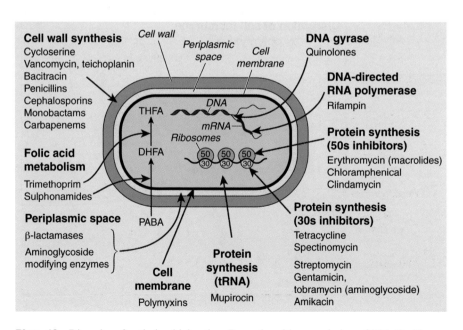

Plate 19 Diversity of antimicrobial action. Reproduced by permission of MA Healthcare.

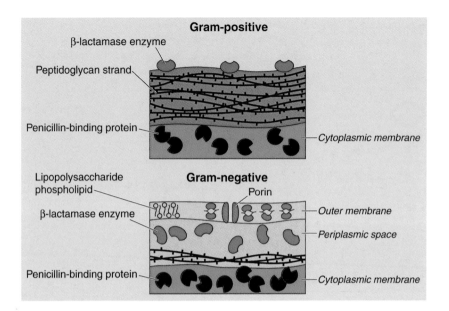

Plate 20 Gram-positive and Gram-negative bacteria. Reproduced by permission of MA Healthcare.

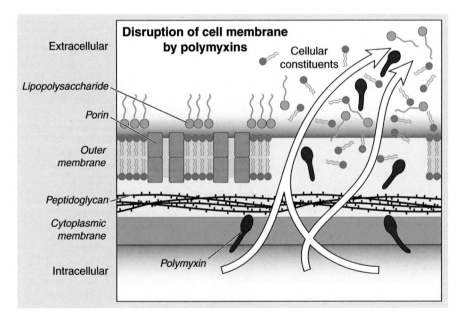

Plate 21 Disruption of the cell membrane by polymyxins. Reproduced by permission of MA Healthcare.

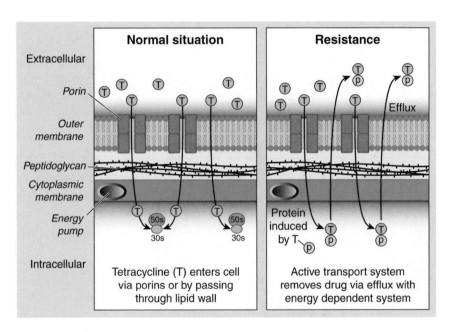

Plate 22 Development of efflux pumps. Reproduced by permission of MA Healthcare.

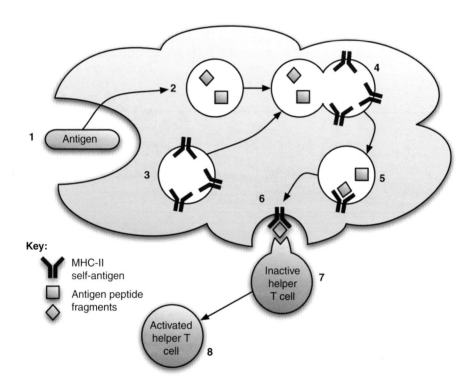

Plate 23 Antigen phagocytosis by antigen-presenting cells. Subsequent processing results in antigen–MHE–II complexes being inserted into the plasma membrane, which activates the T cell.

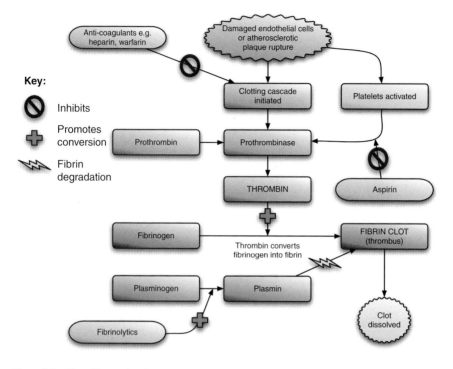

Plate 24 The effects of anticoagulants, aspirin and fibrinolytics on the coagulation cascade.

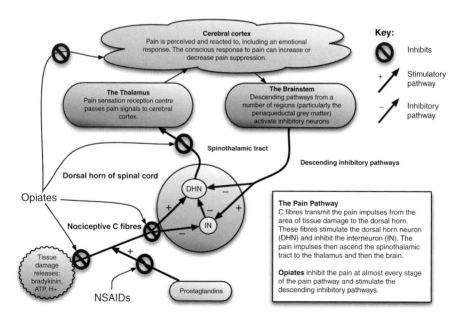

Plate 25 The pain pathway. Sites of action for opiates and NSAIDs are shown

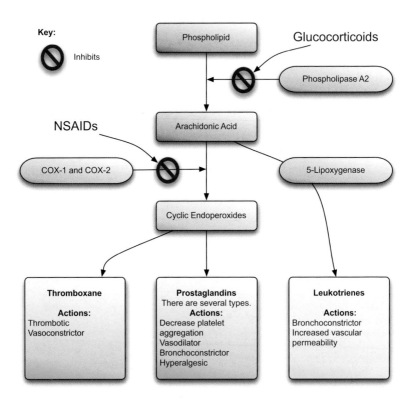

Plate 26 The arachidonic acid cascade and its blockade by glucocorticoids and NSAIDs

5 A Practical Guide to Clinical Governance for Non-Medical Prescribing

RUTH GOLDSTEIN AND RUTH REILLY

The purpose of this chapter is to provide a framework within which all prescribing needs to take place to ensure that it is:

- appropriate to patient's needs
- current in terms of clinical choices
- safe in terms of achieving improved health while minimising patients' risk of adverse events.

The term 'clinical governance' encapsulates all these issues and hence has been adopted by healthcare practitioners and managers. It is frequently referred to in both strategic and practical papers that you will come into contact with during your day-to-day activities and therefore it is essential that you understand the term, its requirements and what it means to your workload.

This chapter will seek to:

- Define clinical governance.
- Provide a background to clinical governance – why it is necessary.
- Expose the different domains of clinical governance.
- Determine who is responsible for clinical governance.
- Explore ways of applying clinical governance to a prescribing role.

DEFINING CLINICAL GOVERNANCE: WHAT IS IT ALL ABOUT?

There are vast quantities of literature available around the concept of clinical governance, some of which needs reading with discernment. You can access information

Towards Prescribing Practice. Edited by J. McKinnon.
© 2007 John Wiley & Sons, Ltd.

from a national, strategic, local or professional point of view. A good place to start assessing what clinical governance is and where it came from is to go to the Department of Health's website and type the term 'clinical governance' into the search engine.

As the NHS approached its 50th anniversary, it was recognised that while services had developed over time there had been no formal structure to ensure the quality of services. Politicians would talk about waiting-list times and the number of operations that were conducted as if these were measures of quality. It was, however, becoming increasingly clear that quality should be concerned with process as well as outcome, hence towards the end of the 1990s it was recognised that these crude measures were not broad or deep enough to ensure the quality of care that was provided. The main political shift through the introduction of clinical governance was the change from making management decisions to that of service provision based on quality and clinical need.

In 1998 the first documents started appearing containing the term 'clinical governance'. The focus of these White Papers was on quality improvement and patient safety. The best-known and most-cited of these publications is *A First Class Service* (Department of Health, 1998). This paper was written from a policy perspective and placed quality improvement at the centre of health policy. Until this point health policy had been more focused on 'getting the job done' rather than a quality/clinical perspective. While each health and social-care practitioner should have taken it upon them to provide a 'quality' service, there was no formal framework to monitor quality and no direction as to what elements would support a quality service. Government policy sought to address these omissions with the inception of clinical governance. The term was devised to emphasise that decisions on patient care were to be made by clinicians using evidence-based practice.

The term clinical governance was used to capture a range of activities that could be applied to numerous clinical settings and situations that would have the potential outcome of improving the overall quality of all healthcare provision. The responsibility of clinical governance was, and still is, considered to be everyone's, this means individuals and organisations. However, clinical governance became the direct responsibility of the Chief Executives of all NHS Trusts. It was considered necessary for all NHS organisations (primary, secondary and tertiary care environments) to develop processes and provide resources for continuously monitoring and improving the quality of the healthcare they deliver and to deliver systems of accountability relating to the quality of the care they provide.

One of the first definitions of clinical governance described it as:

> the system through which NHS organisations are accountable for continuously improving the quality of their services and safeguarding high standards of care, by creating an environment in which clinical excellence will flourish. (Scally and Donaldson, 1998: 62)

For practitioners and patients this means a way of continuously monitoring and improving the standard of care given.

In more detail, one could consider that clinical governance aims to:

- Ensure good communication between patients and healthcare workers and between different services and organisations providing care to patients.
- Involve patients and carers in planning and agreeing their care and involving them (where appropriate) in decisions as to the way in which services are delivered.
- Look out for potential risks before they happen and learn from situations when care and treatment could have been better, in a non-judgemental way.
- Ensure the workforce (at all levels) has the right skills to meet the needs of patients.
- Assess the quality of care given, making changes where necessary and then assessing the care again to see that the changes have had an effect (in other words, carry out audits).
- Share good and bad practice; if something works well it should be shared with colleagues so that more people can benefit, and if it doesn't work it should be shared so other people do not duplicate mistakes!
- Give treatment and care based on good evidence that it will have the best outcome for the patient. This relates to the role of the National Institute for Health and Clinical Excellence (NICE).

As you can tell just from this introduction, the concept of clinical governance has grown and developed considerably since it first emerged as an idea related to quality. What it actually involves and how that relates to day-to-day practice will be explored a little later in this chapter. The next section provides more of an insight into why clinical governance was considered necessary.

WHY IS CLINICAL GOVERNANCE NECESSARY?

For a long while before the term was developed, a culture of quality/errors/blame was developing worldwide. In particular, in the USA there has always been a 'fear' among providers of services that errors in the course of practice or failure to deliver the expected outcome would result in blame and potential litigation. As healthcare in the UK has developed and human nature has demanded more and more from healthcare providers, our expectations of services have grown, almost to the point that they are beyond what is practical. In the 1990s it was no longer considered acceptable just to offer a service, people wanted a high-quality service and, more importantly, the quality of the service was required to be consistent from one area to another. It was no longer acceptable to offer a good service in some parts of the country but not in others. The government was pushing an agenda of equity. Its White Paper *The New NHS, Modern and Dependable* (Department of Health, 1997) specified that service provision would have no barriers due to postcode, class or finance. The government's goal was to ensure minimum quality standards across the country, which when achieved would mean all healthcare provision was of an acceptable and known standard.

Therefore, the clinical governance framework was introduced to:

- Ensure that quality was placed at the centre of healthcare.
- Ensure that the highest quality of care was provided nationwide.
- Prevent mistakes and reduce the number of repeated errors that occurred.
- Improve patients' confidence in the healthcare they received.

THE DIFFERENT DOMAINS OF CLINICAL GOVERNANCE

One of the easiest ways to understand what clinical governance actually means in practice is to break it down into specific areas that relate eventually to tasks. There have traditionally been considered to be seven domains of clinical governance; in other words, seven areas that are thought to contribute to the provision of safe, appropriate, high-quality healthcare. These are:

- clinical audit
- patient and public involvement
- risk management
- clinical effectiveness (standards)
- staffing and staff management
- education, training and continuing professional development
- use of information management and technology to improve the delivery of healthcare.

It is important to realise that the separation between the domains is something that is done for convenience's sake. It does not necessarily mean that in practice these areas are discrete. For example, clinical audit is an aspect of clinical effectiveness, as you may be required to audit how well you are prescribing in accordance with clinical guidelines. Evidence or results of clinically effective practice and audit may rely on information or education and training sessions for developing improved care. Clinical governance therefore represents a holistic system that embraces the seven domains, but not necessarily individually.

Later on in this chapter we shall explore what prescribers should be incorporating into their day-to-day practice to ensure that they have absorbed the concept of clinical governance into practice. For now we shall take these seven domains and briefly describe what is meant and what impact they have for a prescribing role.

CLINICAL AUDIT

It is important that prescribers are up to date with their prescribing choices and implement the national guidance on prescribing for certain conditions in their practice. A clinical audit is an ideal way of reviewing prescribing, updating knowledge and implementing change if necessary. For example, if you are working in general practice you should be prescribing within the latest guidance for patients with hypertension. The easiest way to assess this is to review 100 prescribing choices you have made for patients with hypertension and assess if they are in accordance with current evidence-based practice. If so, then your audit has confirmed your good practice; if not, then you need to update your knowledge and alter your prescribing patterns accordingly.

PATIENT AND PUBLIC INVOLVEMENT

Central to clinical governance is involving patients and carers. If you are trying to deliver a high-quality service you need to know what patients consider as contributing to the quality of care they receive. A patient satisfaction survey is one way of assessing the quality of your service and also identifying issues that are important to patients that you may have overlooked. Using the Expert Patient programme is another way of involving patients in the delivery of services. Local Patient Advice and Liaison Services (PALS) are a further way of involving patient views in your service delivery. It is worthwhile contacting your local PALS coordinator to determine how the PALS service functions within your locality.

RISK MANAGEMENT

This is concerned with reducing the number of errors and subsequent adverse events from occurring in practice. It is based on the idea that if you can identify a potential problem, then you are likely to resolve it before it actually becomes a problem. It includes a focus on responding to errors and incidents in a positive way, first of all by identifying when things go wrong, logging the issues and then reviewing the processes that led up to the incident. Furthermore, if you can learn from someone else's errors then it may prevent you from carrying out the same error.

For this reason risk management is also about sharing others' experiences, both good and bad. At a local level, primary and secondary care trusts have systems in place for staff to report in their errors, incidents and near misses and then these are shared among other members of staff working for the trust. It is all generally done on an anonymous basis and fundamental to the success of such initiatives is that they are carried out in a no-blame culture. Risk management in a no-blame culture is not about punishment. It is about identifying the root causes of error and putting proactive systems in place, sharing the experience with others. Prescribing practitioners must work within their local trust's guidance for risk management and error/incident reporting. They need to identify the processes used locally to report incidents and make sure they are also included in the feedback cycle once incidents have been reported. In this way they learn from others' mistakes before they are forced to learn from their own!

At an even more remote level, there is a national scheme that is overseeing a number of risk management issues: the National Patient Safety Agency (NPSA). All trusts have a responsibility to report incidents to the NPSA, which reviews the incidents that are reported, looks for categories among them and sends out summaries that are an amalgamation of all incidents it receives. This spreads the learning more widely than within one trust and ensures that all relevant professional groups are aware of potential risk areas. An example of this is the risk of using methotrexate for a chronic illness at the dose for acute treatment. There have now been several incidents reported to the NPSA about this issue and subsequent guidance from the NPSA includes the need for prescribers to have an alert on their computer whenever they prescribe the drug, and also for pharmacists to have an additional check on their computer when they dispense the medication.

CLINICAL EFFECTIVENESS (STANDARDS)

Clinical effectiveness is the part of clinical governance that is most easily related to a prescribing role. It is all about ensuring that the most appropriate treatments are offered to patients, and this includes prescribing choices. The National Institute for Health and Clinical Excellence (NICE) was set up to support this aspect of clinical governance. Publications such as the *British National Formulary* also contain contemporary evidence-based clinical guidelines. We shall examine further the range of sources and initiatives available to the prescriber to support clinical effectiveness later in the chapter.

STAFFING AND STAFF MANAGEMENT

If the correct staffing levels are not present and staff have no positive management culture within which to work, then there is a direct impact on the quality of care that is provided. Guidance may not be explicit as to exactly what constitutes adequate staffing levels, however within trusts there is a focus, through clinical governance, to ensure that staffing levels are appropriate to ensure that patients are not delayed in accessing treatments due to staffing shortages. Furthermore, it is important that staffing levels are adequate to ensure that practitioners who are working are not put under unnecessary pressure in terms of increased workload.

EDUCATION, TRAINING AND CONTINUING PROFESSIONAL DEVELOPMENT

Once upon a time there was no requirement for any practitioner to remain informed by a current evidence base. On reflection, this is absurd. Scientific progress moves forward at breathtaking speed and new treatments and therapies are being continuously developed. It is essential that patients benefit from practice that is fuelled by current research rather than outdated directives and/or ritual. With this in mind, this domain became embedded in the concept of clinical governance, and now there is an obligation for all people working in healthcare to remain up to date and take part in relevant and continuous training and education. This can take many guises, for example attending conferences, professional update meetings, reading articles or embarking on obtaining a higher degree. We shall look more into what this means for prescribers in the later sections of this chapter.

USE OF INFORMATION TECHNOLOGY

The past 20 years have seen an explosion in the use of information technology and this has been included in clinical governance, as it was considered to be central to the delivery of a quality service. The opportunities offered in terms of speed of communication and access to up-to-date information are such that practitioners struggle to function adequately without utilising modern systems such as e-mail and the World Wide Web. For a number of people, the need to utilise information has dovetailed into their training and education needs and the two strands of clinical governance have become interwoven.

Providing seven areas of clinical governance helps remove the mystery from the term. The categories aid identification of aspects of practice deserving attention and in turn assist practitioners to align their practice with clinical governance framework requirements. They also give organisations a building block to develop strategies and support for their staff.

These seven pillars have been somewhat superseded by the definitions and structure provided by the *Standards for Better Health* (Department of Health, 2006), which have been developed to provide organisations with a comprehensive framework to work within and to be monitored against to ensure adequate clinical governance arrangements are in place. These standards also have seven domains, namely safety; clinical and cost effectiveness; patient focus; accessible and responsive care; care environments and amenities; and public health. Each domain has been broken down into specific issues that can be used as a 'checklist' by organisations. However, for the purpose of this chapter we shall continue to consider clinical governance in the original seven domains that have become the foundations of today's evolving systems. As these are the bedrock of the new system, they will remain relevant and appropriate even as the framework around them becomes more sophisticated.

DETERMINING WHO IS RESPONSIBLE FOR CLINICAL GOVERNANCE

Earlier in this chapter I commented that clinical governance was considered to be everyone's responsibility, including individuals and organisations. By this I mean that while an individual practitioner, be it a nurse, pharmacist, doctor or dentist, is responsible for the way in which they conduct their professional responsibilities, the organisation within which they are working has a responsibility for ensuring that the correct resources and support are available to ensure that the individual can perform safely and offer a high-quality service. With this remit in mind, all organisations have developed their own clinical governance frameworks. It is worthwhile looking on the Internet at this stage to see what is provided by organisations you are working for (or have worked for) in terms of their clinical governance framework.

If you look at several examples you will see a similar pattern emerging. They will all generally start with a very brief overview of what clinical governance is, and then set out a framework for its delivery within their organisations. There will be a set of areas addressed, including risk, audit, staff training, incident reporting/error management and clinical effectiveness. Finally, there will be an organisational structure to support clinical governance. This will often involve one umbrella clinical governance group with sub-groups set up to address all the other areas mentioned above. How these function in practice and furthermore how they relate to practitioners is varied and you will need to explore what is happening within your locality. But for the purpose of this chapter, you need to be aware that your organisation will have a clinical governance framework within which your practice is required to fit. You are likely to find that they have resources such as training events, reporting systems, minimum staffing levels and audit advice that help you fulfil your own personal clinical governance activities.

APPLYING CLINICAL GOVERNANCE TO A PRESCRIBING ROLE

One of the easiest ways of seeing what practitioners need to do in order to embed clinical governance into their practice is to consider the original seven domains and then develop procedures that support those areas and that are carried out in everyday work. Clinical governance activities should not be done separately from your day-to-day role, but they should be part of daily practice. This is not always as easy as it sounds.

The seven domains, as we have seen, are:

- clinical audit
- patient and public involvement
- risk management
- clinical effectiveness (standards)
- staffing and staff management
- education, training and continuing professional development
- use of information technology.

We shall consider these again from a practical standpoint.

CLINICAL AUDIT

Audits are cyclical events that are a way of looking at what is done, comparing it to what should be done, seeing if there are any areas where improvement should be made, making those improvements and then re-evaluating the activity. Prescribing activities lend themselves to audit cycles, as a great deal of prescribing is governed by guidelines and protocols, so these provide the standards against which you conduct your review and adapt your practice accordingly.

The National Prescribing Centre (NPC) has an audit support unit that is a useful resource to review to illustrate how audit can support the clinical governance activities of prescribers. There are also a number of audit templates available from the Royal Pharmaceutical Society of Great Britain that can be used to support the prescribing activities of pharmacists. NICE (2002) produced *Principles for Best Practice in Clinical Audit*, which is the Department of Health's gold standard.

The important aspect about carrying out an audit is that it needs to be useful for your day-to-day work. Therefore, if you prescribe for children then choose an audit topic such as asthma treatment in minors, or the prescribing of sugar-free medicines. If your role is based within chemotherapy, then auditing your prescribing of anti-emetics may be worthwhile. If an audit is not of interest or use to you then you will gain nothing from it and have a 'bad' audit experience that may put you off audit for life.

PATIENT AND PUBLIC INVOLVEMENT

As mentioned before, this is all about accepting that professionals do not always know the best way for services to be developed and delivered. It is important that in your role as a prescriber you get patients' views and feedback on, for example, the location and timing of clinical services, whether there is a need for a domiciliary service, or the best appointment system to ensure that patients suffering with both acute and chronic conditions have fair and appropriate access to services. There are a number of ways to do this, of which the simplest is to carry out a Patient Satisfaction Survey. Many primary and secondary care trusts have templates for patient surveys and are happy to share them with professionals who want to conduct a survey to help inform their service development. It is worthwhile doing an Internet search of your local trust to see what advice and examples it has for you to access.

It is interesting to note that obtaining feedback on services has been considered so central to the quality of a service that the monitoring of GP practices, currently known as the Quality and Outcomes Framework, contains a set of indicators referring to patient involvement and surveys.

A further way to engage the public in your service development is to access the views of 'expert patients'. These are patients who have become involved in the Expert Patient programme, which is a scheme that supports patients with long-term conditions to help them self-manage their condition and to make appropriate use of the health and social-care professionals offering advice and support. The views of these patients are often very insightful and can be used as a resource in terms of service development.

RISK MANAGEMENT

This is one area where a professional needs to reflect on their own and others' experiences as a way of learning from mistakes and reducing the likelihood of repeating errors and incidents. There is a national framework to work within; as previously mentioned, the National Patient Safety Agency has developed a national reporting scheme where incidents are reported and alerts sent around health communities to try to encourage professionals to learn from each other. While the national programme is useful, it should be supported by local initiatives that start with each professional keeping a diary or log of any incidents that they think are relevant as a learning point for the future. These can be good and bad incidents.

Keeping a log of incidents is a good starting point, but this is not the end of risk management. It is important to reflect on what is recorded and develop actions where appropriate to reduce the likelihood of adverse incidents being replicated. Consider a very simple example. If a pharmacist contacts you because he cannot read a prescription written during a home visit, then you need to devise a strategy to ensure that when you write prescriptions you have a solid object to lean on rather than leaning on your knee and making your writing illegible. You may therefore choose to obtain a small clipboard to which you attach your prescription pad. By reflecting on the incident and devising a strategy, you have 'managed the risk' of a similar incident happening again. In 2006 the NPSA launched the Root Cause Analysis tool kit (National Patient Safety Agency, n.d.), which is aimed at identifying the issues; and for managers there is the Incident Decision Tree, which helps to inform what action is necessary following an incident.

You can link your risk management activities to your audit and your continuing educational activities. For example, some practitioners keep a personal log of incidents and near misses they are involved in and then once a year they audit their log to identify common issues. They then identify any training or education needs, obtain relevant training material, review their logs a further six months down the line and measure the impact of their learning.

Learning from your own mistakes is a positive experience, but what if you don't record many incidents? Develop a way of working with colleagues to learn from one another's experiences. This means setting up a sort of 'swap shop' for adverse incidents with your colleagues. You must remember it is not about criticising one another, but learning from both local and national experience. Some areas have evening meetings to discuss incidents; others add a 10-minute slot onto all their local professional meetings to discuss such issues. Try to find out what happens locally and if the answer is nothing, then think about setting up such a scheme. The reduction of clinical risks and learning from mistakes is a cornerstone of clinical governance. A great deal of effort has been made to ensure patients and staff are safe in the NHS, but this is an activity that can always be improved.

Clinical supervision is a further way in which risk can be managed within a professional and ethical framework. This can be done in groups or on a one-to-one basis. It is important to choose the model with which you feel most comfortable. Knapman and Morrison (1998) argue that it is only when there is real partnership within an organisation that supervision becomes a powerful tool for sustaining and developing you as a professional and your practice. Practitioners, managers and employers must all play a part and recognise their responsibility to support the process.

Clinical supervision is a useful exercise for both the supervised and the supervisor. Both have an opportunity to discuss positive and negative issues or incidents, which can provide an insight to both parties involved. Having a positive and effective clinical supervision relationship can be a very supportive process and is part of your personal and professional risk management strategy.

Risk management is also not just a personal issue, but should involve the whole team with which you work. Therefore, if you are working in general practice, for example, it may be appropriate to discuss incidents with all your practice staff, or if you are a pharmacist you may want to discuss incidents with all members of staff in the dispensary. Just remember, the more you share, the greater the risk reduction is.

CLINICAL EFFECTIVENESS

Every person who prescribes either treatments or medication has a professional responsibility to make sure that their prescribing is current, appropriate and safe. However, many practitioners have a tendency to fall into 'patterns' of prescribing, where we have our top 10 favourites for each condition and may rotate between the items on our list. This is not a problem, until the list becomes out of date. With prescribing this can happen very quickly. So you need to develop strategies to help you remain clinically effective and informed by current theoretical understanding. Table 5.1 contains a list of strategies with their advantages and disadvantages. In reality, you will find that you need to choose a mix of approaches.

STAFFING AND STAFF MANAGEMENT

Within any healthcare setting it is important to have the correct mix of skills to ensure the patient's journey is supported throughout. Although you may be the prescriber, it is important that you have staff to support you, such as reception staff, prescription staff and people to manage patient records. Have a look around where you work and identify all the support staff. If you observe your setting on a typical working day, you can determine level of skill mix and whether you have any gaps in service provision arising from this. Reviewing staffing levels needs to be a routine exercise as workload can change, staff move jobs and holiday and sickness cover can have an impact on staffing levels. Here again, a log of events/issues relating to staff levels over a few months can provide a useful tool to support this domain.

Table 5.1 Strategies to maintain clinical effectiveness in a prescribing role

Strategy for keeping up to date	Advantage	Disadvantage
Talk with colleagues	Local, no need to travel Can be quick Can focus on personal goals	Limited by colleagues' knowledge Hard to ask for help in front of colleagues
Talk to representatives from the industry	Up-to-date research and development data available May be hard to organise locally	Biased to own products
Attend conferences Consult professional organisation resources	Can access 'expert' views Time away from practice can aid reflection	Time consuming Costly if not local May not focus on own needs
Read journal articles Form a journal club	Easy to access	Can raise more questions than answers May be biased by author's experience
Take advantage of clinical supervision	Maintains professional integrity and accountability	Unwillingness of your employer to allow time for clinical supervision and lack of supervisor.

Some professional groups have taken it upon themselves to reflect this in their contracting arrangements, for example for pharmacies, an adequate workforce for the demands of the business is part of their essential contract.

For other healthcare practitioners staff management is not a priority and this does not need to be a barrier to fulfilling this part of clinical governance. What is essential is that someone within your work locality does have responsibility for staff management, is aware of the necessary staff levels and can monitor staff issues appropriately.

EDUCATION, TRAINING AND CONTINUING PROFESSIONAL DEVELOPMENT

This area again is about staying in touch with the current evidence base and not relying on your education up to qualification to carry you through a developing and changing role. As with clinical effectiveness, you can conduct your continuing professional development (CPD) in a variety of ways, some of which are listed in Table 5.1. However, the processes you choose may reflect the topic you are studying, your own learning styles or what material is available.

You should also be aware that your continuing professional development may not always cover a topic that is solely linked to your prescribing role. For example, you may identify that you need some support on time management or stress management as well as requiring an update on the treatment of epilepsy.

It is important that any continuing professional development in which you take part is recorded and logged in the way your professional body suggests. It is not just a matter of collecting up loads of certificates and keeping them in files. Continuing professional development should be a cyclical process that starts with identifying a need and goes on to evaluate if that need is fulfilled and, if not, what more needs to be done. By reflecting on your continuing educational needs you can utilise your training time more effectively, as you don't spent time updating material that you don't need. Here again, maintenance of a reflective log in which you identify the need for further learning from gaps in your knowledge that arise in practice can provide a useful starting point.

The National Prescribing Centre has provided some useful advice for practitioners regarding this domain of clinical governance. It acknowledges that an individual prescriber is primarily responsible for their own CPD, and that they must highlight their CPD needs and meet these effectively in order to be professionally accountable and maintain their duty of care. However, the prescriber's employer still holds some responsibility in confirming that the individual is fit for practice, hence organisations that employ prescribers will often have a list of accredited prescribers and will have some CPD requirement for entry on the list. It is worthwhile identifying what system your local organisation is operating and what local support is available.

General practitioners have developed their training and education focus in line with their contract requirements and these are subject to annual appraisal and personal development plans (PDPs). This is monitored as part of their Quality and Outcomes Framework.

Pharmacists are also well supported in terms of education and training. Although their advice is not specifically oriented to a prescribing role, the principles can be related to all areas of practice.

USE OF INFORMATION TECHNOLOGY

It is becoming less common for prescriptions to be handwritten and this has the advantage that prescribed treatment is legible. Also, as technology is so advanced, the items prescribed are often only able to be selected from items that have NICE approval and are on a local formulary. This is one way in which information technology supports clinical governance. Other advantages are electronic access to resources such as libraries, journals, the National Electronic Library for Health, PRODIGY, conference abstracts and disease-specific support groups. Some of these have been included in the further reading and electronic resources sections of this chapter. However, they are only a sample. Always check that all sources are academically credible. Remember that anyone can set up a website.

Furthermore, the development of the 'electronic patient record' system will mean that all prescribers should have full access to a patient's clinical records at the point of prescribing. This supports risk reduction when prescribing for a patient who may also have other practitioners prescribing for them. It is important, therefore, that as prescribers you keep up to date with technological developments that may affect your role and are able to use the developments as they are embedded into your practice.

CONCLUSION

Prescribers need to embed clinical governance into their day-to-day practice by:

- Involving patients and carers in their care and in developing service provision.
- Remaining up to date with prescribing and other professional issues.
- Auditing personal practice to identify prescribing patterns and informing them-selves of education and training needs.
- Ensuring that information is recorded, stored and used in a confidential manner.
- Ensuring that staffing levels are appropriate to workload.
- Having a robust system to record and learn from incidents.

REFERENCES

Department of Health (1997) *The New NHS, Modern and Dependable*. London: The Stationery Office.
Department of Health (1998) *A First Class Service*. London: The Stationery Office.
Department of Health (2006) *Standards for Better Health*. London: The Stationery Office.
Knapman, J & Morrison, T (1998) *Making the Most of Supervision in Health and Social Care*. Brighton: Pavilion.
National Institute for Clinical Excellence (2002) *Principles for Best Practice in Clinical Audit*. Oxford: Radcliffe Press.
National Patient Safety Agency (n.d.) *Root Cause Analysis Tool Kit*. http://www.npsa.nhs.uk/health/resources/root_cause_analysis/conditions. [accessed 26 June 2006]
Scally G & Donaldson, LJ (1998) Looking forward: Clinical governance and the drive for quality improvement in the new NHS in England. *British Medical Journal* **317**(7150): 61–65.

FURTHER READING

Chambers, R & Wakely, G (2000) *Making Clinical Governance Work for You*. Oxford: Radcliffe Medical Press.
Chambers, R, Boath, E & Rogers, D (2005) *Clinical Effectiveness and Clinical Governance Made Easy* (3rd edition). Oxford: Radcliffe Medical Press.
Department of Health (1999) *Saving Lives: Our Healthier Nation*. London: The Stationery Office.

Department of Health (2005a) *Research Governance. Framework for Health and Social Care*. London: The Stationery Office.

Department of Health (2005b) *A Patient-Led NHS: Implementing the NHS Improvement Plan*. London: Department of Health.

Lilley, R (2000) *Clinical Governance: A Workbook for Doctors, Nurses and Managers*. Oxford: Radcliffe Medical Press.

Lugon, M & Secker-Walker, J (eds) (1999) *Clinical Governance: Making it Happen*. London: Royal Society of Medicine Press.

McSherry, R & Pearce, P (2001) *Clinical Governance: A Guide to Implementation for Healthcare Professionals*. Oxford: Blackwell Science.

Pickering, S & Thompson, J (2003) *Clinical Governance and Best Value*. Oxford: Churchill Livingstone.

Roland, M & Baker, R (1999) *Clinical Governance: A Practical Guide for Primary Care Teams*. Manchester: University of Manchester.

Sale, D (2005) *Understanding Clinical Governance and Quality Assurance: Making it Happen*. Basingstoke: Palgrave Macmillan.

Swage, T (2002) *Clinical Governance in Healthcare Practice*. Oxford: Butterworth Heinemann.

ELECTRONIC RESOURCES

British Medical Association – Quality and outcomes framework
http://www.bma.org.uk/ap.nsf/Content/focusqualityoutcomes0903#Indicators

British National Formulary
http://bnf.org/bnf/

The Centre for Evidence-Based Nursing
The Centre for Evidence-Based Nursing works with nurses in practice, other researchers, nurse educators and managers to identify evidence-based practice through primary research and systematic reviews, and promotes the uptake of evidence into practice through education and implementation activities in areas of nursing where good evidence is available. The Centre is also researching factors that promote or impede the implementation of evidence-based practice. The University of York has established a Centre for Evidence-Based Nursing as part of the national network of Centres for Evidence-Based Clinical Practice (which includes the Centre for Evidence-Based Medicine at Oxford and the Centre for Evidence-Based Child Health in London).
http://www.york.ac.uk/healthsciences/centres/evidence/cebn.htm

The Cochrane Reviews
http://www.nelh.nhs.uk/cochrane.asp

The Expert Patient programme
http://www.expertpatients.nhs.uk/about_faq.shtml#1

The Healthcare Commission
http://www.healthcarecommission.org.uk/ Homepage/fs/en

This has replaced the Commission for Health Improvement, however that site is still maintained as an archive.
http://www.chi.gov.uk

Leicestershire Primary Audit Group
http://www.leicester-pcag.org.uk/index.htm

The National Electronic Library for Health
http://www.nelh.nhs.uk

The National Institute for Health and Clinical Excellence (NICE)
http://www.nice.org.uk/

National Patient Safety Agency: Incident Decision Tree
http://www.msnpsa.nhs.uk/idt2/(quvrderoubixy2uxdtxtdd45)/help.aspx?
JS=1&notusedbefore=1

NHS Informatics home page
http://www.informatics.nhs.uk/index.html

Patient Advice and Liaison Services (PALS)
http://www.dh.gov.uk/PolicyAndGuidance/OrganisationPolicy/PatientAndPublicInvolvement/
PatientAdviceAndLiaisonServices/fs/en

PRODIGY
Funded by the Department of Health, PRODIGY has been developed by the Sowerby
Centre for Health Informatics at Newcastle (SCHIN). PRODIGY is the result of a unique
collaboration between SCHIN, the Department of Health and the suppliers of clinical
computing software to general practice. PRODIGY was started as a research project in 1995
and underwent two major development phases before the government announced, at the end
of 1998, its general release to all interested GPs in England.
http://www.prodigy.nhs.uk/

The Royal Pharmaceutical Society of Great Britain
http://www.rpsgb.org.uk/

ScHARR database – Netting the Evidence
http://www.shef.ac.uk/scharr/ir/trawling.html

Standards for Health
http: //www.dh.gov.uk/PublicationsAndStatistics/Publications/PublicationsPolicy
AndGuidance/PublicationsPolicyAndGuidanceArticle/fs/en?
CONTENT_ID=4086665&chk=jXDWU6

Wisdom Centre for Networked Learning Institute of Primary Care & General Practice
Sheffield
http://www.wisdomnet.co.uk/clingov.asp

York Effectiveness bulletins
www.york.ac.uk/inst/crd

6 Collaborative Working and Clinical Management Plans

JOHN McKINNON

This chapter will discuss how the wide variety of strengths of skill and specialised understanding that exist across the spectrum of health professions may be formally and informally harnessed to optimise prescribing practice, holistic care and seamless services. A reflective model for collaborative working between disciplines is discussed. The clinical management plan, originally introduced as the cornerstone of supplementary prescribing, will be shown to house the principles that guide good practice in any field of prescribing and its use is recommended in any therapeutic setting.

ENSHRINING TRADITIONAL EXPERT SKILLS AND PRACTICES

Judging purely by the heat and colour of some of the less-informed debate relating in particular to issues of risk management that accompanied the advent of comprehensive non-medical prescribing, an impartial observer from another world could have been forgiven for thinking that the health professionals at the centre of the proposals had little knowledge of drugs and had hitherto played no part in therapeutic planning and decision making. This could not be further from the truth.

For decades, nurses in trauma and critical care units have advised junior doctors on drug and treatment choices in critical episodes of care and engaged in debate with senior medics about the appropriateness of aspects of treatment. They have both administered and titrated drugs within preset intracranial and haemodynamic parameters (Javacone and Dostal, 1992). Although these practices were both commonplace and essentially risk managed, they were no more risk laden nor commonplace than other non-drug-related nursing practices in trauma care, such as the management of a patient on assisted ventilation (Walters, 1995). These may be some of the

Towards Prescribing Practice. Edited by J. McKinnon.
© 2007 John Wiley & Sons, Ltd.

reasons why following implementation of nurse prescribing in the acute sector of her trust, Green (2004) found that her medical staff were already both informed and convinced about the nurses' ability to prescribe.

In primary care, nurses have long recommended drug treatments in chronic disease management that have merely been endorsed by general practitioners. It was Julia Cumberledge's recognition of this uneconomical 'de facto' prescribing situation in the 1980s that set in motion the non-medical prescribing momentum that brought us to where we are today (Department of Health and Social Security, 1986).

Historical skill and expertise of this kind is not limited to nursing. Midwifery has always been a profession of autonomous practitioners with special prescribing powers (Marshall et al., 2005). Paramedics are experienced in rapid assessment, care and treatment of patients in traumatic situations. Their responsibilities include the prescribing of drugs within a formulary linked to an exemption clause in the 1968 Medicines Act (Benner and Bledsoe, 2005). Furthermore, while more research is needed, paramedic practice has been credited by a number of authorities with reducing pre-hospital mortality (Johnson et al., 2006). Pharmacists daily use their in-depth knowledge of drugs in health and illness to give measured sensitive advice to the public on pharmacy-only medicines and other healthcare products (Rutter, 2004). Physiotherapists work with patients in rehabilitation using a depth of applied knowledge of the neuromusculo-skeletal system easily comparable to the level of pharmacology required to prescribe safely. Such practice has been shown to produce positive outcomes (Goldby et al., 2006).

These perspectives on healthcare practice indicate that a prescribing role for a range of healthcare professionals has not been the huge practical or intellectual leap in the dark that some have implied. Instead, non-medical prescribing has consolidated, liberated and formalised expert skills and practices that have always existed (Department of Health, 2002). This in part explains why research (Latter et al., 2005) has found high levels of confidence in non-medical prescribing among the public, the medical profession and non-medical prescribers themselves. Prescribing skills have been assimilated within well-honed healthcare behaviour rather than the reverse.

Skills and practices have been consolidated in that prescribing studies integrate existing nursing and allied health professionals' knowledge of therapeutics with skills of medicines management and pharmacology.

Skills and practices have been liberated to the extent that the absence of prescribing power constrained holistic care and delayed appropriate treatment prior to medical referral or intervention. Non-medical prescribing provides a platform on which to build better patient access to care.

Skills and practices have also been formalised in that prior to the introduction of phased non-medical prescribing legislation, a host of systems existed in which no formal training was given, ranging from patient group directions to local protocols, with doctors providing vicarious liability that permitted nurses to supply and administer patients with medicines as part of care. These were heterogeneous systems that often lacked legal integrity and potentially placed the practitioners concerned at risk.

The value of legally potent prescribing powers can be demonstrated through the use of the clinical management plan concept set against the principles of the prescribing pyramid (National Prescribing Centre, 1999).

CLINICAL MANAGEMENT PLANS

STATUTORY ORIGINS

Clinical management plans (CMPs) were introduced as the central feature of supplementary prescribing in 2003 (Department of Health, 2003). Supplementary prescribing can be defined as a voluntary partnership between an independent prescriber (a doctor or a dentist) and a supplementary prescriber (SP) to implement an agreed individualised clinical management plan with the patient's agreement for the purpose of treating a specific condition or range of conditions (Cook, 2002).

The supplementary prescriber was originally required to be a registered nurse, a registered midwife or a registered pharmacist, but a number of other allied health professionals such as physiotherapists were later added to this list. The independent prescriber (IP) and the supplementary prescriber are required to have access to and use of a shared record. The nature of the prescribing relationship means that although the IP and the SP may not practise in the same location, they should be able to take part in ad hoc communication to allow consultation and support for the SP to take place with ease. It has always been acknowledged that supplementary prescribing involving an IP and an SP in locations that are remote from one another might only be feasible where electronic shared records are in use.

Within the supplementary prescribing legislation, the clinical management plan is mandatory (Table 6.1). It is a legal document that has two roles:

- It is an endorsement of SP practice by the IP and the limits within which that practice may take place.
- It is a patient-specific therapeutic plan of care.

Tables 6.2 and 6.3 give examples of clinical management plans used in practice.

There is no restriction on the drugs that can be prescribed by nurses and pharmacists as part of this non-medical prescribing mode, with the proviso that they can be prescribed by the IP from an NHS budget. This includes off-label prescribing, black triangle drugs, controlled drugs and drugs marked 'less suitable for prescribing' in the *British National Formulary*. Unlicensed drugs may also be prescribed as part of supplementary prescribing in specified circumstances. Other health professional supplementary prescribers have some additional restrictions. In Chapter 8, Jo West discusses some of these issues in more depth.

Table 6.1   Clinical management plan

Clinical Management Plan

Functions

- Essential foundation stone of supplementary prescribing
- Facilitates all non-medical prescribing practice
- Patient centred
- Houses evidence-based therapeutics
- Formalises concordat and review
- Tool for collaborative working
- Prescribing safety net

Includes

- Name of patient
- Diagnosis, condition or range of conditions being treated
- Dates for commencement and review
- Warnings re allergies/sensitivities/difficulties
- Parameters for treatment and referral to independent/more experienced prescriber
- Arrangements for notification of Committee for Safe Medicines/Medicines and Healthcare Products Agency

Should refer to

- Reference to class or description of medicines/type of appliances included
- Reference to national or local evidence-based guidelines

The role of the patient as a partner is emphasised in that the supplementary prescribing arrangement cannot proceed without the patient's express consent to both the arrangement and the role identity of the SP. Notification of the agreement between the patient, the IP and the SP must be given on the clinical management plan. The supplementary prescribing arrangement must be renegotiated should the identity of the IP or SP change. In circumstances in which a team of prescribers work together, any junior member of the IP's team may represent her/him. In such cases the IP team members' names should all appear on the clinical management plan.

There is a clear delineation of responsibility between the IP and the SP. The IP is responsible for:

- Clinical assessment, diagnosis formulation and scope of the CMP, although the document itself may not necessarily be drawn up by him/her.
- Reaching an agreement with the supplementary prescriber as to the scope and terms of supplementary prescribing practice.
- Providing advice and support to the supplementary prescriber as requested.
- Measuring the need for review against the health status of the patient.
- Reporting of adverse reactions via the yellow card scheme.

Table 6.2   Clinical management plan, suspected and confirmed DVT

THE ROYAL BEST HOSPITAL – CLINICAL MANAGEMENT PLAN SUSPECTED AND CONFIRMED DEEP VEIN THROMBOSIS

Name of Patient: Barry White	Patient medication sensitivities/allergies: Penicillin

Patient identification e.g. ID number, date of birth:
S243856, Date of Birth: 01/04/1973, 14 Soul Way, Music Town, Bogshire

Independent Prescriber(s): Dr Diane Platelet (Consultant Haematologist)	Supplementary Prescriber(s) Mr John Corpuscle (Haemostasis & Thrombosis SCNS)

Condition(s) to be treated Suspected and confirmed deep vein thrombosis (DVT)	Aim of treatment To ensure the patient receives the most appropriate anticoagulation treatment, promptly and safely.

Medicines that may be prescribed by SP:

Preparation	Indication	Dose schedule	Specific indications for referral back to the IP
Enoxaparin sodium pre-filled syringes (all strengths), low molecular weight heparin.	Thromboprophylaxis & treatment of DVT.	Dependent on patient's weight in kilograms (see BNF 50, September 2005, section 2.8.1 and/or dose calculation poster).	Incidences of excessive bruising and/or bleeding. Platelet count < 150 or falls by more than 50% from baseline.
Warfarin sodium tablets (1mg, 3mg & 5mg strengths), oral anticoagulant.	Treatment of confirmed DVT (see supply, administration & dose adjustment of oral anticoagulants & LMWH PGD for inclusion / exclusion criteria – page 1).	Refer to the QMC Anticoagulation Service loading-dose guide. Titrate to INR. Refer to DAWN AC system for maintenance doses. Also see BNF 50, September 2005, section 2.8.2.	Incidences of excessive bruising and/or bleeding. Where recognised side effects occur (see BNF 50, September 2005, section 2.8.2).

Table 6.2   (Continued)

Preparation	Indication	Dose schedule	Specific indications for referral back to the IP
Phytomenadione (vitamin K_1) Konakion MM paediatric injection. **(For oral administration.)**	Reversal of over anticoagulation with warfarin oral anticoagulant (see administration of vitamin K PGD inclusion / exclusion – page 1).	INR > 8 but < 12 = 2mg INR > 12 = 4mg Refer to the vitamin K PGD for inclusion / exclusion criteria (page 1). Also see BNF 50, September 2005, section 9.6.6.	Evidence of major bleeding complications.

Guidelines or protocols supporting clinical management plan:

Guidelines on Oral Anticoagulation 3rd Edition, British Journal of Haematology 1998, 101: 374–387.
Guidelines on Oral Anticoagulation (warfarin): 3rd Edition, 2005 update, BCSH.
The supply, administration & dose adjustment of oral anticoagulants & LMWH. QMC protocol/PGD 2005.
The administration of oral vitamin K. QMC protocol/PGD 2005.
Enoxaparin sodium dose selection poster. QMC 2005.
Warfarin oral anticoagulant loading dose guide. QMC 2005.
British National Formulary, Number 50, September 2005.

Frequency of review and monitoring by:

Supplementary prescriber:	Supplementary prescriber and independent prescriber:
As appropriate according to patient's INR but no greater than 3 monthly. Next review no later than **20/04/2006**.	Annually. Next review no later than **20/01/2007**.

Process for reporting ADRs:

The supplementary prescriber should complete a British National Formulary (BNF) suspected adverse drug reaction 'yellow card' and report the ADR(s) directly to the independent prescriber for review.

All ADRs should also be reported on the DAWN AC computerised decision support software (patient's electronic anticoagulation record) and in the patient's paper medical records.

Shared record to be used by IP and SP:

DAWN AC computerised decision support software (patient's electronic anticoagulation record).
The patient's Royal Best Hospital paper medical records where appropriate.

Agreed by independent prescriber(s)	Date	Agreed by supplementary prescriber(s)	Date	Date agreed with patient/carer
D. Platelet	20/01/2006	J. Corpuscle	20/01/2006	B. White 200106

Source: Steven Davidson, Consultant Nurse, Queens Medical Centre Nottingham.

Table 6.3 Clinical management plan for control of back pain

CLINICAL MANAGEMENT PLAN FOR CONTROL OF BACK PAIN

For teams that have full co-terminus access to patient records

Name of Patient: Mr Sad Man	Patient medication sensitivities/allergies: None known

Patient identification 13/1/70	

Independent Prescriber(s): Dr B Teamworker	Supplementary Prescriber(s) Mrs I Getyoubetter – Physiotherapist

Condition(s) to be treated Musculoskeletal pain – (acute simple low back pain)	Aim of treatment To control pain and encourage mobility

Medicines that may be prescribed by SP:

Preparation	Indication	Dose schedule	Specific indications for referral back to the IP
Co-codamol 8/500mg or Co-codamol 30/500mg tablets	Pain	1–2 tablets every 4–6 hours (maximum 8 tablets daily)	Poor pain control Condition deteriorating Medication side effects To prescribe outwith plan Patient request
Diclofenac sodium 50mgs e/c tablets	Pain	50–150mg daily in 3 divided doses with or after food	

Guidelines or protocols supporting clinical management plan:
BNF 52 (2006) Section 10.1.1

PRODIGY guidelines for back pain www.prodigy.nhs.uk/back_pain (as at Nov 2006)

Frequency of review and monitoring by:

Supplementary prescriber Weekly or as clinically indicated	Supplementary prescriber and independent prescriber 8 weeks

Process for reporting ADRs:
Document in patient records
Report to independent prescriber
Yellow card system

Shared record to be used by IP and SP:
Shared computer records

Agreed by independent prescriber(s)	Date	Agreed by supplementary prescriber(s)	Date	Date agreed with patient/carer
B Teamworker	Date of agree	I Getyoubetter	Date of agree	**Date of agreement**

Source: Petra Clarke, Non Medical Prescribing Academic Lead, University of Lincoln.

The SP is responsible for:

- Prescribing and amending prescriptions within the limits of the CMP.
- Monitoring and assessing patients' progress.
- Working within clinical competence.
- Accepting professional accountability for prescribing practice.
- Returning prescribing responsibility to the independent prescriber if patient need breaches CMP parameters.
- Contemporaneous recording in shared record.
- Distinguishing prescribing roles (i.e. legal freedom to prescribe within supplementary prescribing in comparison to what may be less prescribing latitude under the auspices of some other prescribing mode such as the nurse formulary).

Finally, clinical management plans must give dates for review by the SP and the patient and must be reviewed with the IP once every 12 months. Where it is decided that an annual review may safely be postponed, a rationale as to why this is so must be documented.

USING CLINICAL MANAGEMENT PLANS BEYOND SUPPLEMENTARY PRESCRIBING

The early preoccupation with the link with one particular prescribing mode has served as a distraction from the real value of clinical management plans across all prescribing practice. The discussion that follows will show that all the seven principles that promote safe and effective prescribing are housed within this recording tool. It therefore follows that the use of CMPs can be recommended as a framework in any non-medical prescribing situation, demonstrating best practice and providing a safety net in therapeutics.

Individual Patient-Centred Assessment

The individualised nature of a CMP reinforces the patient-centred approach and the need for expert history taking and assessment (Department of Health, 1998). Identifying the prescribers also follows the 'named carer' approach. Patients can never be merely transferred directly unassessed from a patient group direction on to a CMP. Patient specificity is tokenism without the patient's needs being first identified, measured and cited as the rationale for care. Non-medical prescribing, whether independent or supplementary, demands an individual assessment and individual management from a prescribing practitioner acting within identified boundaries of competence.

Evidence Base for Safe Effective Practice

Therapeutics should be based on the best available evidence (National Prescribing Centre, 1999). Efficacy, appropriateness and acceptability for the patient's condition, age and lifestyle, compatibility with medication history and current medication profile are all active issues. Cost effectiveness is also important (National Prescribing Centre and National Primary Care Research and Development Centre, 2002). Clinical management plans that cite the source(s) of evidence for treatment and/or include local guidelines as an appendix ensure that while the plan itself is a simple, concise document, the guidelines on which prescribed medication is based are easily available for retrieval, inspection and review.

Safety Netting

The guidelines for implementation of supplementary prescribing have been transparent on the mandatory inclusion of clear parameters within which the SP could function and the points at which they would refer back to the independent prescriber. These parameters and points of referral vary depending on the breadth of competence of the prescriber and the complexity of the condition(s) being treated (Baird, 2003).

However, following such a model of accountability need not be limited to one mode of prescribing. All prescribing practice is safer and more effective when clear points of referral, parameters that recognise the limits of practitioner competency and signal the need for support, are established. There is no shame in this for the non-medical prescriber. Referring to higher levels of expertise when there is doubt regarding the best way forward in therapeutic management or when the expertise of a frontline practitioner is exhausted has always formed part of good medical practice. When CMPs are used as a framework in independent non-medical prescribing and point lines of deferral as well as referral in case management are clearly agreed and documented, a safety net is supplied that permits freedom in practice yet protects both prescriber and patient.

Concordance

There will be no reiteration here of the explorative discussion relating to concordance conducted in Chapter 2. Suffice to say that the emphasis on a triangular partnership between prescribers and a patient is a direct endorsement of the concordat culture. This formalises and is fully consistent with the ethos in which a patient is consulted and involved in planning their own care at every stage of treatment (Cook, 2002).

A Central Shared Record

The vision of a shared record as a tool for safe and effective practice is well documented (Department of Health, 1998). These principles are embodied within a CMP, which should be accessible to everyone who contributes to the patient's care plan (including the patient). In this way the record demonstrates interdisciplinary working and prescribing as part of a seamless approach.

Clinical management plans used in conjunction with independent non-medical prescribing showcase collaborative working across professional demarcation lines. It is interesting that the Department of Health stated (2003) at the introduction of clinical management plans that the approach would work best with practitioners among whom mutual respect and trust already existed. Non-medical prescribing therefore requires practitioners to own a certain attitude towards collaborative working.

A Model to Promote Positive Interdisciplinary Practice

Referring to other areas of expertise (dietician, nurse, bereavement counsellor, addiction centre, physiotherapist etc.) is instrumental to collaborative working at patient level. However referrals, whether vertical or horizontal, part of a protocol or issuing spontaneously from practice, are most effective when the practitioner is acting on conscious knowledge of the worth of the contributory role of the referee and can recommend this to the patient as an enhancement of their care. This is important if patient confidence in the care plan is to be maintained. Sustained concordance arises out of such confidence (Little et al., 2001).

The seamlessness of patient care is related to the quality of collaborative working. Referrals deliver tacit messages about the spirit of collaboration between practitioners. There are a number of questions on which the prescriber may reflect to test their commitment to collaborative working:

- Who are they?
- What is it that they do?
- Why can't I do it?
- If I *can* do it, why can they do it better?
- How is patient care enhanced?

Who Are They?

'You'll find that he is a very good listener as well as being experienced with this type of problem. He is very understanding.'

Goding and Cain (1999) argue that knowledge by acquaintance is a distinct way of knowing. In the context of a referral, personal knowledge of a colleague penetrates beyond what can be conveyed by a professional title or curriculum vitae. This personal knowledge means that the prescriber is not just aware of a colleague's quality of practice, but also the qualities that the colleague brings to practice. When this knowledge by acquaintance is shared with the patient, they are able to anticipate the referral positively and concordance with the referral pathway is more likely to be maintained. This is also true when the referral is made to a service user or voluntary group member.

Communication technology, excessive workloads and diaries awash with double bookings mean that knowledge by acquaintance is neglected in favour of e-mails, telephone calls and standardised referral forms. This is unfortunate, as a short time spent observing a colleague at work and joining in their reflective practice means that the prescriber is better equipped to recommend them to a patient by virtue of having witnessed their personal 'signature' on their practice. Personal observation exercises also promote appreciation of specialist knowledge.

What Is It That They Do?

'Mr Daniels studied how to treat pain and how the body moves and has worked at university for several years.'

Specialist practice describes much more than the parameters of a particular discipline. It refers to specialist knowledge. Pound et al. (2001) speak of the experience, research base, factual knowledge, personal and professional interpretive skills that contribute to practice. For example, in the course of assessment of a patient, a physiotherapist will simultaneously utilise skills and draw on areas of knowledge, some of which overlap with other professions such as nursing, but many of which are unique to their field. Building on the patient history, the practitioner works with passive and active movement, observing and testing agility and resistance and using palpation to locate pain and the injury that lies at its source. In doing so they draw on pathophysiological knowledge of the central nervous and musculo-skeletal systems to reach a diagnosis (Porter, 2003).

When prescribers reflect on the nature and level of study required of a colleague to achieve specialist acumen, there are two outcomes. First, they work against stereotypes and prejudices that can be associated with certain professional disciplines and break down potential barriers to interprofessional practice. Second, they begin to articulate the rationale for the referral in a way that will be more meaningful for the patient.

Why Can't I Do It?

'Because her qualification and practice are all about how food and drink fuel the body, she is able to give you more help with your diet than I can and she can make it all suit your personal needs.'

This question is particularly useful for testing the validity of the referral. A major part of good prescribing practice is the link between the limits of our own competence and the need to refer to other professionals (Nursing and Midwifery Council, 2006). Awareness of the skills of a practitioner to whom we refer helps distinguish the role of that practitioner from that of our own. Professional humility and professional inertia are two very different characteristics. Articulating the need for interdisciplinary involvement helps the prescriber to determine whether patient care is actually enhanced by this, or whether merely selfish purposes are being served by passing the responsibility for that care on to someone else. Patients are often able to discern the latter and this may adversely affect concordance. If the prescriber can articulate this difference in specialist skill and knowledge for themselves, they will also be able to do so for the patient.

If I Can Do It, Why Can They Do It Better?

> 'You've come a long way in a short time but I think you need expert help with your
> addiction that I can't give you on my own.'

The skills and areas of knowledge that are either generic or more focused and
specialised vary between professional areas of practice. For example, a nurse might
consider herself as having theory-based counselling skills, but not consider herself a
counsellor who has an in-depth knowledge of cognitive, behavioural and psychother-
apeutic frameworks. A counsellor might be able to discern that a patient has an
altered mood state, but this does not necessarily imply mental healthcare expertise,
which requires both a knowledge of mental illness and skilled insight into the disposition and frame of reference of the individual together with the appropriate range
of therapies. Mental health practitioners may have a sound knowledge of dietary
health principles, but not at the level of a dietician who is able to tailor nutritional
values to the individual needs of a patient's disease state and lifestyle. Where there
is 'knowledge overlap', legitimate referrals are made on the basis of the appreciation of the gap between the basic skill of the prescriber and the advanced skill of
the practitioner to whom the patient is referred. In such cases, the prescriber may
be able to act competently, but understands that patient need is more sensitively
and expertly served by someone else.

How Is Patient Care Enhanced?

> 'I go back to the surgery again to see about my asthma in six weeks. I have a prescription
> for patches so by that time I'll hopefully be a non-smoker! I'm nervous about attending
> the self-help group, but I'm going to give it a go because I think it will help me realise
> that I'm not on my own and the nurse told me I may pick up tips on coping.'

The endpoint of collaborative working should be improved outcomes for patient
care. Prescribers need to be able to predict how such improved outcomes can be
achieved by the referral of choice. How will referred treatment benefit the patient
and how will that benefit complement treatment by the prescriber?

Review

A review in the context of prescribing can be described as a structured critique of a
patient's medication profile, with the aim of agreeing a way forward with the patient
to maximise efficacy, minimise the number and severity of medication-related
difficulties and reduce waste. The use of a clinical management plan formalises a
higher quality of review and evaluation process and, once again, the inclusion of
the patient is significant. The Task Force on Medicines Partnership (2002) makes
the distinction between several different types of medication review:

- Reviews that are conducted in an unstructured, opportunistic way.
- Prescription reviews in which lists of medicines prescribed for each patient are
  reviewed.

- Reviews of medication using the patients' case notes.
- Practitioner and patient meeting personally to holistically review the patient's condition and medication.

The latter style of review is the only one in which the patient is an active participant. This is the one to which prescribing practitioners need to aspire. Indeed, it is difficult to imagine how concordance can be sustained, efficacy determined and safety optimised using any other system. It is interesting that Janet Krska and her colleagues (2005) found that 30 % of pertinent prescribing issues were identified as a direct result of patients' personal involvement in medication reviews.

The quality as well as the structure of the review is relevant. An evaluation of medication review systems already in place (Celino et al., 2005) showed that while some examples of good practice exist, considerable progress needs to be made in actual engagement by practitioners with the principles of concordance. There is a difference between being present at a review and having active participation. For example, many patients called to review did not always have the aim of the exercise explained to them. A number of patients felt interrogated. For some patients, the review process was not a useful one as they were given no opportunity to ask questions. In a few cases this led to feelings of suspicion that the review was merely part of a cost-cutting exercise rather than an initiative designed to benefit them.

Table 6.4 gives the core characteristics of a patient-centred medication review.

It seems that pharmacists, doctors and nurses all bring different strengths and weaknesses of evaluation to medication reviews. Pharmacists are reputed to spend more time discussing the medicines and have been observed to be more 'treatment focused'. Pharmacists also tend to target patients with large medication profiles and others whom research would indicate are most at risk. Doctors are, by comparison, more patient oriented, but sometimes lose focus on the purpose of the review, conducting something more closely resembling a consultation. Doctors also have been shown to omit record-keeping details such as dosage issues along with issues of cost effectiveness. Nurses are also patient focused, but are not as skilled as doctors at identifying issues of poor drug efficacy or poorly tolerated medicines (Krska et al., 2005).

Celino et al. (2005) recommend that human and time resources are used most efficiently when medication reviews are shared across prescribing disciplines that

Table 6.4   The patient and medication reviews

- Explain the rationale for the review to the patient
- Give the patient time to prepare for the review
- The 'most appropriate' practitioner should conduct the review
- Avoid 'interrogating' the patient
- Encourage the patient to talk about their condition and medicines
- Encourage the patient to ask questions
- Keep a written record of the review process and the outcome
- Agree how any amendments to the medication profile will be monitored

work together, matching the appropriate strengths of reviewer to the needs of a particular case. The authors qualify this by adding that training for medication review should form part of continuing professional development.

Clinical management plans encourage best practice in medicines management through the formal requirement for case review, the involvement of the patient from the outset and their interdisciplinary format.

Reflection

Reflection as 'a process of reviewing an experience in order to describe, analyse and evaluate and so inform learning about practice' (Reid, 1993: 305) has been at the heart of continuing professional development for many years (ENB, 1991), although Reid's paper from which this definition is taken questions how much honest and structured reflection occurs in professional life. The place of reflection among the prescribing principles is one that seeks to draw meaning from an episode of care. Critical questions should be asked about:

- The level of consistency in messages conveyed by the patient's facial expression, vocal tone, body language and spoken word.
- Social, cultural and ethical considerations.
- The evidence base for decision making.
- The personal, political and commercial influences on prescribing behaviour.

This degree of critical reflection on prescribing seeks to test how much our practice matches the values we claim to own. To the extent that a clinical management plan is built on an individual assessment, that plan will aid reflection.

CONCLUSION

There is a large body of work to show the depth of expertise across a range of allied health professions to recommend them to prescribing practice. Collaborative working between these professions serves to augment the quality of patient care that accompanies prescribing. Optimum collaborative working takes place when practitioners are aware of the personal and professional strengths, specialist knowledge and expertise offered by other disciplines in comparison to their own. Clinical management plans embrace the seven principles of prescribing and can be recommended as tools for safeguarding good practice.

REFERENCES

Baird, A (2003) How to write a clinical management plan. *Nurse Prescribing Journal* **1**(2): 93–94.
Benner, R & Bledsoe, BE (2005) *Critical Care Paramedic: Principles and Practice*. Harlow: Prentice Hall.

Celino, G, Dhalla, M & Levenson, R (2005) *Implementing Medication Review: An Evaluation of the Impact of 'Room for Review'*. London: The Medicines Partnership.

Cook, R (2002) A brief guide to the new supplementary prescribing. *Nursing Times* **98**(49): 26–27.

Department of Health (1998) *The New NHS, Modern and Dependable*. London: The Stationery Office.

Department of Health (2002) *Liberating the Talents*. London: The Stationery Office.

Department of Health (2003) *Supplementary Prescribing by Nurses and Pharmacists with the NHS in England, A Guide for Implementation*. London: The Stationery Office.

Department of Health and Social Security (1986) *The Cumberledge Report: Neighbourhood Nursing, A Focus for Care*. London: The Stationery Office.

English National Board (1991) *The Professional Portfolio*. London: English National Board.

Goding, L & Cain, P (1999) Knowledge in health visiting practice. *Nurse Education Today* **19**(4): 299–305.

Goldby, LJ, Moore, AP, Doust, J & Trew, ME (2006) A randomized controlled trial investigating the efficiency of musculoskeletal physiotherapy on chronic low back disorder. *Spine* **31**(10): 1083–1093.

Green, H (2004) Nurse prescribing in the acute sector: One trust's experience. *Nurse Prescribing Journal* **2**(1): 9–14.

Jacavone, J & Dostal, M (1992) A descriptive study of nursing judgment in the assessment and management of cardiac pain. *Advances in Nursing Science* **15**(1): 54–63.

Johnson, S, Brightwell, R & Ziman, M (2006) Paramedics and pre-hospital management of acute myocardial infarction: Diagnosis and reperfusion. *Emergency Medicine Journal* **23**(5): 331–334.

Krska, J, Ross, SM & Watts, M (2005) Medication reviews provided by GPs and nurses: an evaluation of their quality. *International Journal of Pharmacy Practice* **13**(2): 77–84.

Latter, S, Courtenay, M, Maben, J, Myall, M & Dunn, N (2005) *An Evaluation of Extended Formulary Independent Nurse Prescribing*. Southampton: School of Nursing and Midwifery and School of Medicine, University of Southampton.

Little, P, Everett, H, Williamson, I, Warner, G, Moore, M, Gould, C, Ferrier, K & Payne, S (2001) Observational study of patient-centredness and positive approach on outcomes of general practice consultations. *British Medical Journal* **323**(7318): 908–911.

Marshall, J, Sullivan A & Raynor, M (2005) *Decision Making in Midwifery Practice*. Edinburgh: Churchill Livingstone.

National Prescribing Centre (1999) Signposts for prescribing nurses – general principles of good prescribing. *Prescribing Nurse Bulletin* **1**(1): 1–4.

National Prescribing Centre & National Primary Care Research and Development Centre (2002) *Modernising Medicines Management, A Guide to Achieving Benefits for Patients, Professionals and the NHS*. London: National Prescribing Centre.

Nursing and Midwifery Council (2006) *Standards of Proficiency for Nurse and Midwife Prescribers*. London: Nursing and Midwifery Council.

Porter, S (2003) *Tidy's Physiotherapy* (13th edition). Oxford: Butterworth Heinemann.

Pound, R, Davis, M, Gammon, K, Martindale, J, Page, C & Stapleton, J (2001) Practice and knowledge: An action research approach. *Community Practitioner* **74**(3): 104–106.

Reid, B (1993) 'But we're doing it already!' Exploring a response to the concept of reflective practice in order to improve its facilitation. *Nurse Education Today* **13**(4): 305–309.

Rutter, P (2004) *Community Pharmacy: Symptoms, Diagnosis and Treatment.* Edinburgh: Churchill Livingstone.

Task Force on Medicines Partnership and the National Collaborative Management Services Programme (2002) *Room for Review, A Guide to Medication Review: The Agenda for Patients, Practitioners and Managers.* London: Medicines Partnership.

Walters, AJ (1995) A Heideggerian hermeneutic study of the practice of critical care nurses. *Journal of Advanced Nursing* **21**(3): 492–497.

7 Consultation and Decision Making

CLARE ALLEN

The continual development and evolution of healthcare roles means more professional groups taking total responsibility for the management of patients. This responsibility now includes deciding treatment options and prescribing appropriate medication without deference to medical authority. Achieving this safely necessitates developing new skills, which although not new within healthcare, may be new to the professional groups whose roles are expanding. Consultation skills are among these; traditionally, consulting has sat uncomfortably outside the medical model.

You may think that professionals consult all the time on many different levels, so is there really a need to learn how to do it?

The answer to this is yes! Consulting safely and effectively requires a breadth and depth of knowledge and skills, including those that relate to communication, interviewing, history taking, hypothesis formation and decision making. It is much, much more than just talking to the patient. Developing sound consultation skills is an effective way to help synthesise the vast range of information sources and is not easy when the information given may be incomplete or even contradictory. Furthermore, a patient-centred approach to the consultation is essential for the formation of a therapeutic relationship that will achieve greater adherence to treatment and self-care options.

Yet these are not skills that can be taught effectively through written methods: they involve observation, consistent practice, clinical mentorship and ongoing critical reflection to ensure that experience-based learning is taking place. What can further confuse the practitioner is a tendency to use terms like consultation, communication, interviewing and history taking interchangeably. But as you will read, there are differences that, when understood, will enhance your practice as a prescriber.

The purpose of a consultation may seem obvious, yet patients seek help for a myriad of reasons that have been well documented for many years; see Matarazzo (1984) and the description of behavioural pathogens and immunogens, or those described earlier by Kasl and Cobb (1966) as 'healthy' behaviours – preventive; 'illness' behaviours – seeking professional help; and 'sick role' behaviours – aimed at returning to health through interventions. Centrally it is a belief in the presence or risk of an illness state that is detrimental to the patient's wellbeing, the resolution of which requires the intervention of a professional. Patients seek help to identify problems that may be manifest or hidden, professionals seek to resolve or stabilise

Towards Prescribing Practice. Edited by J. McKinnon.
© 2007 John Wiley & Sons, Ltd.

them to the patient's satisfaction – and to achieve this within the ability of the professional and the limitation of available resources.

Despite the possibility that the patient is unwell, the act of seeking help is in itself traumatic. Patients may fear confirmation of what they perceive as serious. This may be actual (symptoms are present), possible (they have had exposure to a particular illness or disease) or probable (there is a strong hereditary link within their family). In addition, the patient will consider that there are at least moderate, if not severe, consequences from the risk. They will also feel that seeking help will secure beneficial results – for example, that the professional can either make them better or reassure them as to the outcome. Finally, they will perceive that any disadvantages (e.g. unpleasant treatments) do not outweigh the benefits of being well again at the end of the episode. Each of these orientations to advice seeking demonstrates that individual perception of illness is not necessarily a rational process. The situation is complex from the onset. Conducting a consultation becomes like a detective seeking the clues to solve the problem.

While a consultation itself contains several elements, this chapter will concentrate on the verbal and cognitive skills used to make prescribing decisions, not including in any detail the role of physical examination skills or information technology in decision support. The rationale for this is seen in Epstein et al. (2000), who state the commonly agreed fact that 80 % of diagnoses can be made from health history and interviewing alone and in primary care this may be higher still. This chapter will seek to give you some frameworks and techniques that will enable you to become more efficient in conducting your consultations with individuals you encounter, and to collate this information into some meaningful form that promotes safe and effective prescribing.

CONSULTATION THEORY

Consultation theory is not new. Indeed, the last fully established model to be developed within medicine is about a decade old, but for those new to consultation theory, an established framework or model is a good place to start. Many of the references within this chapter relate to medical consultation. The reason for this is that with the exception of CAIIN, the Consultation Assessment and Improvement Instrument for Nurses (Redsell, 2002), consultation theory from the perspective of other healthcare professionals is scarce (Paiguana, 1997a, 1997b), so models from medicine remain highly relevant. CAIIN was developed specifically to support new roles in nursing through helping to identify consultation strengths and weaknesses, thus helping to develop improved levels of consultation capability.

There are generally four basic types of consultation to which the models may be applied and these vary in the extent to which history taking and interviewing are necessary in order for them to be effective. These are briefly detailed below.

- *The comprehensive health interview* is valuable for any patient who is entering the healthcare system for the first time, or has not been seen in the recent past. The purpose is to establish the status of the current problem and establish baseline data allowing for future changes to be compared and evaluated.

- *The problem-focused interview* is where you have information available but are focusing on the patient's present concern. This does not take the place of a comprehensive assessment. It occurs when a viable database exists, and consists of a thorough evaluation of the presenting condition. It may not include holistic evaluation of other systems unless that is indicated as part of the questioning undertaken.

- *The ongoing review or partial health assessment* focuses on monitoring the patient's existing conditions. It is a mini review of existing information as a follow-up on health status. Information gathered is assessed to determine improvement or deterioration.

- *The emergency assessment*, in response to an acute or life-threatening health need, is a rapid and focused assessment aimed at sustaining life or preventing acute deterioration.

The discipline of medicine has developed several useful models for consultation. While the dates may seem old, they are the seminal theories in this field.

Chronologically, the primary models are those listed in Table 7.1 and, although this is not a comprehensive list, they are much cited in contemporary consultation literature. The full references are given at the end of this chapter.

Table 7.1   Chronology of popular consultation models

Date	Principal author(s)	Title
1957	M Balint	The Doctor, the Patient and the Illness
1964	E Berne	Games People Play
1975	J Heron	Six Category Intervention Analysis
1976	P Byrne & B Long	Doctors Talking to Patients
1977	Royal College of General Practitioners	Definition of general practice
1979	NCH Stott & RH Davis	The exceptional potential in each primary care consultation
1981	CG Helman	Disease versus illness in general practice
1984	D Pendleton et al.	The Consultation: An Approach to Learning and Teaching
1987	R Neighbour	The Inner Consultation
1987	RC Fraser	Clinical Method: A General Practice Approach
1989	J Middleton	The exceptional potential of the consultation revisited
1991	S Cohen-Cole	The medical interview: The three function approach
1996	S Kurtz & J Silverman	The Calgary-Cambridge Observation Guides
2002	SA Redsell	Consultation Assessment and Improvement Instrument for Nurses (CAIIN)

Reproduced by permission of Julie Smith, SYSHA.

In all the theories, the aim of the consultation is to discover the patient's concern and effect a suitable treatment. The way this is undertaken varies, so examples of the differing approaches need more consideration.

In the first theory to consider, Byrne and Long (1989) categorise the consultation into six stages:

- relating to the patient
- discovering the reason for attendance
- conducting a verbal or physical examination
- considering the patient's condition
- detailing treatment
- terminating.

As you can see, this model centres around what is wrong today and the reason for attendance. It also considers the range of dialogue used, from professional centred to patient centred. It does not, though, diversify further into co-morbidity or health promotion.

A different viewpoint is offered by Pendleton et al. (1984), who see the consultation more as a series of tasks for the professional to perform. Notably, however, they take a far wider perspective, seeing the opportunity offered by the patient attending. In this model we see a more holistic approach. Importantly, the patient is seen as a partner in care. There is consideration of ongoing problems, not just the presenting ones; the patient is involved in deciding treatment options in order to maximise concordance; and thought is given to future health through relationship building. In contrast to Byrne and Long, whose model initially appears directive, Pendleton et al. offer a facilitative style in which the power is shared between professional and patient.

Their schema is as follows:

- Define the reason for attendance, including the nature and history of the problem, aetiology, patient ideas and expectations, and effects of the problem.
- Consider other continuing problems.
- Choose an appropriate action in agreement with the patient.
- Achieve a shared understanding of the problem with the patient.
- Involve the patient in management and encourage them to accept responsibility.
- Use the time and resources appropriately.
- Establish and maintain a relationship in order to allow completion of other tasks such as attendance at screening.

Thirdly, Heron (1975) gives a six-category intervention analysis:

- *Prescriptive*: giving advice and being directive.
- *Informative*: imparting new knowledge.
- *Confronting*: challenging restrictive behaviours.

- *Cathartic*: seeking to release emotion, for example by encouraging crying.
- *Catalytic*: encouraging the patient to self-discover in terms of their illness.
- *Supportive*: offering the patient approval, comfort and support.

All sections are interlinked to the consultation as a whole and do not follow the end-to-end sequence of the others, rather offering the types of interactions that may occur.

Now consider again the contrasting focus of Middleton (1989). Middleton's format is:

- Discovering the patient's agenda.
- Considering the patient's database (risk factors, continuing problems, dormant problems).
- The doctor's (health professional's) own agenda (external pressure, practice considerations etc.).

This schema highlights the economic perspective, including external pressures and practice considerations, as well as the professional's personal agenda.

Latterly consultation theory has moved to a problem-based learning approach, as seen in the Calgary-Cambridge guide (Kurtz & Silverman, 1996). This approach considers the consultation from the stance of problem-based learning. Its main substantive theme is that successful outcomes, in terms of concordance, under-standing and even speed of recovery, depend on patients feeling that their knowledge and perceptions about their illness are addressed and valued by the professional. The steps are as follows:

- Initiating the session.
- Gathering information.
- Building a relationship.
- Giving information – explaining and planning.
- Closing the session.

The five broad categories are expanded within the framework, which gives the details of each task as a way to maximise the interaction.

Each perspective draws our attention to different issues that we need to address when considering the consultation. Yet despite their contrasting focus, all are centred on discovering both why the patient has sought help and how to effect a solution. We might therefore regard as the main area for debate the expectation that patients are able to express themselves adequately, communicate effectively and understand the information given. Getting the information you want without getting a lot that you don't is where the skills of interviewing and health history taking come to prominence.

It is sometimes thought, mistakenly, that interviewing and health history taking are one and the same thing, when in fact there are subtle yet distinct differences.

It is possible for patients to be interviewed at length by healthcare professionals without pertinent parts of their health history being obtained. Similarly, a health history can be taken, yet vital elements of the presenting condition can be missed as the interviewing techniques have failed to elicit all the pertinent information.

Together, health history taking and interviewing form dynamic components of the consultation. They are skills that any prescriber can develop in order to prevent or minimise the dysfunctional elements creeping in. They are crucial to gaining the important and supplementary information required in order to make a differential diagnosis. This can be called need to know, nice to know and nuts to know! The pivotal process is, therefore, the accurate collection of data.

Clearly, for effective consultation outcomes, patients and professionals need to be able to communicate effectively on a variety of levels that reflect patient need and ability to understand. There is evidence that interpersonal skills determine patient satisfaction, so the aim of any consultation should be shared understanding. However, the message received is not always the message intended. Both parties therefore need to be clear about what is being communicated. Brereton (1995) found evidence to suggest that in nursing, for example, communication is not as effective as it should be. This is reinforced by communication issues being the number one of the most common causes of complaints received by the NHS (Department of Health, 2005).

EFFECTIVE PATIENT INTERVIEWING AND HISTORY TAKING

The goal of an effective interview in this context is to gather enough relevant information to form a patient database for the episode and prescribe the appropriate medication.

Eliciting is a key skill within interviewing and one that requires practice in order to use it to its full potential. Asking questions and getting the required information are different things and can require differing approaches. Giving the patient the opportunity to express their concerns is therefore key. Evidence suggests that patients often have more than one problem and that the severity of the problem, to them, is not linked to the order in which they disclose it. Indeed, evidence from a US study by Beckman and Frankel (1984) found that in only 23 % of consultations was the patient allowed to complete their opening statement of concerns. Furthermore, of the 52 patients who made up this 23% in the study, only one actually managed to complete their whole complaint! The average interruption took place after only 18 seconds.

Where consultations are time restricted, there can be a temptation to concentrate on objective health data and the gathering of facts at the expense of more subjective information, yet it is this that will tell you how the presenting problem is affecting the patient's day-to-day life and is therefore highly significant. Within a holistic assessment, it is important that both types of data are treated with equal importance, but for patients, disclosing information about a physical set of symptoms may be easier and therefore introduced earlier in the conversation. This again illustrates why allowing the patient to explain their concern fully is important. Either way, impressions form from the information elicited that will strongly influence how patients and professionals respond to each other. Subjective health data can also only be verified by the patient and as such may influence any prescribing decisions by the professional and provide an indication of likely concordance.

Whatever data you collect, your approach should be systematic and logical, including information gathered from your very first sighting of the patient. The use of a simple mnemonic framework can help in focusing open and closed questioning, providing a basis on which to use eliciting skills to gain the information you need. There are many in current use within healthcare. A common example is SWIPE: When did it Start? What makes it Worse? What causes Improvement? Is there a Pattern? What is the Evaluation (what is being done to make it better)?

More detailed are TROCARSSS (Time, Rapidity, Occurrence, Characteristics, Associations, Relief, Site, Spread, Severity) and OPQRSTU (Onset, Provocation/palliative factors, Quality, Region/radiation, Severity, Time, U – how does it affect you?). All follow the same basic sequence and help focus the interviewing, thus minimising the chance of forgetting to ask about an aspect of the condition, and give the best possible opportunity to identify the cues given.

Validating the data ensures that what you have collected is correct. In some instances this is easy to do, such as re-checking a measurement taken using instruments. In others, the validation comes from the patient in the form of repeating information back, for example 'So what you are telling me is that the pain is only there when you exercise. . .' gives the patient a clear opportunity to affirm or refute what is said. Always be sure to exclude any factors that influence the accuracy and never assume that because data is abnormal your measurement was wrong.

Validation also provides the patient with opportunities to expand on the information they give: 'Now you come to mention it I do have. . . but didn't think anything of it . . .'

DECISION MAKING FOR SAFE PRESCRIBING

Decision making is the portion of the consultation in which the synthesis of all information takes place and the prescribing decision is primarily made. It is a combination of clinical/diagnostic reasoning and hypothesis formation. Historically, this aspect of care has been within the medical domain. This is despite the fact that many people, professionals and lay persons alike, use information to make a diagnosis almost without realising it. For example, 'I have a cold' is a valid diagnosis. The processing of information linked to signs and symptoms gives us the information we have to deduce what is wrong: temperature, runny nose, headache and so on.

All clinical reasoning methods depend on depth and breadth of knowledge – recognition of what the problem is, what the diagnosis is, what is to be done and how to do it. As an experienced practitioner you will have considerably more knowledge to call on than will a beginner. The use of heuristics based on knowledge and experience allows for rapid processing of cues, signs and symptoms without the need to gather all information and then deduce and disregard the non-relevant. In order to be successful in making a diagnosis, the professional must interpret information gained from the patient, clinical signs and symptoms, and relate these to the three areas of knowledge and skill detailed below:

- Evidence-based knowledge gained from professional training.
- Current and past clinical experience (including the ability to differentiate when what you are told by the patient does not accord with what you observe).
- Clinical knowledge and performance of techniques.

These three elements, combined with the patient's history, make up the foundation on which to base clinical/diagnostic reasoning.

Diagnostic reasoning may be understood as a hypothetico-deductive reasoning approach. In this approach, an initial hypothesis (not a diagnosis at this stage) is made based on initial presentation and patient-led information, coupled with the information from diagnostic tests and physical examination. Remember, tests that are diagnostic such as blood tests, monitoring tests or treatment tests all have a contribution to diagnostic reasoning in providing new information, showing the progression of existing conditions or assessing the efficiency of treatments. Abnormal results obviously require careful assessment; it should be acknowledged that technical error can exist; and results should be checked against existing records to identify trends or emerging patterns. Test results may give partial confirmation of the already formed hypothesis or may refute it. They may also indicate pathology not immediately detectable from history or physical examination. You will need to make a professional judgement in each case.

The additional information gathered centres on expanding the possibility that this is the correct notion, or refuting it by gaining information that cannot possibly fit with what is known about the pattern of the presenting problem. Recognition of patterns is therefore a key skill, which again sets experienced practitioners apart from novices. Taking this a level higher, recognition of pathognomonic signs and symptoms, where what you see can be indicative of a specific condition, can be of use. However, commonality of symptoms may only lead to differential diagnostic states. The following case studies will illustrate this.

Julia is 31 and is complaining of frequency and pain on micturition. You use your patient interviewing skills to take a full history and find that she also has supra-pubic pain, and malodorous urine.

This has been going on for a couple of days prior to coming to the surgery. At this stage your working hypothesis is of a urinary tract infection. From Julia's notes you see she has had this before.

What further information/investigations do you think will give you the conclusive information on which you can make a diagnosis and develop a treatment plan?

Susan is 39 and comes to the surgery for a routine smear. As part of the conversation she complains of feeling tired all the time. She has two teenage children and had another baby 11 months ago. She initially put her tiredness down to a hectic lifestyle and recently returning to work two mornings a week.

You review her notes and take a health history. You note that she has put on weight since her postnatal appointment nine months ago and when you ask when her last period was she is unsure.

Your experience of this type of history is limited and you do not immediately recognise any patterns, but you recognise that there are some cues from the history that this may be something to be concerned about.

What further information do you need to ask Susan? What investigations or examinations do you think may be needed in order to make a diagnosis?

Maria is a 36-year-old breastfeeding mother to a 9-month-old child who attends clinic with left shoulder pain. She is having difficulty sleeping and experiencing problems managing her child, who is now trying to pull himself to stand.

Three months ago Maria grasped a hot saucepan handle and a sudden withdrawal of her left hand injured the left shoulder. Maria complains of left shoulder pain, intermittent ache in the C5 area, aggravated by any outward or backward movements of the left arm. There is no pain at rest. There is no medical history of note and Maria is not on any current medication.

Maria is of slim, petite build and around 5 feet tall. Examination reveals thoracic spine scoliosis from childhood and you observe muscle wasting of the left infra-spinatous area. Resisted lateral gleno-humeral rotation of the left shoulder reproduced the pain. Movement was weak and there was loss of end range of elevation.

What is your diagnosis and how is it reached? What treatments would you recommend? What medication would you prescribe?

Paul and Heaslip (1995) state that all reasoning has nine common elements. If we understand these, they argue, we are well positioned to use and monitor reasoning in clinical practice. They are:

- *The purpose, goal or end product.* The question of 'what do we want to achieve to meet the patient's needs?' must always be kept in mind.
- *The question or issues to be solved or dealt with.* When we apply diagnostic reasoning it is in relation to a problem set. The patient has a concern; what can be done to identify and resolve or stabilise it? The question must relate to the goal.
- *The professional perspective or frame of reference.* Whenever we reason professionally we do it from the standpoint of the professional perspective. Having a narrow perspective or one based on fallacious reasoning may be detrimental to the reasoning process.
- *The empirical dimension.* Deficits in experience, data or evidence on which to base our reasoning can be problematic. From our vast knowledge and experience we must choose the most appropriate elements.
- *The conceptual dimension.* All reasoning uses some concepts but not others at any given time. Deficits in knowledge of those concepts and theories that drive professional practice leave us with insufficient knowledge on which to base interpretation of what the patient tells us.
- *Assumptions.* All reasoning has a starting point. But this point can be fact or assumption. Failure to acknowledge this distinction leads to confusion as to what is fact and what is not – with the potential for reasoning to be based on assumption rather than fact.
- *Inferences.* Reasoning proceeds by steps called inferences: 'Because this has happened, it means that this has also occurred.' Information alone does not determine what we deduce, and lack of scope in knowledge and practice must be acknowledged. Safe prescribing practice requires vigilance and critical reflection. Without these and an ongoing development of self-awareness and emotional intelligence, it can be possible to develop prejudices and patterns of prescribing practice that are false.
- *Implications and consequences.* No reasoning is static; it works to an endpoint. There are possible consequences beyond those the professional has considered and an undesirable outcome could potentially be seen as a problem in reasoning.
- *Implicit and explicit elements.* These allow us to justify what we did and why – for example, why this course of action was chosen in preference to another.

Diagnostic reasoning allows for differential diagnosis: the combination of symptoms described by the patient, signs, laboratory data, illness profiles, knowledge of demographics and social influences that added together give the widest scope on which to reach a conclusion. While much of consultation theory depends on the gathering and interpretation of facts, the contribution of intuition should be considered in the diagnostic reasoning process. Intuition has been defined as 'the immediate apprehension that something is so without the benefit of conscious reasoning' (Guralnik, 1972). Having a concept that by its nature does not fit within scientific study and a body of evidence-based practice is difficult. However, it can be argued that intuition is not really problematic in this respect. Rather, it may be seen as the unconscious drawing on the vast knowledge and skills gained from clinical practice and the commonality of situations, which simply makes it possible to recognise a patient condition without going through the whole of the diagnostic reasoning process.

This process is a major aspect of clinical experience. It involves the skilful combination of deep understanding of underpinning theories; thorough knowledge of clinical theories, facts and skills; and personal understanding of oneself as a professional and the ability to assimilate these areas to solve complex problems.

By using conscious and unconscious knowledge, the end of interviewing should see the gathering of sufficient health history information on which to base diagnostic reasoning, hypothesis formation and decision making. If this has been comprehensive the information will be both objective and subjective, and cover the following categories:

- physiological
- psychological
- biographical
- sociocultural
- developmental
- spiritual.

Having gathered the information and detected the cues, deciding what to do with this information becomes the central skill within the consultation. Without this, it is not possible to make a sound prescribing decision.

A danger here, of course, is 'jumping to conclusions' without fully assessing the facts. In particular, practitioners with a limited scope of expertise should be aware of the possibility of concentrating on cues they have knowledge of and failing to eliminate irrelevant cues from the process. Alongside time constraints, the possibility of bias – thinking we know enough to make a decision – needs to be acknowledged as a key reason for premature closing. Gathering information from a patient can be time consuming, and having a patient database avoids duplicating this process. However, inappropriate use can lead to professionals assuming that a patient repeatedly presenting with the same symptoms always has the same problem. Likewise, knowledge of an existing condition or co-morbidity can lead to assumptions about the patient's current presentation. Concluding and decision making too early in the consultation can lead not only to dissatisfaction but also to dissonance in the immediate future. The influence of time cannot be overestimated from either the patient's or the professional's perspective. Professionals may have many patients to see and patients want rapid resolution or stabilisation of their current health problem. While it is not feasible to have consultations with no time limit, closing too soon may lead to that vital piece of information being missed.

When all reasonable explanations have been gathered for the initial cues, each hypothesis should be evaluated in order to make the final decision. Since data to reject one hypothesis may support another, it is important to consider the possibility of co-existing conditions; the possibility with the most supporting evidence is the most probable and allows for decision making to take place.

As we have seen, decision making is the end process of information gathering, rationalisation and assimilation of the presenting facts. There are different theories of decision making that relate to different situations and what their intended outcome is to be. There is also the tendency for differing disciplines to view their own decision making theory as unique. While it can be argued that many professionals possess the ability to gather and interpret that information, the healthcare sector has been slow in granting the authority to do so to professionals other than doctors. However, the NHS Plan, which you can find at www.doh.gov.uk/nhsplan, details ten key roles for nurses, relating to some of the vital components of the decision-making process.

In prescribing there are two primary categories of decision making: autocratic, which is professional led; and collaborative, which involves a consensus between patient and professional.

One way of reaching decisions about a patient is to devolve the process to the expert who is deemed to have the knowledge needed to choose the right course of action. It must be acknowledged that professional-led decisions do have a place within prescribing. A key advantage of this method is speed – quick decisions are obviously necessary in an emergency situation. Outside emergencies, this method is also used where only the expert has the necessary knowledge, or where no other professional with greater knowledge or skill is available.

The downside, however, is that patients can feel they have had no input into decisions about their health. This may have a negative impact on concordance. Further, one professional cannot be assumed to be the best expert. While some non-medical prescribers will be generalists, expertise in all domains of practice is unrealistic. More importantly, perhaps, instances of professional errors of judgement provide added impetus for us to examine and challenge the notion of 'professional knows best'.

In contrast to the expert autocratic decisions are decisions by collaboration. This may include the patient, the professional, relatives and the GP, and is the most effective way of ensuring that treatment is acceptable and concordance is high. Collaborative decisions can:

- improve the quality of the decision
- improve the patient's 'ownership' or feeling of participation in the decision
- increase the chances of compliance with treatment or advice.

Although full consensus may be difficult to achieve, a shared opinion on the major factors can be enough to maintain satisfaction for both professionals and patients. Key to achieving a successful outcome are avoiding 'zero-sum' approaches (the notion that someone needs to 'win') and establishing effective communication. The latter, in particular, ensures that assumptions are dealt with and that both sides have the opportunity to air opinions and fears.

These points are especially pertinent given the emergence of notions of the 'expert patient'. At the same time, the current ethos of the NHS to provide a bottom-up, patient-led service, centred on need and delivered by consensus of professional and patient, acknowledges the need to respect the patient's perspective as valid and of worth to the decision-making process. See www.doh.gov. uk/involvingpatients/positionstatement.htm.

The following extract from the *British Medical Journal* (Coulter, 1999: 219) sums up this perspective succinctly:

> Partners work together to achieve common goals. Their relationship is based on mutual respect for each other's skills and competencies and recognition of the advantage of combining these resources to achieve beneficial outcomes. Successful partnerships are non-hierarchical and the partners share decision making and responsibility. The key to successful doctor–patient partnerships is therefore to recognise that patients are experts too. The doctor is, or should be, well informed about diagnostic techniques, the causes of disease, prognosis, treatment options, and preventive strategies, but only the patient knows about his or her experience of illness, social circumstances, habits and behaviour, attitudes to risk, values, and preferences. Both types of knowledge are needed to manage illness successfully, so both parties should be prepared to share information and take decisions jointly.

At this point, there may be a possibility of using computerised decision support. While several early studies including Massel et al. (2000), Qamar et al. (1999) and Jonsbu et al. (1993), found their usefulness to be limited by their narrow scope and concentration on life-threatening conditions, decision support systems have a significant role, especially in supporting new prescribers. The support is not just as a diagnostic aid but also an excellent safety net tool, as more non-medically trained practitioners provide front-line services, for example in NHS Direct, and is recommended by the National Prescribing Centre (http://www.npc.co.uk/). Algorithms and software have been developed to improve decision making, but the key here is to remember they are for '*decision support*', not a substitution for the development of key clinical and cognitive skills. PRODIGY (http://www.prodigy.nhs.uk) provides knowledge that is practical and reliable to support safe and effective clinical practice and is funded by the Department of Health. It aims to provide an up-to-date source of clinical knowledge to help the multiprofessional healthcare workforce and patients to manage common conditions seen in primary care. Around 200 topics are covered using various formats, including full guidance, quick reference guides and patient information leaflets.

The development of any effective management plan resulting from the collaborative approach requires agreement on the following areas: what the patient's problem is, the purpose of treatment, and the roles of professional and patient. Although there is evidence that collaborative decisions are more effective than individualised ones, factors that can hamper collaborative decisions also need to be considered.

The most common reason for problems in collaboration lies in conflicting goals between the patient and the professional. Parties bring differing agendas, which may include self-oriented needs that are not best served by the most appropriate decision. Secondly, we need to consider power differences. Sharing of information does not always mean equal collaboration. The perception of the professional as expert can be both positive and negative. On the positive side, there is trust that the knowledge will be used to help the patient. On the negative side, the patient may not feel that their views will be taken seriously. The feeling of disempowerment at not being able to challenge the views of a professional may exclude the patient from hearing information fully and/or they may allow themselves to be persuaded against their will. While collaborative decisions tend to be most acceptable to patients, there is no magic formula for getting the level of collaboration and professional direction right. The egocentric views of professionals may lead them to disregard patients' feelings and perceptions about their illness. And even where this is not the case, patients may not have the necessary social skills to communicate their views effectively. The professional must manage each consultation so as to facilitate a collaborative approach.

DYSFUNCTIONAL CONSULTATIONS

No chapter on consultation skills would be complete without an acknowledgement that things do not always go to plan, even for the most experienced and skilled practitioner! Consultations can close in a manner that is unsatisfactory to the patient or the professional, or both. These consultations can be said to be dysfunctional. Much of the study on dysfunctional consultation comes from medicine. However, the reasons cited have relevance to all professionals dealing with patients and are therefore relevant to prescribing.

A consultation can be said to be dysfunctional from the patient perspective if: the objectives of the patient are not met or are altered without their consent. An example of this is a patient who presents with one problem that concerns them, but the professional directs them to another, possibly ongoing, complaint about which the patient is not concerned. The patient feels the initial complaint is being trivialised. This has links to both health-seeking behaviour and health locus of control. The individual questions whether their health is under their own control or that of others.

Goffman (1990) suggests that people give others the kind of impression that will lead them to act voluntarily in accordance with their objectives. Therefore, not all self-presentations are positive. In some cases, the impressions people try to convey are far from desirable, such as in the pursuit of medication that is not needed.

A consultation can be said to be dysfunctional from the professional perspective if: the objectives of the professional are not met or are altered; the professional recommends a course of action that the patient refuses; or the professional gives a less effective treatment for the sake of maximising concordance, but feels frustrated that their recommendations are rejected.

By applying attribution theory, we can view dysfunction in three ways:

- *Consensus* – would all professionals faced with this situation act in the same manner?

- *Consistency* – is it the professional's interviewing style that is the issue?
- *Distinctiveness* – is it only when certain conditions apply (e.g. the professional is busy) that this occurs?

For both patients and professionals, satisfaction, compliance and concordance can be considered indicators of dysfunction. Marinker (1997, 1998) suggests that only about 50 % of patients with chronic disease take their prescribed medication or treatment in the effective therapeutic dose. With the traditional model of compliance, the patient brings a problem to the professional, who recommends a treatment based on evidence of the disease; the patient's beliefs and values are seen to distract from the 'science' of treatment and cure. Within concordance, dysfunction can be minimised by patient and professional who, though holding differing standpoints, form a therapeutic alliance. This reaffirms the evidence of Stewart et al. (1979), who found a positive relationship between professional and patient and a patient-centred approach the most likely to ensure concordance. In relation to general practice, Larson and Lars (1991) found that failure to comply with treatments was directly linked to the failure to explore the patient's expectations of the consultation; the patient's perception of their presenting health problem; information about the advice given to the patient; and the relevance of the advice given to the patient.

In addition, Byrne and Long (1989) cite the following behaviours as contributors to dysfunctional consultations:

- rejecting patient offers ('we'll talk about that next time')
- reinforcing self-position ('this will be best for you')
- denying the patient ('that is not relevant')
- refusing the patient's ideas ('that will not help your condition')
- evading questions or changing the subject
- not paying attention or doing something else
- not responding to feelings
- talking over or interrupting the patient.

As a professional there are several useful areas you can consider to minimise dysfunction. These include how you give advice: while needed in some cases, it can imply that the patient is not capable of handling their own problems, or can result – albeit unintentionally – in the patient not considering the full range of treatment options. Likewise, you may give a social response rather than a therapeutic one. The patient tells of an injury sustained while gardening, and the practitioner pursues the gardening theme rather than exploring the injury fully. The following are phrases and approaches that may sound very familiar!

- *Giving false reassurance*: the 'you will be fine', 'this won't hurt', 'I'm sure it's nothing' response.
- *Overloading*: bombarding the patient with questions in order to get the data or giving too much of a response without clarification.

- *The halo effect*: steering clear of tricky questions because you think the patient 'looks all right'.
- *Biased questioning*: 'You practise safe sex, don't you?' Patients may be too embarrassed to admit non-adherence.

It is also possible as a professional to introduce bias without realising it, for example the potential cultural differences in communication. Some languages have no equivalent word for common conditions such as depression; while maintaining attention through eye contact is perceived as important in western cultures, it can be perceived as rude in other cultures. Likewise, touch can be both comforting and threatening. The inability of patients to receive and interpret information can be due to unintentional language, terms, jargon and abbreviations, but also variations in the interpretation of body language. Patients may be reluctant to give personal information to a stranger, even a health professional; this may be viewed as being 'difficult'. Gender issues may be an undetected concern by some professionals, which may mean that patients do not disclose fully to one or the other gender, likewise variations in willingness to express pain or distress. Remember also that professionals have their own language that can surreptitiously creep in.

So there are several ways in which dysfunction can happen. Some can be introduced without intention and having awareness will help you minimise these possibilities, thus adding to the soundness of the prescribing decisions you make.

CONCLUSION

It is part of the process of lifelong learning to develop new professional skills and use them to enhance professional practice and give excellent patient care. It has been the intention of this chapter to offer practitioners new to consulting an insight into some of the areas involved. We have looked at consultation models, hypothesis formation and decision making from a theoretical standpoint. The introduction to theories and models has given a framework against which you can critically analyse your current approach to consultation in professional practice. Prescribing decisions cannot be made on one set of data alone. By developing the skills involved, this can help in many aspects that together will help you to become a safe and effective prescriber.

REFERENCES

Balint, M (1986) *The Doctor, the Patient and the Illness*. Edinburgh: Churchill Livingstone.

Beckman, HB & Frankel, RM (1984) The effect of physician behaviour on the collection of data. *Annals of Internal Medicine* **101**(5): 692–696.

Berne, E (1964) *Games People Play: The Psychology of Human Relationships*. New York: Grove Press.

Brereton, ML (1995) Communication in nursing: The theory–practice relationship. *Journal of Advanced Nursing* **21**(2): 314–324.

Byrne, P & Long, B (1989) *Doctors Talking to Patients*. London: Royal College of General Practitioners.

Cohen-Cole, S (1991) The medical interview, the three function approach. In Cohen-Cole, S & Bird, J (eds) (2000) *Mosby Year Book* (2nd edition). St Louis: Mosby Inc.

Coulter, A (1999) Paternalism or partnership? Editorial *British Medical Journal* **319** (18 September): 719–720.

Department of Health (2005) *Report of the Independent Complaints Advocacy Service*. London: The Stationery Office.

Epstein, O, Perkins, GD, Cookson, J & de Bono, DP (2000) *Clinical Examination*. London: Moseby.

Fraser, RC (1987) *Clinical Method: A General Practice Approach*. London: Butterworths.

Goffman, E (1990) *The Presentation of Self in Everyday Life*. Harmondsworth: Penguin.

Guralnik, DB (ed.) (1972) *Webster's New Word Dictionary*. Toronto: Nelson, Foster and Scott.

Helman, CG (1981) Disease versus illness in general practice. *Journal of the Royal College of General Practitioners* **31**(230): 548–552.

Heron, J (1975) *Six Category Intervention Analysis*. Guildford: Human Potential Research Project, University of Surrey.

Jonsbu, J, Aase, O, Rollag, A, Liestol, K & Erikssen, J (1993) Prospective evaluation of an EDB-based diagnostic program to be used in patients admitted to hospital with acute chest pain. *European Heart Journal* **14**(4): 441–446.

Kasl, V & Cobb, S (1966) Health behaviours, illness behaviour and sick role behaviour. *Archives of Environmental Health*. **12**: 532–541.

Kurtz, S & Silverman, J (1996) The Calgary-Cambridge Observation Guides: An aid to defining the curriculum and organising the teaching in communication training programmes. *Medical Education* **30**: 83–89.

Larson, CHR & Lars, L (1991) Connections between the quality of consultations and patient compliance in general practice. *Family Practice* **8**(2): 154–160.

Marinker, M (1997) Personal paper: Writing prescriptions is easy. *British Medical Journal* **314**(8 March): 747–748.

Marinker, M (1998) Compliance is not all. *British Medical Journal*. **316**(7125): 151.

Massel, D, Dawdy, JA & Melendez, LJ (2000) Strict reliance on a computer algorithm or measurable ST segment criteria may lead to errors in thrombolytic therapy eligibility. *American Heart Journal* **140**(2): 221–226.

Matarazzo, JD (1984) Behavioural health. In Matarazzo, JD, Miller, NE, Weiss, SM & Herd, JA (eds) *Behavioural Health: A Handbook of Health Enhancement and Disease Prevention*. New York: John Wiley & Sons, Ltd.

Middleton, J (1989) The exceptional potential of the consultation revisited. *Journal of the Royal College of General Practitioners* **39**: 383–387.

Neighbour, R (1987) *The Inner Consultation*. Lancaster: MTO Press.

Paiguana, H (1997a) Consultations: The process. *Practice Nursing* **8**(7): 18–20.

Paiguana, H (1997b) Consultations: In practice. *Practice Nursing* **8**(8): 20–22.

Paul, RW & Heaslip, P (1995) Critical thinking and intuitive nursing practice. *Journal of Advanced Nursing* **22**(1): 40–42.

Pendleton, D, Schofield, T, Tate, P & Havelock, P (1984) *The Consultation: An Approach to Learning and Teaching*. Oxford: Oxford University Press.

Qamar, A, McPherson, C, Babb, J, Bernstein, L, Werdmann, M, Maskic, D & Zaich, S (1999) The Goldman algorithm revisited: Prospective evaluation of a computer-derived algorithm versus unaided physician judgment in suspected acute myocardial infarction. *American Heart Journal* **138**(4): 705–709.

Redsell, SA (2002) *Consultation Assessment and Improvement Instrument for Nurses (CAIIN)*. Leicester: Department of General Practice and Primary Health Care, University of Leicester.

Royal College of General Practitioners (1977) Definition of general practice. *Journal of the Royal College of General Practitioners* **27**: 117.

Stewart, MA, McWhinney, IR & Buch, CW (1979) The doctor/patient relationship and its effect on outcome. *Journal of the Royal College of General Practitioners* **29**: 77–82.

Stott, NCH & Davis, RH (1979) The exceptional potential in each primary care consultation. *Journal of the Royal College of General Practitioners* **29**: 201–205.

8 Legislation, Regulation and Accountability in Prescribing

JO WEST

Medical legislation is a very complex area. It is the aim of this chapter to address some of this legislative complexity to both aid the understanding of the prescriber and facilitate safe, appropriate practice. So why has our legal system invested so much time and energy into devising an almost incomprehensible process when it comes to the supply of medicines?

The reasoning behind this complex and expensive legal system is public safety. Without these legal constraints, access to all medicines could be inappropriately obtained and their use unrestricted. The use of medicines is a huge public health issue, one that needs control, and we address this control by regulation. Regulation is our answer to reducing medicine-assisted suicide, antibiotic resistance, substance misuse; the list goes on. While public health is discussed in Chapter 4, it is the aim of this chapter to discuss the legislation itself, the accountability of prescribers in practice, and the regulation of the pharmaceutical industry in terms of drug licensing and advertising. We shall also consider the legal requirements for writing a prescription.

Let us consider that regulation is the answer to public safety. We have a regulatory system for the medication products themselves, both in terms of their make-up and effectiveness and their supply chain. We also have regulation of the professionals that are involved with the use of medicinal products. We need to define the classification of medicines in the first instance, and how this classification links to the prescribing and availability of medicines to the general public. This brings us to the Medicines Act 1968, and to the Misuse of Drugs Act 1971 – two major pieces of legislation with which prescribers need to be familiar (Dimond, 2005).

The Medicines Act 1968 and European Community Council Directives and Regulations together provide the regulatory framework for medicines. The primary purpose of the legislation is to safeguard public health by controlling the production and distribution of medicinal products. We shall be focusing on the legislative framework solely in relation to medicines for human use.

Towards Prescribing Practice. Edited by J. McKinnon.
© 2007 John Wiley & Sons, Ltd.

LICENSING OF MEDICINES

Prior to any medicinal product becoming available on the market, a marketing authorisation, formerly known as a product licence, must have been granted. This is a licence that is granted based on the safety, quality and efficacy of the medicinal product. The labelling of the medicine, however, is covered within the legislation along with requirements for good manufacturing practice. The process for obtaining a marketing authorisation for a medicine for human use comprises both a centralised system and a national system (Appelbe and Wingfield, 2005). The centralised system is administered by the European Medicines Agency and is used for new active substances and certain high-technology and biotechnology products. Other products are handled within the national system, which involves the Medicines and Healthcare Products Regulatory Agency (MHRA). Marketing authorisations may be recognised by other European member states.

Any application for a marketing authorisation must be accompanied by certain information, some of which is contained within a Summary of Product Characteristics (SPC). Each year a Medicines Compendium is produced by the Association of the British Pharmaceutical Industry (ABPI) listing the SPCs in current use, these are also available at www.medicines.org.uk. An SPC is a very informative document, one that contains useful information for the prescriber. This then leads us to an understanding of the term 'prescribing unlicensed medicines'; that is, products that do not have a marketing authorisation.

UNLICENSED MEDICINES

The prescribing of unlicensed medications is restricted with regard to non-medical prescribers. This will be covered later in the chapter. Children are one patient group where it may be necessary to use a drug outside the limits of its licence. The *BNF for Children* (British Medical Association et al., 2005) states that a drug or formulation that is not included within a marketing authorisation can be supplied against a prescription. Often the unlicensed medicine has to be specially obtained direct from a pharmaceutical company, imported by a specialist importer, manufactured by a specialist manufacturing unit – either hospital or commercially based – or prepared extemporaneously. If unlicensed medicines are prescribed, then they should be used with great care as limited information is available on their use. The *BNF for Children* provides supportive information to prescribers, many medicines being included with their unlicensed dosages.

CLASSIFICATION OF MEDICINES

The Medicines Act 1968 also covers the registration of retail pharmacies to ensure that certain medicines may only be supplied to the public from retail pharmacies under the supervision of a pharmacist. Some medicines, however, can be sold with relative safety from retail premises other than a pharmacy, without the supervision of the pharmacist. This leads us to consider the classification of medicines within the Medicines Act 1968.

A clear knowledge and understanding of the classification of medicines is necessary in order that the prescriber can signpost and inform the patient as appropriate. There are three classes of medicinal product under the Medicines Act 1968: general sales list (GSL) medicines, pharmacy (P) medicines and prescription-only medicines (POMs). The legal classification of a product is contained within the product's SPC. The classification in practice is an indication of the availability of a medicinal product and to some extent an indication of the product's safety. More information on the classification of medicines can be found in *Medicines, Ethics and Practice: A Guide for Pharmacists*, published annually by the Royal Pharmaceutical Society of Great Britain.

GENERAL SALES LIST MEDICINES

General sales list (GSL) medicines are those that have been granted a marketing authorisation as a GSL medicine or are listed in the General Sales List Order and can be sold from retail premises other than a pharmacy. In reality, this means that sales of GSLs are seen from various locations such as petrol stations and supermarkets. A good example of a GSL medicine is paracetamol 500mg tablets in a pack size of 16 for the treatment only of adults. Another example is Nicorette patches, an aid to stopping smoking.

PRESCRIPTION-ONLY MEDICINES

Prescription-only medicines (POMs) are those that can only be sold or supplied from pharmacies in accordance with a prescription provided by an 'appropriate' practitioner and are specified in the Prescription-Only Medicines Order or are classified as a POM within the product's marketing authorisation. An example of a POM is a pack of 100 paracetamol 500mg tablets. Another example is the antibiotic amoxicillin.

To clarify this further, let us consider how the definition of the term 'appropriate practitioner' has developed to today's understanding. The legal definition of an appropriate practitioner has developed dramatically over the last few years, initially with the Medicines Act 1968 classifying doctors, dentists and veterinary practitioners as appropriate practitioners, and then with the Medicinal Products: Prescription by Nurses, etc. Act 1992 classifying certain registered nurses, midwives and health visitors complying with certain conditions as appropriate practitioners. The definition of an appropriate practitioner was added to yet again by the Health and Social Care Act 2001, which introduced the concept of a supplementary prescriber. From April 2003 amendments to the Prescription-Only Medicines Order and NHS regulations allowed supplementary prescribing by suitably trained nurses and pharmacists. The prescribing rights of supplementary prescribers have since been extended to include first-level nurses, pharmacists, registered midwives, chiropodists/podiatrists, physiotherapists and radiographers (Department of Health, 2005).

The latest legislative change, The Medicines and Human Use (Prescribing) (Miscellaneous Amendments) Order SI 2006/915, addresses independent prescribing by pharmacists and nurses for those professionals who have successfully completed an independent prescribing course and are registered as such with their respective professional bodies (Department of Health, 2006d). We address this in more detail later in the chapter when we consider what can actually be prescribed on an NHS prescription.

Hence for members of the general public to obtain a prescription-only medicine, they need to have a prescription from an appropriate practitioner before they can be supplied by a pharmacy or dispensing general practice.

PHARMACY MEDICINES

The third classification of medicinal product is the pharmacy (P) medicine and this includes medicinal products that are not classified as either general sales list or prescription-only medicines. Pharmacy medicines can only be sold from registered retail pharmacy premises under the supervision of a pharmacist. An example of a P medicine is paracetamol 500mg in a 32 tablet pack size.

So what this complex legal classification of medicines means is that GSL and P medicines are available for sale from pharmacies under the supervision of a pharmacist, and GSL medicines are more readily available from other retail premises for sale to the public for self-care. It is perhaps reasonable to think of GSL medications as very safe medicines and appropriate for self-selection. This view could be challenged, nevertheless. With P medicines safety is somewhat more of a concern and hence the input of a pharmacist is appropriate. POMs are subject to tighter control and need a prescriber to write a prescription prior to supply. Prescribers can, however, prescribe the majority of GSL and P medicines, which is covered in more detail later.

Understanding this legal classification of medicines allows a prescriber to direct a patient to purchase P and GSL medicines rather than providing a prescription. This may be useful if the patient is not exempt from NHS prescription charges. Perhaps more importantly, the prescriber needs to be fully aware of the medicines available for purchase and the potentially very dangerous interactions with prescribed medicines. There is also the potential for symptoms to be masked by the inappropriate use of over-the-counter medicines. Hence during the consultation the prescriber must identify all other medicines being administered and other medications that the patient has tried prior to the consultation.

CONTROLLED DRUGS

We have considered the legal classification of medicines and the need to legislate in order to ensure public safety. This brings us on to the second very important piece of legislation, the Misuse of Drugs Act 1971, which aims to prevent the misuse of controlled drugs by placing controls on substances that are 'dangerous or otherwise harmful drugs' (Royal Pharmaceutical Society of Great Britain, 2005) relating to their export, import, possession, manufacture and supply. The Misuse of Drugs Act 1971 divides controlled drugs into three classes, A, B and C, based on decreasing order of harmfulness. The classes are used solely to indicate the penalty on conviction for an offence. The Misuse of Drugs Regulations 1985 lists controlled drugs in schedules, 1 to 5, indicating abuse potential/therapeutic value according to different levels of control. It is the Misuse of Drugs Regulations 2001 that covers the use of controlled drugs in medicine. We shall consider the different schedules of controlled drugs and also further into the chapter we shall address the additional requirements when writing a prescription for a controlled drug.

SCHEDULE 1 (CD LIC)

The drugs listed in schedule 1 have no medicinal use, and include such items as LSD and ecstasy.

SCHEDULE 2 (CD POM)

The drugs listed in schedule 2 include more than 100 substances, mainly opiates, such as diamorphine, methadone etc.

SCHEDULE 3 (CD NO REGISTER)

This schedule contains most of the barbiturates such as phenobarbitone, and also includes temazepam, buprenorphine etc.

SCHEDULE 4

The drugs in this schedule are split into two parts. Part I (CD Benz) contains most of the benzodiazepines such as diazepam, and Part II (CD Anab) contains most of the anabolic and androgenic steroids, along with clenbuterol and some growth hormones.

SCHEDULE 5 (CD INV)

This schedule contains preparations of certain controlled drugs. Examples here include codeine and pholcodine. There are no restrictions on the prescribing of these controlled drugs.

Later in the chapter we shall consider the issues regarding writing a prescription for a controlled drug and who can do this legally.

ROLE OF THE MHRA

While we have already mentioned the Medicines and Healthcare Products Regulatory Agency (MHRA) with regard to its role in issuing marketing authorisations for medicinal products, its regulatory role is much broader.

The MHRA is the government agency that has the responsibility for ensuring the safety and efficacy of medical devices and medicines. We have already discussed how medicines are issued with a marketing authorisation following direct approval by the MHRA itself. However, medical devices are handled slightly differently, with the MHRA having a responsibility to audit the performance of 'notified bodies', which are private organisations that can approve medical devices. Once on the market, both medicines and medical devices are handled similarly. The MHRA also licenses manufacturers and distributors directly.

Within its responsibility of ensuring the safety of medicines the MHRA administers the Adverse Drug Reaction Scheme, which is also known as the yellow card reporting scheme (British Medical Association and the Royal Pharmaceutical Society of Great Britain, 2006). Any drug has the potential to cause unwanted adverse reactions and this scheme enables these unwanted effects to be monitored and addressed. All prescribers have a responsibility to report suspected adverse reaction, either online via the MHRA website or via the yellow cards that can be found at the back of the *BNF*.

Medicines that are being intensively monitored because they are either new on the market or have recently been licensed for new indications are annotated with a black triangle (▼) and all suspected reactions to these 'black triangle drugs' should be reported. However, for established drugs and herbal remedies, all serious reactions in adults and all serious and minor adverse reactions in children under 18 years of age should be reported.

The *BNF*, produced in March and again in September each year, provides important information to prescribers on the prevention of adverse reactions. Ways to prevent adverse reactions are stated as:

- Use a drug only where there is a good indication for its use; if the patient is pregnant then only use the drug where it is absolutely necessary.
- Always establish whether the patient has had previous allergic or idiosyncratic reactions to the drug.
- Always establish whether the patient is taking other drugs, including purchased medicines and complementary medicines, to prevent drug interactions.
- Address age and genetic issues, along with hepatic and/or renal disease, where these may alter the metabolism or excretion of drugs.
- Always prescribe as few drugs as possible and ensure the patient understands the dosage instructions.
- Always prescribe drugs that you are familiar with and be aware of adverse drug reactions when prescribing new drugs.
- Alert the patient to any potential adverse reactions associated with the use of the drug.

Any concern regarding actual or suspected defects in medicinal products for human use must be reported to the Defective Medicines Report Centre at the MHRA. An example where this pathway should be used is where medicines are suspected of being counterfeit. The structure is in place at the MHRA to alert health professionals and recall the product where the defect is considered to be a risk to public health.

WRITING AN NHS PRESCRIPTION

There are a number of issues to consider when writing a prescription, many of which are related to the capacity in which you are prescribing, for example as supplementary prescriber, independent nurse prescriber or GP. We shall only consider here prescriptions for human use and the focus will be on NHS prescriptions.

THE NHS PRESCRIPTION FORM

It is imperative that the prescription pad that is being used is the appropriate one for the prescriber who is taking responsibility for the prescription. This ensures that the NHS pays for the medicines dispensed in primary care by community pharmacies or dispensing practices. The prescription forms are obtained from the primary care trust. The different prescription types available are shown in Table 8.1, and examples of some of the prescription forms, 0406 versions, are included in Figures 8.1–8.5 for information.

WHAT CAN BE PRESCRIBED?

There is no straightforward answer to this question. What can be prescribed depends once again on the type of prescriber signing the prescription.

General Practitioner Prescribing

Let us consider what a general practitioner can prescribe currently, working to the General Medical Services Contract that was introduced in April 2004 (Department of Health, 2006a). The contract states that:

'a prescriber shall order any drugs, medicines, or appliances which are needed for the treatment of any patient.'

So in theory a GP can order any medication. There is, however, a list of medicines that are not allowed to be prescribed. This list forms Schedule 1 to the NHS (General Medical Services Contract) (Prescription of Drugs etc.) Regulations 2004. These drugs are known as 'scheduled drugs' or the 'black list', as this was the term utilised when it was first introduced in 1985. An up-to-date list of scheduled drugs can be found in the current Drug Tariff in Part XVIIIA (see later in the chapter).

Table 8.1 Different prescription types available

Prescription pad	Used by	Colour	Used for
FP10NC – example included in Figure 8.1	GPs	Green	Usual prescription used for handwritten prescriptions.
FP10SS – example included in Figure 8.2	GPs, hospital-based prescribers, nurses, supplementary prescribers	Green	As for FP10NC but for use with computer system, hence computer- printed prescription.
FP10MDA-SS – example included in Figure 8.3	GPs, hospital-based prescribers, nurses, supplementary prescribers	Blue	A drug misuse instalment prescription. Used for computer-printed prescriptions for controlled drugs – normally methadone. A4 width, normal length. Allows for instalment dispensing.
FP10MDA-S	GPs	Blue	Drug misuse instalment prescription. A4 width, normal length. Used for handwritten prescribing to addicts (usually methadone) and for dispensing by pharmacists in instalments.
FP10HNC	Hospital-based prescribers	Green	For handwritten prescriptions.
FP10HMDA-S	Hospital-based prescribers	Blue	A drug misuse instalment prescription. A4 width, normal length.
FP10D – example included in Figure 8.4	Dentists	Yellow	Yellow prescription used only for dentists.
FP10P – example included in Figure 8.5	Nurses, supplementary prescribers	Lilac	Contains information printed on the prescription form indicating the type of prescriber, e.g. 'Community Practitioner Nurse Prescriber'.
FP10P-Rec	GPs, nurses	Lilac	A prescription receipt form. Used in out-of-hours centres, and in other units not using FP10 prescribing.
FP10MDA-SP	Supplementary prescribers	Blue	A drug misuse instalment prescription, for 'occasional use'. A4 width, normal length. For handwritten controlled drug instalment prescriptions.

'SS' denotes a prescription that is not pre-printed with the prescriber details and address and allows for the prescribers' computer systems to print these details. 'S' denotes a pre-printed prescription where the prescriber details, address etc. are printed by the prescription manufacturer and allows for these prescriptions to be handwritten.

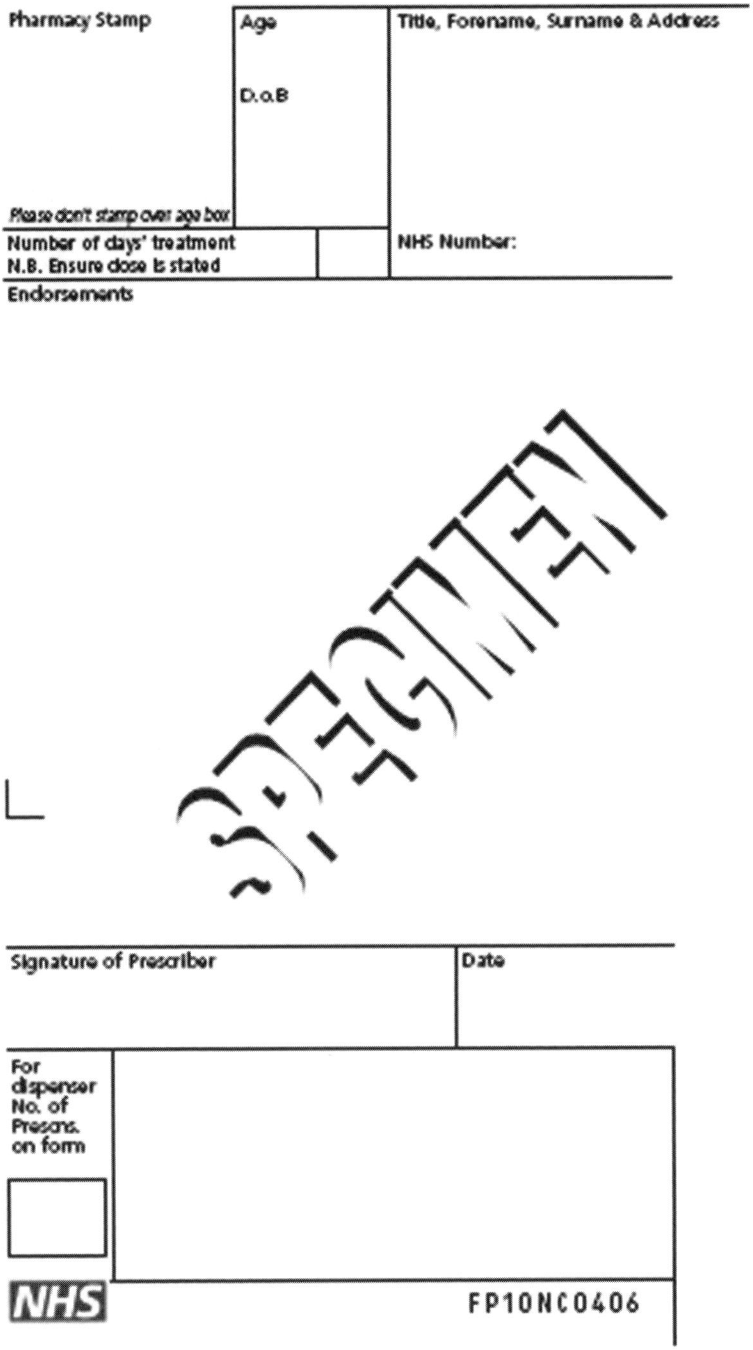

Figure 8.1   Front page of FP10NC

Figures 8.1–8.7 are Crown Copyright material which is reproduced with the permission of the Controller of HMSO and the Queen's Printer for Scotland.

FP10NC0406

| **NOTE** | Patients who don't have to pay must fill in parts 1 and 3 (unless they are exempt on age grounds, and their age is printed on the front of this prescription). Those who pay must fill in parts 2 and 3. Penalty charges may be applied if you make a wrongful claim for free prescriptions. If you're unsure about whether you are entitled to free prescriptions, pay and ask for an FP57 form. You cannot get one later. The FP57 tells you about getting a refund. |

| **Part 1** | The patient doesn't have to pay because he/she: |

			Collectors of Schedule 2 & 3 CDs should sign their name:
A	☐	is under 16 years of age	
B	☐	is 16, 17 or 18 **and** in full-time education	
C	☐	is 60 years of age or over	
D	☐	has a valid maternity exemption certificate	
E	☐	has a valid medical exemption certificate	
F	☐	has a valid prescription pre-payment certificate	*Pharmacy use only*
G	☐	has a valid War Pension exemption certificate	*Evidence not seen*
L	☐	is named on a current HC2 charges certificate	
X	☐	was prescribed free-of-charge contraceptives	
H	☐	*gets Income Support (IS)	
K	☐	*gets **income based** Jobseeker's Allowance (JSA (IB))	
M	☐	*is entitled to, or named on, a valid NHS Tax Credit Exemption Certificate	
S	☐	*has a partner who gets Pension Credit **guarantee** credit (PCGC)	

| *Name: | Date of Birth: | NI no: |

*__Print__ the name of the person (either you or your partner) who gets IS, JSA (IB), PCGC or Tax Credit.

| **Declaration** *For patients who do not have to pay* | I declare that the information I have given on this form is correct and complete. I understand that if it is not, appropriate action may be taken. I confirm proper entitlement to exemption. To enable the NHS to check I have a valid exemption and to prevent and detect fraud and incorrectness, I consent to the disclosure of relevant information from this form to and by the NHS Business Services Authority, the NHS Counter Fraud and Security Management Service, the Department for Work and Pensions and Local Authorities. Now sign and fill in Part 3 |

| **Part 2** | I have paid £ | Now sign and fill in Part 3 |

| **Part 3** | *Cross ONE box* I am the patient ☐ | patient's representative ☐ |

Sign here ✎		Date / /
Print name and address*		
		Postcode

*If different from overleaf

Figure 8.1   Reverse of FP10NC

FP10SS0406

Do you need to pay prescription charges? Read all the statements in Part 1 opposite. You don't have to pay a prescription charge if one (or more) of the exemptions applies to you (the patient) on the day you are asked to pay. Put a cross in the first Part 1 box that applies to you, read the declaration and complete and sign Part 3.

Pension Credit guarantee credit (PCGC) replaced Minimum Income Guarantee (MIG) in October 2003. If you get PCGC tick "aged 60 or over" – line C. If you (the patient) are a partner aged under 60 of someone getting PCGC tick "S – has a partner who gets Pension Credit guarantee credit". Pension Credit savings credit on its own does not entitle you to help.

Proof. Show the person dispensing your prescription valid proof of why you don't have to pay, such as a benefit book, exemption or pre-payment certificate. If you cannot show proof, you can still get your medicine free. But the NHS Counter Fraud and Security Management Service (NHS CFSMS) are more likely to check your entitlement later if you do not show proof.

Paying Prescription charges? You (or your representative) should put in Part 2 the amount you have paid and then sign and complete Part 3.

Want help with prescription charges? You can get information by ringing 0845 850 1166 or by reading leaflet HC11. You may be able to get an HC11 from your surgery or pharmacy. Or, ring 08701 555 455 to get one. Or go to www.dh.gov.uk and enter "HC11" in the search facility.

Not entitled to free prescriptions? Pre-pay. You may find it cheaper to buy a pre-payment certificate (PPC) if you think you will have to get more than 5 items in 4 months or 14 items in 12 months. Phone 0845 850 0030 to find out the cost, or order a PPC and pay by credit or debit card. Buy on-line at www.ppa.org.uk. By cheque – get an application form (FP95) from your pharmacy or go to www.dh.gov.uk and enter "Prepayment" in the search facility – the FP95 tells you what to do.

Unsure whether you should pay? You should pay for this prescription and ask for a receipt form FP57. **You must get a receipt when you pay the charge, you cannot get one later.** If you find you didn't have to pay, you can claim your money back up to 3 months after paying. The FP57 tells you what to do.

Information about the medicine or other items on this form will be processed centrally to pay monies due to the pharmacist, doctor or appliance contractor for items they have supplied to you. The NHS will also use this information to analyse what has been prescribed and the cost. The NHS CFSMS may use information from this form to prevent and detect fraud and incorrectness in the NHS.

Penalty Charges. If you are found to have made a wrongful claim for free prescriptions, you will face penalty charges and may be prosecuted under powers introduced by the Health Act 1999. Routine checks are carried out on exemption claims including some where proof may have been shown. You may be contacted in the course of such checks.

NOTE Patients who don't have to pay must fill in parts 1 and 3 (unless they are exempt on age grounds, and their age is printed on the front of this prescription). Those who pay must fill in parts 2 and 3. Penalty charges may be applied if you make a wrongful claim for free prescriptions. If you're unsure about whether you are entitled to free prescriptions, pay and ask for an FP57 form. You cannot get one later. The FP57 tells you about getting a refund.

Part 1 The patient doesn't have to pay because he/she:

A is under 16 years of age
B is 16, 17 or 18 and in full-time education
C is 60 years of age or over
D has a valid maternity exemption certificate
E has a valid medical exemption certificate
F has a valid prescription pre-payment certificate
G has a valid War Pension exemption certificate
L is named on a current HC2 charges certificate
X was prescribed free-of-charge contraceptives
H *gets Income Support (IS)
K *gets Income based Jobseeker's Allowance (JSA (IB))
M *is entitled to, or named on, a valid NHS Tax Credit Exemption Certificate
S *has a partner who gets Pension Credit guarantee credit (PCGC)

Collectors of Schedule 2 & 3 CDs should sign their name:

Pharmacy use only / Evidence not seen

*Name: _____ Date of Birth: __/__/__

*Print the name of the person (either you or your partner) who gets IS, JSA (IB), PCGC or Tax Credit.

Declaration (For patients who do not have to pay) I declare that the information I have given on this form is correct and complete. I understand that if it is not, appropriate action may be taken. I confirm proper entitlement to exemption. To enable the NHS to check I have a valid exemption and to prevent and detect fraud and incorrectness, I consent to the disclosure of relevant information from this form to and by the NHS Business Services Authority, the NHS Counter Fraud and Security Management Service, the Department for Work and Pensions and Local Authorities. Now sign and fill in Part 3.

Part 2 I have paid £ _____

Part 3 Cross one box [ ] I am the patient [ ] patient's representative†

Sign here: _____ Now sign and fill in Part 3
Print name and address* _____ Date __/__/__
Postcode _____

†If different from overleaf

Figure 8.2 Reverse of FP10SS

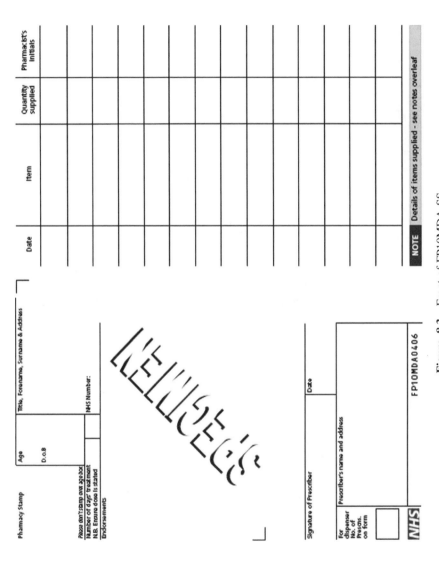

Figure 8.3 Front of FP10MDA-SS

FP10MDA0406

NOTES For patients

1 Free of charge prescriptions. You should put a cross in the first box in **Part 1** that applies to you, read the declaration and complete and sign **Part 3**. Show the pharmacist proof of why you don't have to pay, such as a benefit book, exemption or pre-payment certificate. The proof must be valid on the day you claim exemption from prescription charges.

2 If you pay for your prescriptions, you only pay for your first instalment. You should put in **Part 2** the amount you have paid and then sign and complete **Part 3**.

3 Information about the medicine or other items on this form will be processed centrally to pay monies due to the person who dispensed your prescription. The NHS will also use this information to analyse what has been prescribed and the cost. The NHS Counter Fraud and Security Management Service (NHS CFSMS) may use information from this form to prevent and detect fraud and incorrectness in the NHS.

Penalty charges. If you are found to have made a wrongful claim for free prescriptions, you will face penalty charges and may be prosecuted under powers introduced by the Health Act 1999.

NOTES For prescribers and pharmacists

4 This form can only be used when a prescriber wants to arrange for the instalment dispensing of the drugs diazepam, buprenorphine or any controlled drug listed in Schedule 2 of the Misuse of Drugs Regulations 2001 (as amended). In a hospital the form can only be used for the treatment of outpatients. When used as part of the management of drug dependence, prescribing of diamorphine, cocaine and dipipanone requires a licence from the Home Office.

5 The prescription must be written as required by the Misuse of Drugs Regulations 2001. Computer generated prescriptions are only permitted where the prescriber has a hand writing exemption from the Home Office.

6 This form can also be used for items such as diluents which are related to the drug dependence. This form should not be used for prescribing for other conditions or when prescriptions do not need to be dispensed in instalments.

7 The total quantity prescribed must not exceed the amount sufficient for 14 days consecutive treatment. Please delete unused spaces. The prescriber should take into account weekends and Bank holidays so that 14 days prescribing may be dispensed over a shorter period taking account of Bank holidays and weekends.

8 The pharmacist should record overleaf each separate dispensing which should only be made on the day specified by the prescriber, during the pharmacist's normal opening hours or at such times as agreed by the pharmacist.

NOTE
Patients who don't have to pay must fill in parts 1 and 3 (unless they are exempt on age grounds, and their age is printed on the front of this prescription). Those who pay must fill in parts 2 and 3. Penalty charges may be applied if you make a wrongful claim for free prescription. If you're unsure about whether you are entitled to free prescription, pay and ask for an FP57 form. You cannot get one later. The FP57 tells you about getting a refund.

Part 1 The patient doesn't have to pay because he/she:

Collectors of Schedule 2 & 3 CDs should sign their name

Pharmacy use only
Evidence not seen

A	is under 16 years of age
B	is 16, 17 or 18 **and** in full-time education
C	is 60 years of age or over
D	has a valid maternity exemption certificate
E	has a valid medical exemption certificate
F	has a valid prescription pre-payment certificate
G	has a valid War Pension exemption certificate
L	is named on a current HC2 charges certificate
X	was prescribed free-of-charge contraceptives
H	*gets Income Support (IS)
K	*gets **income based** Jobseeker's Allowance (JSA (IB))
M	*is entitled to, or named on, a valid NHS Tax Credit Exemption Certificate
S	*has a partner who gets Pension Credit **guarantee** credit (PCGC)

* Name: _____ Date of Birth: _____ NI no: _____

* **Print** the name of the person (either you or your partner) who gets IS, JSA (IB), PCGC or Tax Credit.

Declaration
For patients who do not have to pay

I declare that the information I have given on this form is correct and complete. I understand that if it is not, appropriate action may be taken. I confirm proper entitlement to exemption. To enable the NHS to check I have a valid exemption and to prevent and detect fraud and incorrectness, I consent to the disclosure of relevant information from this form to and by the NHS Business Services Authority, the NHS Counter Fraud and Security Management Service, the Department for Work and Pensions and Local Authorities. Now sign and fill in Part 3

Part 2	I have paid £

Part 3
Cross ONE box I am the patient ☐ patient's representative ☐

Sign here ✍ _____

Print name and address* _____ Date / /

Postcode _____

*if different from overleaf

Figure 8.3 Reverse of FP10MDA-SS

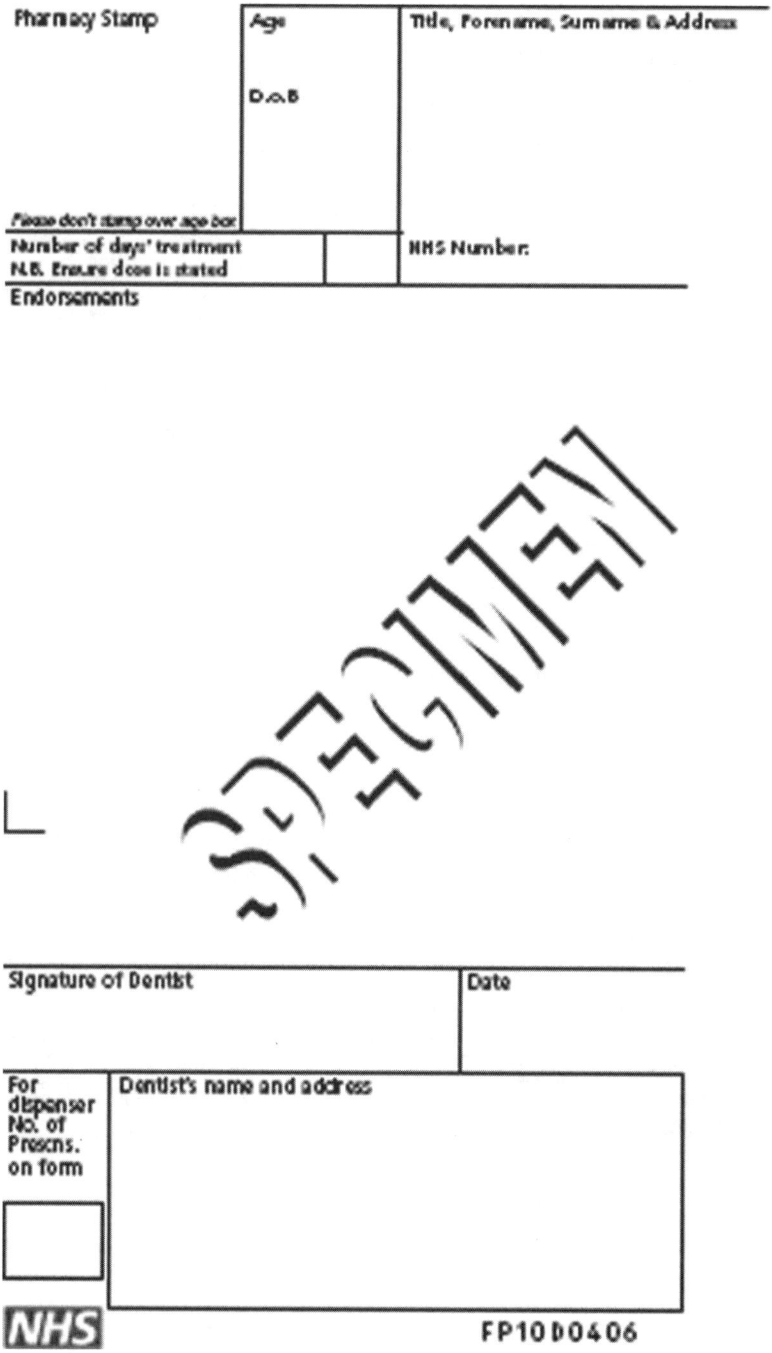
Pharmacy Stamp

Age

D.o.B

Title, Forename, Surname & Address

Please don't stamp over age box

Number of days' treatment
N.B. Ensure dose is stated

NHS Number:

Endorsements

SPECIMEN

Signature of Dentist

Date

For dispenser
No. of
Prescns.
on form

Dentist's name and address

NHS

FP10D0406

Figure 8.4 Front of FP10D

FP10D0406

| NOTE | Patients who don't have to pay must fill in parts 1 and 3 (unless they are exempt on age grounds, and their age is printed on the front of this prescription). Those who pay must fill in parts 2 and 3. Penalty charges may be applied if you make a wrongful claim for free prescriptions. If you're unsure about whether you are entitled to free prescriptions, pay and ask for an FP57 form. You cannot get one later. The FP57 tells you about getting a refund. |

Part 1 — The patient doesn't have to pay because he/she:

Collectors of Schedule 2 & 3 CDs should sign their name:

A ☐ is under 16 years of age

B ☐ is 16, 17 or 18 **and** in full-time education

C ☐ is 60 years of age or over

D ☐ has a valid maternity exemption certificate

E ☐ has a valid medical exemption certificate

F ☐ has a valid prescription pre-payment certificate

G ☐ has a valid War Pension exemption certificate

L ☐ is named on a current HC2 charges certificate

X ☐ was prescribed free-of-charge contraceptives

H ☐ *gets Income Support (IS)

K ☐ *gets **income based** Jobseeker's Allowance (JSA (IB))

M ☐ *is entitled to, or named on, a valid NHS Tax Credit Exemption Certificate

S ☐ *has a partner who gets Pension Credit **guarantee** credit (PCGC)

| *Name: | Date of Birth: | NI no: |

***Print** the name of the person (either you or your partner) who gets IS, JSA (IB), PCGC or Tax Credit.*

Declaration
For patients
who do not
have to pay

I declare that the information I have given on this form is correct and complete. I understand that if it is not, appropriate action may be taken. I confirm proper entitlement to exemption. To enable the NHS to check I have a valid exemption and to prevent and detect fraud and incorrectness, I consent to the disclosure of relevant information from this form to and by the NHS Business Services Authority, the NHS Counter Fraud and Security Management Service, the Department for Work and Pensions and Local Authorities. Now sign and fill in Part 3

Part 2 — I have paid £   Now sign and fill in Part 3

Part 3 — Cross ONE box I am the patient ☐   patient's representative ☐

Sign here ✍		Date / /
Print name and address*		
		Postcode

*If different from overleaf

Figure 8.4   Reverse of FP10D

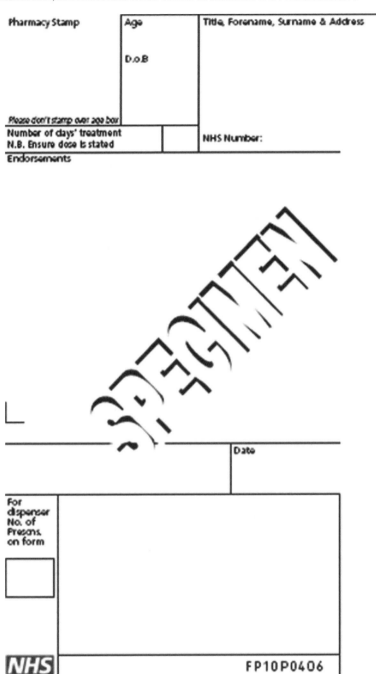

Figure 8.5   Front of FP10P

FP10P0406

NOTE	Patients who don't have to pay must fill in parts 1 and 3 (unless they are exempt on age grounds, and their age is printed on the front of this prescription). Those who pay must fill in parts 2 and 3. Penalty charges may be applied if you make a wrongful claim for free prescriptions. If you're unsure about whether you are entitled to free prescriptions, pay and ask for an FP57 form. You cannot get one later. The FP57 tells you about getting a refund.

Part 1	The patient doesn't have to pay because he/she:

A	☐	is under 16 years of age
B	☐	is 16, 17 or 18 **and** in full-time education
C	☐	is 60 years of age or over
D	☐	has a valid maternity exemption certificate
E	☐	has a valid medical exemption certificate
F	☐	has a valid prescription pre-payment certificate
G	☐	has a valid War Pension exemption certificate
L	☐	is named on a current HC2 charges certificate
X	☐	was prescribed free-of-charge contraceptives
H	☐	*gets Income Support (IS)
K	☐	*gets **income based** Jobseeker's Allowance (JSA (IB))
M	☐	*is entitled to, or named on, a valid NHS Tax Credit Exemption Certificate
S	☐	*has a partner who gets Pension Credit **guarantee** credit (PCGC)

Collectors of Schedule 2 & 3 CDs should sign their name:

Pharmacy use only Evidence not seen

* Name:	Date of Birth:	NI no:

***Print** the name of the person (either you or your partner) who gets IS, JSA (IB), PCGC or Tax Credit.*

Declaration For patients who do not have to pay	I declare that the information I have given on this form is correct and complete. I understand that if it is not, appropriate action may be taken. I confirm proper entitlement to exemption. To enable the NHS to check I have a valid exemption and to prevent and detect fraud and incorrectness, I consent to the disclosure of relevant information from this form to and by the NHS Business Services Authority, the NHS Counter Fraud and Security Management Service, the Department for Work and Pensions and Local Authorities. **Now sign and fill in Part 3**

Part 2	I have paid £	Now sign and fill in Part 3

Part 3	Cross ONE box I am the patient ☐	patient's representative ☐
Sign here ✍		Date / /
Print name and address*		
		Postcode

If different from overleaf

Figure 8.5 Reverse of FP10P

There is another group of medicines where restrictions apply to their prescribing. These medicines are listed in Schedule 2 to the NHS (General Medical Services Contract) (Prescription of Drugs etc.) Regulations 2004. This schedule specifies patient groups who are eligible to receive certain drugs for certain conditions only. This list can also be found in the current Drug Tariff in Part XVIIIB. If one of these medicines is prescribed the prescriber must endorse the prescription with the reference 'SLS'.

The situation is complicated further when we consider the prescribing of appliances by a GP. In this situation only appliances that are included in the current Drug Tariff Part IX can be prescribed.

Part XV of the Drug Tariff includes a list of items that are termed 'borderline substances', that is, items where it is not clear whether it is a medicine or a toiletry, or in some instances a medicine or a food. The list includes all items that have been approved for GP prescribing but the prescription should be endorsed 'ACBS'.

General practitioners are able to write prescriptions for controlled drugs, but must comply with the additional requirements for writing a controlled drug prescription explained below.

Dental Practitioner Prescribing

There is a restricted list of medicines termed the *Dental Practitioner's Formulary* that comprises the only items that a dentist can prescribe on the NHS. This list can be found in Part XVIIA of the Drug Tariff and does contain some controlled drugs. A dental practitioner is legally able to prescribe all prescription-only medicines, including controlled drugs, but prescribing outside the *Dental Practitioner's Formulary* would have to be carried out on a private prescription.

Nurse Prescribing

This area of prescribing has been the focus of much interest and development over the last few years. Legislative changes took place in May 2006 that enable us to consider this area in two parts: community practitioner nurse prescribing and independent nurse prescribing.

Community Practitioner Nurse Prescribing

This group of prescribers consists of registered nurses or registered midwives who have completed the necessary training and subsequent to this have been registered with the Nursing and Midwifery Council as being able to prescribe from the *Nurse Prescribers' Formulary*. These nurse prescribers were formerly district nurses and health visitors, however the legislation changed on 1 May 2006 with Statutory Instrument 2006 No. 915 The Medicines for Human Use (Prescribing) (Miscellaneous Amendments) Order 2006.

Community practitioner nurse prescribers can prescribe only those items appearing within the *Nurse Prescribers' Formulary for Community Practitioners* in the current edition Drug Tariff Part XVIIB(i). This does not allow the prescribing of controlled drugs.

Independent Nurse Prescribing

This is a new category of nurse prescriber introduced in the legislation on 1 May 2006 and replaces the previous term of Extended Formulary nurse prescriber. Along with this change in legislation came the abolition of the *Extended Nurse Formulary*, a list of medications from which the Extended Formulary nurse prescriber could prescribe. Instead, we now have the independent nurse prescriber, defined in the legislation as a person who is a registered nurse or a registered midwife who has completed the necessary training and has registered with the Nursing and Midwifery Council as being able to prescribe drugs, medicines and appliances as an independent nurse prescriber. Let us clarify this further: an independent nurse prescriber is able to prescribe any *licensed* medicine for any medical condition within their competence, including certain controlled drugs for specified conditions, as shown in Table 8.2.

Table 8.2 Controlled Drugs that can be prescribed by Independent Nurse Prescribers along with the corresponding conditions for which they can be prescribed

Controlled drug	Route of administration	Specified condition
Buprenorphine	Transdermal	Palliative care
Chlordiazepoxide hydrochloride	Oral	Symptomatic treatment of withdrawal of alcohol
Codeine phosphate	Oral	
Co-phenotrope	Oral	
Diamorphine hydrochloride	Oral or parenteral	Palliative care, pain relief in suspected myocardial infarction or following trauma, including post-operative
Diazepam	Oral, parenteral or rectal	Palliative care, tonic–clonic seizures, symptomatic treatment of withdrawal of alcohol
Dihydrocodeine tartrate	Oral	
Fentanyl	Transdermal	Palliative care
Lorazepam	Oral or parenteral	Palliative care, tonic–clonic seizures
Midazolam	Parenteral or buccal	Palliative care, tonic–clonic seizures
Morphine sulphate	Oral, parenteral or rectal	Palliative care, pain relief in suspected myocardial infarction or following trauma, including post-operative
Morphine hydrochloride	Rectal	Palliative care, pain relief in suspected myocardial infarction or following trauma, including post-operative
Oxycodone hydrochloride	Oral or parenteral	Palliative care

It is important for the independent nurse prescriber to be aware of the additional requirements necessary when prescribing a controlled drug, and these are addressed in detail later in the chapter.

Independent Pharmacist Prescribing

The legislation that introduced the term independent nurse prescriber also enables independent prescribing by pharmacists. They are able to prescribe all medicines, as for independent nurse prescribers, the only exception being controlled drugs. Currently there is no legislation enabling the prescribing of controlled drugs by independent pharmacist prescribers. An independent pharmacist prescriber is a registered pharmacist registered with the Royal Pharmaceutical Society of Great Britain (RPSGB) as having successfully completed a training programme accredited by the Society, thus qualifying them as an independent prescriber.

Supplementary Prescribers

As mentioned previously, supplementary prescribers can be first-level nurses, pharmacists, registered midwives, chiropodist/podiatrists, physiotherapists or radiographers.

Nurse and pharmacist supplementary prescribers can prescribe any medicine, including controlled drugs and unlicensed medicines, that is included in a clinical management plan that has been agreed by the independent prescriber, which must be either a doctor or dentist, the supplementary prescriber and the patient.

'Allied health professionals' (AHPs) is the term that refers to chiropodists/podiatrists, physiotherapists and radiographers. AHPs are able to prescribe all medicines, including unlicensed medicines, that are included in a clinical management plan that has been agreed by the independent prescriber, who must be either a doctor or dentist, the supplementary prescriber and the patient. There is, however, no legislation in place that allows the prescribing of controlled drugs.

For each of the professionals mentioned above, when becoming a supplementary prescriber, the requirements are that an approved training course is completed and following this the individual professional is registered with their respective professional body as having successfully completed the approved course for supplementary prescribing.

WRITING THE NHS PRESCRIPTION

Clear instructions on prescription writing can be found in the current edition of the *BNF*. This is also covered within the web-based training package 'Prescribers and FP10 prescriptions', produced by the NHS Business Services Authority (NHSBSA). In this section we will address the legal requirements and refer you to other resources for more detailed information.

The legal requirements for prescriptions for prescription-only medicines are as follows and are covered by The Medicines for Human Use (Prescribing) Order 2005, Statutory Instrument number 765.

A prescription:

1. Shall be signed in ink with his own name by the appropriate practitioner giving it.
2. Shall be written in ink or be indelible, unless it is a health prescription which is not for a controlled drug in schedules 1, 2 or 3, in which case it can be written by using carbon paper.
3. Shall contain the following:

   i. the date – this can be the date that the prescription is written if the prescriber is intending the prescription for immediate use. It can, however, be a date intended as the date before which it shall not be dispensed – hence providing a mechanism for post-dated prescriptions as used occasionally with antibiotics.
   ii. the address of the appropriate practitioner – this will be the address of the practice for a general practitioner. For a nurse or other appropriate practitioner employed by the primary care trust this will be the trust's address.
   iii. information whether the prescriber is a doctor, dentist, supplementary prescriber, a community practitioner nurse prescriber, or an independent nurse or pharmacist prescriber.
   iv. the name, address, age – if under twelve – of the person for whose treatment the prescription is written.

4. The prescription is valid for a period of 6 months from the date of the prescription. Prescriptions for controlled drugs in schedules 2 and 3 are valid for 13 weeks from the date of the prescription. Legislation is currently being changed for this to be 28 days.

Figure 8.6 provides an example of an NHS prescription correctly completed for the prescription-only medicine furosemide.

With the implementation of the Electronic Prescription Service (EPS), there are exemptions to requirements 1 and 2 stated above. EPS will allow the transfer of prescriptions from general practice to pharmacy in electronic format; hence hand-written signature requirements are not practically appropriate in this circumstance. Implementation of the EPS is currently expected during 2007. There are many other requirements in terms of good practice when writing a prescription. It is expected that the prescription is written legibly, for example, and the date of birth of the patient should be included. More importantly, in terms of reducing waste of medicines and the need for a multiprofessional approach to improving concordance, it is important to ensure the dosage instructions, along with dosage frequency, are clearly understood and agreed by the patient. The prescription should always include clear instructions, avoiding the use of 'to be taken when required' or 'to be taken as before'.

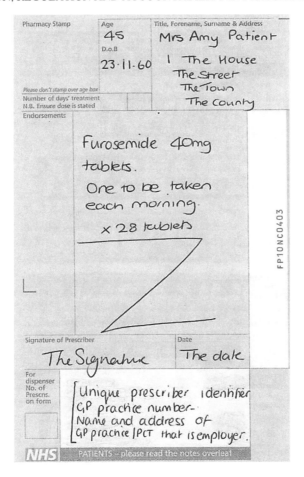

Figure 8.6 Correctly completed NHS prescription for furosemide

WRITING AN NHS PRESCRIPTION FOR A CONTROLLED DRUG

The requirements for writing a prescription for a prescription-only medicine apply here along with some additional requirements. These are:

1. The form and the strength of the preparation must be included.
2. The total quantity of the preparation should be written in words and figures; this can be written as the total number of dosage units.
3. The dose.
4. The words 'for dental treatment only' if issued by a dentist.

The additional requirements for writing a controlled drug prescription apply to schedule 2 and schedule 3 drugs with the one exception of temazepam.

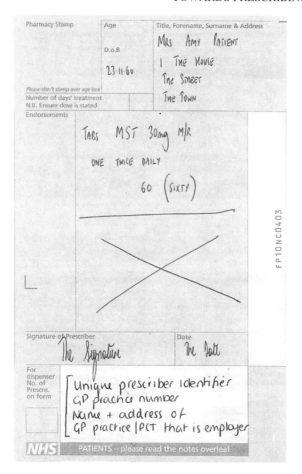

Figure 8.7   Correctly completed NHS prescription for MST

The additional requirements for writing a controlled drug prescription do not apply to schedule 4 and schedule 5 drugs. Figure 8.7 provides a correctly completed example of an NHS prescription for MST tablets.

THE DRUG TARIFF

In the above sections we have mentioned the Drug Tariff on a number of occasions. Let us now explain what the Drug Tariff is and why it is important that it is used correctly.

The Drug Tariff is produced *monthly* by the Pharmaceutical Directorate of the NHSBSA for the Secretary of State for Health. It is imperative that when using the Drug Tariff you use the up-to-date copy; using a copy from the previous month could lead to some expensive mistakes!

The Drug Tariff is a rule book that should be followed by chemist contractors and dispensing doctors when dispensing, including the fees payable to these dispensing contractors. More importantly for prescribers, it states the current drug and appliance costs and what is allowed to be prescribed.

ACCOUNTABILITY, INDEMNITY AND THE PRESCRIBING DECISION

We have covered how to write a prescription and which medicines can legally be prescribed. Now let us consider the accountability of the prescriber.

Prescribers are accountable for their own prescribing decisions and need to have satisfied themselves that the medicines they prescribe are appropriate for the patient in terms of safety and efficacy. The prescriber should also address value for money within the prescribing decision to ensure best use of resources within the National Health Service. In 1999 the government launched the National Institute for Clinical Excellence (NICE), now known as the National Institute for Health and Clinical Excellence. This was set up to ensure fair and fast access to NHS services based on need, and to move away from 'postcode treatment', seen as different treatments being provided as a consequence of where you live. NICE does this by providing up-to-date guidance on the clinical and cost effectiveness of new and existing medicines and technologies. To address variance from rational prescribing, NICE has included prescribing within its guidelines. It is imperative that prescribers be aware of existing and new NICE guidance, as it is produced and where it is relevant to their field of practice and prescribing area.

Another development, this time at local level, to address the lack of cost-effective rational prescribing was the interest being shown at health authority and more recently at primary care trust level in the provision of prescribing advice via prescribing advisers. These people are very useful contacts for prescribers who have specific queries relating to clinically- and cost-effective prescribing.

It has long been recognised that the prescriber is not only subject to but also influenced by various external pressures during the consultation process, such as patient requests, influence via the pharmaceutical industry or indeed their prescribing colleagues. Consider an independent nurse prescriber working within a general practice – do they have the independence to prescribe medicines outside of the practice formulary?

One study carried out by Prosser et al. (2003) has shown that the prescribing decision for new drugs is greatly influenced by the pharmaceutical industry, in particular the pharmaceutical representative, non-peer-reviewed literature, the mass media and to a lesser degree 'respected' hospital consultants. Other influences cited are the failure of current therapy and the adverse effect profile. This study was carried out prior to the establishment of NICE and supports its work to provide up-to-date guidance. Patients' requests for new drugs have also been found to be a powerful influence and this has been shown to be the case in the United States and

New Zealand, the only two countries that allow advertising of prescription-only medicines direct to the consumer (Mintzes et al., 2002).

In the UK, the MHRA justifies the regulation of drug industry advertising in order to protect the public from misleading claims, the argument being that the choice of prescription-only medicine forms part of a complex system of medical care and that such choice should be based on science and professional judgement. NICE supports the professional in making their own clinical decisions.

British regulations covering the advertising of medicinal products to healthcare professionals and the general public are covered in Statutory Instrument 1994 No. 1932. Advertising of prescription-only medicines to the general public is not allowed under this legislation. Some general principles also apply when advertising prescription-only medicines to healthcare professionals. Only products that have a marketing authorisation can be advertised, one exception being registered homeopathic medicinal products, and only information contained within the SPC can be included. Lastly, the advertisement must encourage the rational use of that product and not exaggerate any of the medicine's properties.

The legislation also places restrictions on free samples, inducements and hospitality that, if allowed to be provided by the pharmaceutical industry, could be construed as an 'encouragement' for a prescriber to prescribe a specific product.

All healthcare professionals who are involved with prescribing should make their choice of medicinal product for their patients on the basis of evidence, clinical suitability and cost effectiveness. This view is expressed by each professional regulatory body. It is imperative that prescribers are aware of the influence of the pharmaceutical industry and are clear as to the reasons for their prescribing decision.

General practitioners and dental practitioners have a tradition of working as independent practitioners and have always been responsible for their own professional indemnity insurance. This area has become more sensitive as more professions have moved into the prescribing arena. The accountability aspects must be addressed by the employer of the prescriber, as they would be held vicariously liable for the actions of the employee. In many cases these new prescribers do not have the employment independence of the traditional GP. For example, many prescribing nurses are employees of NHS bodies such as primary care trusts; indeed, we are also seeing more salaried GPs.

All prescribers must have sufficient professional indemnity insurance by means of membership of a professional organisation or trade union that provides this cover. If the prescriber is employed, then the job description should state that prescribing is included within the role.

How important is professional indemnity with regard to the prescriber? We shall address this by considering the issue of medication errors. This is a high priority for the government, which stated in *An Organisation with a Memory* (Department of Health, 2000) its aim of a 40 % reduction in serious error rates along with the establishment of the National Patient Safety Agency, whose remit is to collect, collate, review and analyse error reports and produce and disseminate solutions so that lessons can be learned. *Building a Safer NHS for Patients* was published in 2004 by the Department of Health and states that the actual morbidity and mortality associated with medication errors is unknown. However, 9 % of all incidents reported to the NPSA during a pilot study were found to involve medicines and 20 % of claims reported to the Medical Protection Society involved medicines. The website www.saferhealthcare.org.uk, supported by the NPSA, states that prescribing error rates are within the range of 0.56 % to 9.9 %.

Medication errors are preventable and are mistakes that happen when medicines are prescribed, dispensed or used. Prescribing errors have been found to occur for the following reasons: inadequate knowledge of the patient and their clinical condition, inadequate knowledge of the drug, calculation errors, illegible handwriting, drug name confusion, poor history taking, fatigue and inappropriate workload of the prescriber.

The prescribing error by an American cardiologist (Charatan, 1999), who wrote a prescription for Isordil, an anti-angina medication, that was misread by the dispensing pharmacist because of the poor handwriting and was subsequently dispensed as Plendil, an anti-hypertensive medication, should prey heavily on the minds of prescribers. The patient suffered a fatal heart attack several days later; both the cardiologist and the dispensing pharmacist were fined the equivalent of £140,000.

With more information becoming available on the subject of prescribing errors, responsibility lies with the individual prescriber and the employer in minimising the risk of a prescribing error happening and in having the necessary professional indemnity insurance in place in the unfortunate event that it does. Barber et al. (2003) suggest that, to improve prescribing, interventions are needed at three levels: improving training and testing the competence of prescribers; control the environment in which prescribers perform in order to standardise it, have greater controls on riskier drugs and use technology to provide decision support; and change organisational cultures, which do not support the belief that prescribing is a complex, technical act and that it is important to get it right.

The aim of this chapter has been to provide an overview of the legislation on medicines, their regulation, the pharmaceutical industry and the accountability of prescribers in practice. It will be clear from the discussion that legislation never stands still. By the time this book is published there will have been more legislative changes. It is important that prescribers address these changes as they arise. This chapter hopes to have provided the tools necessary for this to happen.

REFERENCES

ABPI (2006) *Medicines Compendium 2006*. Surrey: Datapharm Communications Ltd.
Appelbe, GE & Wingfield, J (2005) *Dale and Appelbe's Pharmacy Law and Ethics* (8th edition). London: Pharmaceutical Press.
Barber, N, Rawlins, M & Dean Franklin, B (2003) Reducing prescribing error: competence, control, and culture. *Quality and Safety in Healthcare* **12**: i29.

British Medical Association & the Royal Pharmaceutical Society of Great Britain (2006) *British National Formulary 51*. London: BMJ Publishing Group and RPS Publishing.

British Medical Association, the Royal Pharmaceutical Society of Great Britain, & the Royal College of Paediatrics and Child Health (2005) *BNF for Children*. London: BMJ Publishing Group and Royal Pharmaceutical Society of Great Britain and RCPCH Publications.

Charatan, F (1999) Family compensated for death after illegible prescription. *British Medical Journal* **319**(4 December): 1456.

Department of Health (2000) *An Organisation with a Memory: Report of an Expert Group on Learning from Adverse Events in the NHS*. Available from: http://www.dh.gov.uk/ PublicationsAndStatistics/Publications/PublicationsPolicyAndGuidance/Publications PAmpGBrowsableDocument/fs/en?CONTENT_ID=4098184&chk=u1I0ex [accessed 29 June 2006].

Department of Health (2004) *Building a Safer NHS for Patients: Improving Medication Safety*. Available from: http://www.dh.gov.uk/assetRoot/04/08/49/61/04084961.pdf [accessed 26 June 2006].

Department of Health (2005) *Supplementary Prescribing by Nurses, Pharmacists, Chiropodists/Podiatrists, Physiotherapists and Radiographers within the NHS in England*. Available from: http://www.dh.gov.uk/PublicationsAndStatistics/Publications/ PublicationsPolicyAndGuidance/PublicationsPolicyAndGuidanceArticle/fs/en? CONTENT_ID=4110032&chk=c4V6nR [accessed 22 June 2006].

Department of Health (2006a) *General Medical Services*. Available from: http://www. dh.gov.uk/PolicyAndGuidance/OrganisationPolicy/PrimaryCare/PrimaryCareContracting/ GMS/fs/en [accessed 20 June 2006].

Department of Health (2006b) *National Institute for Health and Clinical Excellence (NICE)*. Available from: http://www.nice.org.uk/ [accessed 20 June 2006].

Department of Health (2006c) *NHS English Prescription Forms*. Available from: http:// www.dh.gov.uk/PolicyAndGuidance/MedicinesPharmacyAndIndustry/Prescriptions/NHS EnglishPrescriptionForms/NHSEnglishPrescriptionFormsArticle/fs/en?CONTENT_ID = 4067685&chk=VLhJbW [accessed 22 June 2006].

Department of Health (2006d) *Improving Patients' Access to Medicines: A Guide to Implementing Nurse and Pharmacist Independent Prescribing within the NHS in England*. Available from: http://www.dh.gov.uk/PublicationsAndStatistics/Publications/Publica- tionsPolicyAndGuidance/PublicationsPolicyAndGuidanceArticle/fs/en?CONTENT_ID= 4133743&chk=HSzl1/ [accessed 22 June 2006].

Department of Health NHS Business Services Authority, Prescription Pricing Division (2006a) *Drug Tariff May 2006*. London: The Stationery Office.

Department of Health NHS Business Services Authority, Prescription Pricing Division (2006b) *Prescribers and FP10 Prescriptions*. Available from: http://www.ppa.org.uk// education/f10.htm [accessed 22 June 2006].

Dimond, B (2005) *Legal Aspects of Medicine*. London: Quay Books.

Mintzes, B, Barer, ML, Kravitz, RL, Kazanjian, A, Bassett, K, Lexchin, J, Evans, RG, Pan, R & Marion, SA (2002) Influence of direct to consumer pharmaceutical advertising and patients' requests on prescribing decisions: Two site cross sectional survey. *British Medical Journal* **324**(2 February): 278.

Prosser, H, Almond, S & Walley, T (2003) Influences on GPs' decision to prescribe new drugs – the importance of who says what. *Family Practice* **20**(1): 61.

Royal Pharmaceutical Society of Great Britain (2005) *Medicines, Ethics and Practice: A Guide for Pharmacists* (29th edition). London: Royal Pharmaceutical Society of Great Britain.

9 Prescribing in Palliative Care

YVONNE HOPKINS AND LINDA BRAY

The aim of this chapter is to provide a framework for practice, underpinned by recognised principles that affect the role of nurses when prescribing in palliative care. The emergence of palliative care as a medical discipline in 1987 (Doyle, 1997) will be considered, as will how its development has influenced the way in which palliative care nursing has developed, in particular the role of the clinical nurse specialist.

Key therapeutic areas will be explored using a patient-centred approach to describe prescribing both within drug licences and outside of drug licences, a common practice in palliative care (Ahmedzai et al., 2002).

Before we can explore nurse prescribing in palliative care, it is important to consider related issues that have had an influence on the provision of palliative care.

PALLIATIVE CARE ADVANCES

Palliative medicine was officially recognised in October 1987 following the formation of the Association of Palliative Medicine of Great Britain and Ireland. Work such as the founding of St Christopher's Hospice in London in 1967 by Dame Cicely Saunders provided the early momentum for developments that emerged later and continue to advance.

A core component of the early development of hospices and palliative care was found in the management of pain using opiod drugs and was considered, by Robbins (1998), to have provided the great impetus behind the development of palliative care teams and hospices. The growth in knowledge and the belief in the ability to control the pain of progressive cancer and other symptoms provided the foundations for symptom management in palliative care and this is now seen as a core skill of professionals working in this specialism.

Recognised treatments and medications are now commonly integrated within the palliative care of people with cancer and other life-limiting diseases and also within the realms of chronic disease management. This, however, requires responsive,

Towards Prescribing Practice. Edited by J. McKinnon.
© 2007 John Wiley & Sons, Ltd.

knowledgeable and skilled professionals to provide the optimal level of care to meet the needs of individuals. The National Council for Hospices and Specialist Palliative Care Services (NCHSPCS) (1995) reminds us that a key component of effective palliative care is multiprofessional working.

It is also important to note that the provision of palliative care education and training has only recently been available for the majority of medical practitioners. One example of inadequate education has resulted in some general practitioners being reluctant to introduce syringe drivers for the control of symptoms in the community setting, only seeing them as the last resort. In some instances syringe drivers may be necessary earlier in the disease trajectory to control symptoms such as nausea and vomiting. Other members of the multidisciplinary team such as district nurses and specialist nurses – i.e. Macmillan nurses – should be influential in changing this view of practice. Specialist practitioners have an extensive advisory role within their respective disciplines. Their wide experience and knowledge of disease management equip them for this role by virtue of the volume of patients referred to them for specialist assessment and symptom management. On average, a general practitioner would expect to care for approximately ten patients per annum with an advanced malignant disease. By comparison, a specialist palliative care nurse working in primary care would expect to care for an average of 100 patients in a year with a variety of complex problems.

It has been demonstrated that skilled practitioners working within specialities are safe prescribers and would only prescribe within their own competence following appropriate training (Latter et al., 2004). When patients are seen by an array of providers, there are concerns about the fragmentation of care. This is a concern for practitioners caring for people with palliative care needs because continuity of care is essential to avoid some of the pitfalls that result from inappropriate prescribing. One example of this would be where specialist and generalist nursing and medical staff are caring for a patient in the community. This is illustrated in the example below.

Box 9.1

The specialist practitioner has been asked to assist the PHCT with managing a patient's complex pain. Following the assessment by the specialist nurse, which indicates a neuropathic pain only partially responsive to the prescribed strong opioid, the GP was advised that a tricyclic antidepressant would be beneficial if it was not contraindicated in addition to the fentanyl and oral morphine currently being taken. Amitriptyline 25 mg at night was commenced, but before the medication had reached optimum effect the patient was seen by a community nurse, who contacted a different GP within the practice and requested a home visit to advise about pain control. The GP visited the patient and doubled the fentanyl patch dose. The result of this was adverse opioid side effects owing to the patient having a larger dose of opioid than he required. This was despite information being available about the current pain problem and proposed management plan in the patient's record, both in the surgery and in the patient's home.

THE DEVELOPING ROLE OF CLINICAL NURSE SPECIALISTS IN PALLIATIVE CARE

The expansion in the numbers of clinical nurse specialists in palliative care has increased apace during the past 20 years. These clinical nurse specialists are now present in many areas of patient care in both the primary and secondary care settings. There is an expectation that clinical nurse specialists have achieved a certain level of expertise underpinned by extended knowledge and experience. Castledine (1992) refers to the early development and evolution of clinical nurse specialists following the Royal National Commission on the National Health Service (Merrison, 1979). This proposed a clinical career structure for nurses who were experienced but did not want to advance their career through the management route.

The development and evolution of nurses specialising in palliative care dates back to the mid-1970s, when roles were established in hospital, community and voluntary settings. Initial support for these posts was often provided by the charity Macmillan Cancer Support, as it is now named. Over time these roles have expanded into contemporary clinical nurse specialists with a specific responsibility for the care of terminally ill patients and their families. The role of the clinical nurse specialist has developed in response to social, technological and political changes that have influenced the delivery of healthcare. Although clinical nurse specialists need autonomy to enhance their role, it must be seen within the context of team working to ensure that continuity of care is maintained for the patient (Cutts, 1999).

There is a suggestion by Clark et al. (2002) that it is essential to clarify the role of the clinical nurse specialist in palliative care if their expertise is to be used effectively and efficiently. It is paramount that they adapt to the rapidly changing landscape of healthcare policy, research and initiatives being presented to them. Current important influences are practice-based commissioning, hospital avoidance and the care management model that is developing in the primary care setting. This may mean that in the future clinical nurse specialists working in palliative care may operate differently, and a variety of models may emerge reflecting local needs. The drivers of these influences on ways of providing care are finance, efficiency, equity, the changing dynamics between commissioners and providers of care, and lastly the notion of striving to deliver a patient-led NHS.

End-of-life care initiatives such as the Gold Standards Framework, the Liverpool Care Pathway for the Dying and Preferred Place of Care instil quality in the provision of care and can act as a benchmark for commissioning future care.

GENERAL NURSES

The role of nurses providing general palliative care to patients and their families, both in the community and in hospital, is crucial in that they are members of the multidisciplinary team caring for patients. Some have a wide and varied knowledge of palliative nursing practice. This group of health professionals provides a high proportion of palliative care with no need for the involvement of specialist palliative care providers.

However, when patients or their families have complex problems or issues that need to be addressed, the patient should be offered specialist intervention. One of the skills of generalist nurses working with patients with palliative care needs is in their insight and acknowledgement of when to refer to specialist services for the benefit of the patient. In this instance communication and team working are paramount. Joint consultations between the specialist and generalist nurse to patients can be very supportive, not only for the patient but also for the generalist nurse. An opportunity for increasing knowledge by working alongside the specialist nurse can be invaluable.

PALLIATIVE CARE MEDICATION

As the role of the clinical nurse specialist in palliative care has developed, their involvement in symptom management has become more sophisticated and complex. Within the hospital and primary care settings, they assess and oversee the management of complex symptoms, providing advice and support to clinical staff.

The patient assessment undertaken by the clinical nurse specialist plays a major part in informing the symptom management plan. Particular features of this assessment are:

- Whole-patient assessment examines a range of issues that may cause suffering.
- How symptoms are perceived by and affect the patient and their families in their everyday life.
- The use of a variety of tools for measuring symptoms, e.g. visual analogue scales, numerical scales, body charts, time for discussion and acknowledgement.

Body charts are used routinely in practice to assess and evaluate the site and nature of pain. They may also highlight that the patient has more than one site of pain and more than one type, all of which should be addressed and may require a combination of approaches (Bennett et al., 2005). Visual analogue scales (VAS) enable the patient to score the pain usually on a continuous line, either horizontal or vertical. Some VAS have no numbers and the patient decides where along a continuum they would rate their pain. Other scales use numbers from 0 = no pain with up to 4, 5 or 10 for the worst pain, depending on which scale is being used in a locality. The benefit of using VAS for the patient is that they are simple, reproducible and reliable. Some patients find it difficult, however, to give their pain severity a numerical score. In this case the use of categorical scales may be more meaningful to the patient. Some examples of tools used to measure pain are provided in Tables 9.1 and 9.2.

Pain questionnaires are used in conjunction with the above to offer a comprehensive assessment of a patient's pain history. They provide descriptors, meanings and describe the effect the pain is having on their quality of life. Pain is a uniquely personal experience for the patient and it requires skill and an understanding of the totality of pain, its physical, emotional, social and spiritual dimensions.

An example of a behavioural pain assessment used in the elderly is the Doloplus-2 Scale, which records behaviour; somatic reactions (e.g. protective body postures, expression and sleep pattern); psychomotor reactions (e.g. washing, dressing and general mobility); and psychosocial reactions (e.g. communication, social life and problems of behaviour).

This emphasises the importance of investing time in this process to attain the most beneficial way for the patient to communicate their pain to the clinician. A particularly challenging group of patients is those with communication difficulties, such as people with dementia and those with learning difficulties.

Successful pain management relies on careful assessment to allow differentiation between the variety of pain syndromes. Careful assessment helps the clinician to identify the type of pain and subsequently the best approach to alleviating it.

Table 9.1 Outcome measures scales

- Verbal rating scale, e.g. McGill Pain Questionnaire (Melzac, 1975)
  No pain; mild; discomforting; distressing; horrible; excruciating.

- Numerical rating scale, e.g. Brief Pain Inventory (Daut et al., 1983)

  A. Pain intensity
  0   1   2   3   4   5   6   7   8   9   10
  No pain   Pain as bad as you can imagine
  B. Pain relief
  0%   10%   20%   30%   40%   50%   60%   70%   80%   90%   100%
  No relief   Complete relief

- Visual analogue scale, e.g. Memorial Pain Assessment Card (Fishman et al., 1987)

  A. Pain intensity _____
  LEAST   WORST
  possible pain   possible pain
  B. Pain relief _____
  NO   COMPLETE
  relief of pain   relief of pain

Source: Davies (2002)

Table 9.2　Body maps help the patient accurately locate their pain

PAIN SCALE

If the pain changes position, mark it on the figure.

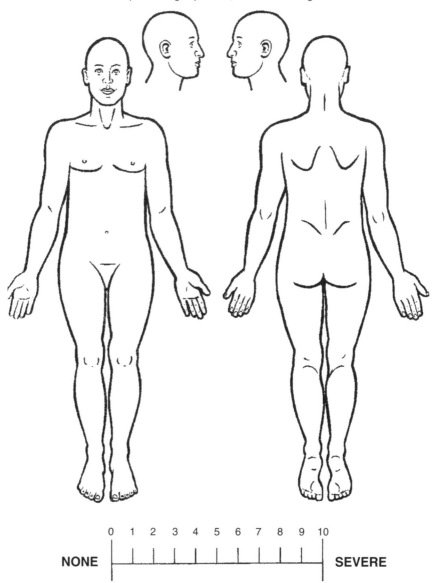

There are seven well-known approaches to the management of all pain. These are:

- Explanation
- Raise the pain threshold
- Modify lifestyle
- Modify the pathological process
- Modify pain perception
- Interrupt pain pathways
- Psychological intervention.

Following the initiation of treatment, the patients' symptoms are continually monitored and interventions are evaluated. There has been much debate about the benefits to the patient of non-medical prescribing. While some nurses view nurse prescribing as a positive step, some will regard it as time consuming with no benefit to patients, especially in rural practices where practices dispense medications directly to the patients. The practice of nurse prescribing in palliative care may reduce the contact that specialist nurses would have with the patient's GP. Communication and contact with the primary healthcare team (PHCT) is an essential part of team working, particularly important for patients with palliative care needs. Contact with the PHCT often results in the sharing of information and knowledge, thus confirming the educative role of the specialist for the generalist, which has an impact on patient care.

The clinical nurse specialist will provide information to clinical staff on a range of interventions that they might not have considered. Some of the following will require the intervention of an oncologist, specialist palliative care physician or a pain consultant. For examples see Table 9.3.

RADIOTHERAPY FOR BONE PAIN

Symptoms of bone pain include a constant ache and pain on movement. Local radiotherapy is the treatment of choice if there are painful bone metastases. A single dose of radiotherapy given on one day will achieve pain relief in 60–80 % of

Table 9.3   Approaches to symptom management

- Radiotherapy for bone pain.
- Bisphosphonate therapy – for tumour-induced hypercalcaemia, bone pain and prophylactic use to reduce the incidence of skeletal-related events in patients with cancer involving bone.
- Complementary therapies – touch therapies and psychological interventions.
- Nerve blocks for neuropathic pain – usually recommends the involvement of specialist palliative care physicians or a pain consultant.
- Non-opioid treatment for neuropathic pain – such as the use of corticosteroids, tricyclic antidepressants such as amitriptyline and/or anticonvulsants such as gabapentin and carbamazepine.
- Syringe drivers for symptom control – e.g. anti-emetics for established nausea or vomiting early in the disease process if necessary.

patients, with total relief in 30 % (Barton, 2005). Radiotherapy treatment involves the use of ionising radiation, usually X-rays that cause damage at the cellular level. When radiation passes through a living cell there is both a direct and an indirect effect on the reproductive component of the cell. Direct damage results in the form of deletions and breaks to the DNA chain. Indirect damage, which is probably the most important effect of the radiation, is the reaction by the radiation with water molecules in individual cells, which results in the release of toxic free radicals. Normal cells have the capacity to repair and recover from radiation damage, but the repair mechanism in malignant cells is often deficient. The death of the cell resulting from radiotherapy is, therefore, either due to reproductive failure as a result of DNA damage or apoptosis through the impact of the radiation on the cell regulatory mechanisms (Hoskin, 2004). The mechanism of the relief of bone pain using radiotherapy is not clear. There is a suggestion in Hoskin (2004) that local effects on bone tissue possibly affect the release of pain-mediating humoral agents and osteoclast/osteoblast interactions. These factors together are important in achieving and maintaining pain relief.

A short case study is provided to illustrate some of the issues that patients with bone pain may present with.

Box 9.2

A 64-year-old man with prostate cancer and evidence of bone metastases on a recent bone scan consulted his GP about severe pain in the right hip. The pain was so great that he was unable to work and had difficulty walking. He had been reviewed by the urologist two weeks prior to the GP's decision to refer him to a Macmillan nurse for assessment and advice regarding pain management. He was also referred to a physiotherapist and crutches were provided to assist with walking. His current analgesia regime consisted of co-codamol 30/500 2 tablets four times daily.

- **What would be a realistic plan to manage this patient's pain?**
- **Who should he be referred on to?**
- **What alternative treatments may be required?**

BISPHOSPHONATE THERAPY

Bisphosphonates can be used to treat malignant bone pain, particularly in patients with myeloma, breast, lung and prostate cancers with bone involvement. This therapy is usually administered intravenously every four weeks, with the patient attending an outpatient facility. The response rate in solid tumours is 40 %, but in myeloma this rises to 80 % (Barton, 2005). The intravenous route is preferable owing to its efficacy, tolerability and predictability, whereas oral preparations have been shown to be poorly and variably absorbed (Back, 2001).

Bisphosphonates have a role in prophylaxis against bone pain, fractures and hypercalcaemia. This long-term strategy should reduce skeletal complications. They are also used to treat established malignant bone pain. At the present time bisphosphonates such as pamidronate, sodium clodronate and ibandronic acid need to be administered every three to four weeks, but zoledronic acid has a longer duration of four to six weeks. Analgesic effect is usually achieved within 14 days (Watson et al., 2005). Bisphosphonates target areas of bone where osteoclast activity is high. Osteoclasts are known to destroy old bone and osteoblasts build new bone. Bisphosphonate therapy helps to restore the normal balance of osteoclasts and osteoblasts by inhibiting osteoclast resorption. This occurs when bisphosphonates bind hydroxyapatite crystals with a high affinity and affect osteoclast recruitment and activation. This results in a reduction in pain, strengthening of bone and reduction in the amount of calcium lost from the bone.

Usual doses of the bisphosphonates commonly used in palliative care are:

- Zoledronic acid – 4 mg i/v over 15 minutes.
- Disodium pamidronate – 90 mg i/v diluted to 500 ml in sodium chloride 0.9 % (minimum 375 ml), infuse over 2–4 hours (Watson et al., 2005).

Side effects of intravenous bisphosphonate therapy include transient pyrexia and flu-like symptoms on the day after administration, thrombophlebitis (especially after rapid administration), hypocalcaemia, urticaria and angio-oedema (Stannard and Booth, 2004). It is important that the side effects of bisphosphonates are discussed and made clear to the patient and their carer. If patients are expecting to experience malaise as a result of their treatment, the anxiety that will result will be reduced.

There have been recent concerns about a complication of osteonecrosis of the jaw. Reports in 2004 identified this problem as a rare side effect in some patients who were receiving bisphosphonate therapy. It has been acknowledged, however, that measures need to be taken to prevent osteonecrosis in patients with a history of receiving bisphosphonate therapy prior to dental treatment. It is recommended that patients should have a dental check prior to commencing treatment. With patients already receiving bisphosphonates who require major dental treatment such as extractions or implants, some doctors may consider suspending treatment for two to four months prior to treatment. The benefit of this is not yet certain, but patients need to be given the choice (Cancer Research UK, 2006).

COMPLEMENTARY THERAPIES IN CANCER AND PALLIATIVE CARE

The evidence base for the use of complementary therapies in the care of people with cancer is relatively small. This may be a reflection of the limited resources invested in this area of practice. The two therapies for which best scientific evidence exists are:

- Acupuncture for chemotherapy-induced nausea (Thompson and Filshie, 1993).
- Visualisation/meditation for improved quality of life.

Table 9.4

Physical	Psychological	Others
Aromatherapy	Relaxation	Diets/vitamins
Reflexology	Guided imagery	Homeopathy
Massage	Meditation	Chinese herbs
Shiatsu	Healing	Naturopathy
Osteopathy	Yoga	Essiac
Chiropractic	Art therapy	Iscador
Acupuncture	Hypnosis	Shark's cartilage

Source: Bell and Sikora (1996)

Psychological interventions resulting in an intimate connection between the body and mind are increasingly being seen as benefiting physical and mental ailments.

Few clinical trials have been conducted in the past, and those that were have been of poor methodological quality, mainly due to the constraints around the nature of the control group in such studies (Kohn, 1999). Kohn undertook a study of complementary therapies in cancer care for Macmillan Cancer Relief in 1999. As one would expect, there are a variety of opinions about the place of such therapies for people with cancer and other long-term conditions. Therapies can be classified by mode of action, as illustrated in Table 9.4.

Complementary therapies form an integral part of general palliative care, with many people finding them particularly useful in the management of stress and pain and for dealing with negative emotions. The hospice movement in particular offers a wide range of complementary therapies to its patients, which are provided to improve the quality of their lives.

In 2003, national guidelines were published for nine of the better-known complementary therapies to encourage the development of best practice: acupuncture, aromatherapy and hypnotherapy (NCHSPC, 2003). Increasing numbers of regulatory professional bodies are being established for complementary therapies and currently there are plans to establish such a body for herbal medicine.

It is imperative that prescribing practitioners have a good knowledge of guidelines and relevant organisations and they must keep themselves up to date with the latest supporting research. When assessing a palliative care patient the following issues need to be considered in relation to complementary therapies:

- Is the complementary therapy a potential source of adverse reactions?
- Is the patient already using a complementary therapy that they find helpful?
- Is that complementary therapy being practised according to national guidelines?
- Is the complementary therapy being used contraindicated with any current/ planned medication?
- Could a new or alternative complementary therapy be introduced that has the potential to enhance the impact of current/future medication?

The NHS Trusts Association has compiled and now manages *The NHS Directory of Complementary and Alternative Practitioners* for use by NHS healthcare professionals. The directory provides listings of all practitioners who, by a process of self-selection, have put themselves forward to work either directly in NHS practices or from their own practice on a referral basis.

As the use of complementary therapies within mainstream healthcare continues to increase, so does the related research activity. There is still very little evidence to support the use of complementary therapies within palliative care. Some evidence, however, points to the fact that patients find them valuable (Wilcock et al., 2003).

It is important to add a word of caution around the use of herbal remedies. Practitioners should be meticulous in taking a history that includes a profile of all prescribed medications and those acquired by patients from other sources such as health shops, pharmacies, supermarkets, herbalists and other retail sources. Herbal remedies are viewed by the general public as 'healthy', but they do contain active ingredients that may have an adverse effect on the individual.

NERVE BLOCKS FOR NEUROPATHIC PAIN

Nerve blocks are appropriate for nerve pains and are described as:

- regional local anaesthetic blocks
- sympathetic blocks
- cordotomy.

Regional local anaesthetic blocks are effective when used to relieve nerve injury pain. Sympathetic blocks may involve local anaesthetic blocks of the stellate ganglion or the lumbar sympathetic chain.

Percutaneous cordotomy is the procedure of choice in palliative care and is usually performed at the level of C1 or C2. A unilateral cordotomy carries a relatively low morbidity risk, but is only suitable for unilateral pain (Sinnott, 1997).

NON-OPIOID APPROACHES FOR NEUROPATHIC PAIN

Early recognition and treatment of nerve pain are crucial to the success of managing this type of pain. Nerve pain can present in a variety of ways. It may occur as a direct result of stimulation, which may be quite slight but evoke an exaggerated response such as allodynia, when a feather touch of an area of the patient's skin results in a painful response. There may be an increasingly painful response to a painful stimulus, or a delayed but prolonged response after the stimulus has ceased. There may also be continuous pains or paroxysmal pains in the absence of any stimulus. This is illustrated in Table 9.5.

The three main common approaches used for this difficult pain syndrome are antidepressants, anticonvulsants and corticosteroids. Table 9.6 provides a list of some of the above drugs and includes classifications and some of the common side effects of the individual medications.

Table 9.5 Abnormal sensations associated with neuropathic pain

Spontaneous pains that arise in the absence of stimuli
- Continuous pain (dysaesthesias)
- Paroxysmal

Evoked pains
- Allodynia: a painful response to a non-painful stimulus
- Hyperalgesia: increased painful response to painful stimulus
- Hyperpathia: delayed and prolonged response to stimulus

Table 9.6 Non-opioid approaches to neuropathic pain

Medication commonly used in neuropathic pain	Classification of drug	Side effects
Amitriptyline	Tricyclic antidepressant	Dry mouth, sedation, blurred vision, constipation, nausea, arrhythmias, postural hypotension, tachycardia and syncope, sweats, rash and tremors
Gabapentin	Anticonvulsant	Dizziness, drowsiness, ataxia, fatigue
Carbamazepine	Anticonvulsant	Nausea and vomiting, dizziness, headache, ataxia, constipation or diarrhoea, anorexia and rash
Dexamethasone	Corticosteroid	Gastro-intestinal effects, musculo-sketal effects, endocrine effects, neuropsychiatric effects and ophthalmic effects

Antidepressants

Antidepressants work by blocking the presynaptic reuptake of serotonin and noradrenaline, which may modulate pain signalling in the spinal cord. It has been assumed in the past that antidepressants worked by altering the patient's mood, however there is good evidence that antidepressants have a separate analgesic effect (Sinnott, 1997).

When a tricyclic antidepressant such as amitriptyline is prescribed for neuropathic pain, the therapeutic approach varies from that used in people who are depressed. When taken as an antidepressant the dose is much greater; that is, a starting dose of 30–75 mg in adolescents or the elderly, increasing to 200 mg if necessary. Amitriptyline is commonly used in palliative care at a dose of 10–25 mg at night, increasing slowly to 150 mg daily. Thus doses required for neuropathic pain may be lower, and the speed of onset is faster (1–7 days) than for depression (McQuay et al., 1996).

Patients occasionally experience early morning drowsiness or take a long time to settle at night. By advising them to take their amitriptyline two hours prior to going to bed instead of at bedtime, this effect may be resolved. Early morning drowsiness naturally concerns the patient and their carer when they often have a multiplicity of problems and this could affect their quality of life. Through addressing this the practitioner will not only resolve the drowsiness, they will also provide reassurance for the patient and their carer, which all have an impact upon maximising concordance.

Anticonvulsants

There is a standard view that this group of drugs work as membrane stabilisers, resulting in the diminution of abnormal neuronal hyperexcitability and the suppression of paroxysmal discharges.

An anticonvulsant used in some centres is gabapentin. Some anti-epileptics act as peripheral sodium-channel blockers, while others mainly have an impact in the dorsal horn. The *BNF* recommends 300 mg on day 1, 300 mg BD on day 2, and 300 mg TDS on day 3, then titrate according to response in 300 mg steps to a maximum of 1800 mg a day. Caution should be used in the elderly and those with poor renal function. It is also important to avoid abrupt withdrawal (withdraw over one week) if stopping use of the drug.

Corticosteroids

The use of steroids for nerve pain is based on the theory of the reduction of oedema and inflammation surrounding the compressing tumour mass. In addition to this action, there is a view that steroids act as analgesics by other mechanisms, including a direct influence on electrical activity in damaged nerves.

The use of corticosteroids has been shown to reduce pain in various situations, with a number of possible mechanisms for their analgesic activity:

- A reduction in spontaneous discharge in injured nerves.
- Inhibition in prostaglandin synthesis leading to reduced inflammation.
- A reduction in capillary permeability and peri-tumour oedema.
- A reduction in injury-induced nerve sprouting.
- A reduced calcitonin gene-related peptide and substance P content of sensory fibres, which is possibly a central effect related to improved mood (Tiernan, 1997).

The dose of corticosteroids varies between centres and across symptoms. Dexamethasone doses relating to particular indications are illustrated in Table 9.7.

Adverse effects of cortcosteroids need to be balanced by their benefits. The usefulness of this class of drug is best described as exaggeration of the normal physiological action of corticosteroids. Practitioners should be mindful of adverse side effects, particularly when dosages increase.

Table 9.7   Indications and doses for dexamethasone usage

Average dose of dexamethasone	Indication
2–4 mg/day	To increase appetite
2–4 mg/day	To improve sense of wellbeing
2–4 mg/day	Non-specific pain relief
2–4 mg/day	Anti-emetic action
2–4 mg/day	Weakness
4–8 mg/day	Co-analgesic for nerve compression pain
4–8 mg/day	Pain due to hepatomegaly
Up to 16 mg/day	Cerebral tumours – raised intracranial pressure
Up to 16 mg/day	Spinal cord compression
Up to 16 mg/day	Superior vena cava obstruction
Up to 16 mg/day	Intestinal and ureteric obstruction

Source: Back (2001)

Oropharyngeal candida is a common side effect of corticosteroid therapy and develops within a few days. Proximal myopathy may occur after only ten days, but the usual peak period of onset is two to three months. Other complications associated with corticosteroids include hyperglycaemia, peptic ulceration, cushingoid features and psychotic reactions. It is, therefore, important for practitioners to prevent, monitor and respond to patient symptoms and concerns.

An important rule for corticosteroids is to use the lowest possible dose for the shortest period of time that is clinically effective. In patients requiring long-term corticosteroid therapy, the dosage should be reduced to the lowest effective level to maintain therapeutic benefit (Tiernan, 1997).

SYRINGE DRIVERS FOR SYMPTOM CONTROL

The ingestion of anti-emetic tablets can often be a potent emetic stimulus; this is considered to be a reversible cause for vomiting and is illustrated in the following case study.

Box 9.3

A 50-year-old man with advanced carcinoma of the pancreas presented with gradual onset of vomiting and constipation. There was no tenderness of his abdomen, which was also soft on examination. He was unable to keep down his tablets, so he was commenced on a subcutaneous (SC) infusion containing an anti-emetic. His bowels were managed with rectal preparations to relieve the constipation until the vomiting was controlled.

The nausea and vomiting gradually settled over the course of a week to the extent that his 24-hour dose of anti-emetic could be administered as oral tablets in three divided doses in addition to regular oral laxatives, titrated to prevent further episodes of constipation.

Other indications for subcutaneous infusions of medication by a syringe driver include:

- dysphagia
- intestinal obstruction
- semi-comatose or comatose states
- profound weakness
- poor absorption of drug in the GI tract.

NON-MEDICINAL INTERVENTIONS

The clinical nurse specialist would work alongside the patient and their family/carer to reduce symptomatology by providing a range of non-medicinal interventions. This may require working in partnership with physiotherapists and occupational therapists to actively help patients to manage dyspnoea, fatigue and mobility problems.

Ways in which clinical nurse specialists may be required to support and advise patients include:

- relaxation techniques
- advanced psychosocial support
- diversional guidance
- self-help remedies, e.g. for sweating, anorexia and dyspnoea management.

SWEATING

This is a common symptom experienced particularly by people with Hodgkin's disease, leukaemia and tumours with liver metastases. It is particularly distressing for patients and results in fatigue due to lack of sleep and low mood. It is important, therefore, to establish the cause of the sweating and correct if possible. If this is not possible, then general measures are often discussed with the patient and carer to give them some control over the situation, in addition to recognising the impact this symptom is having on the patient in association with reassurance from the clinician.

It is important to exclude infection as a possible cause of sweating and treat appropriately. Fever is not always present if the patient is taking steroids or has a reduced white cell count. Other causes of sweats include:

* chemotherapy treatment such as bleomycin
* blood transfusions
* hormone treatments
* menopause
* anxiety.

General remedies to reduce sweating include the use of fans, sponging, regular washing, encouraging the intake of oral fluids and the use of aids such as Chillow Pillows, which dissipate heat from the patient's head or body.

Drug options include aspirin, NSAIDs, thioridazine, propantheline, cimetidine and megestrol.

ANOREXIA

Anorexia is a problem common to people with cancer and is often associated with cachexia and fatigue. It may be due to the site of the tumour, the side effects of treatments such as chemotherapy, radiotherapy, medications or psychological factors such as low mood or anxiety.

Self-help strategies usually include eating small and frequent snacks, or eating whatever the patient desires, however strange. Other helpful tips include using a small plate to encourage the patient to try small portions, avoiding cooking smells until ready to eat, avoiding isolation at mealtimes and seeking advice about fortifying food and drinks. Carers often require reassurance and support for this problem; nurturing and providing food and drink form a basic demonstration of caring on behalf of the carer.

A trial course of dexamethasone, 2–4 mg daily, can be helpful if there are no contraindications, and the effect of steroid therapy should be apparent within one week. If no improvement is noted, steroids should be discontinued.

DYSPNOEA

Breathlessness is one of the most challenging symptoms of advanced cancer and end-stage respiratory disease. It is often managed with a range of medications including oxygen, nebulisers, anxiolytics and opioids. Pharmacological approaches are often not without side effects. A sense of control is important to patients with difficulties in breathing. They usually choose to remain at home and to stay as active as their disease will allow to enhance their quality of life (Syrett and Taylor, 2003).

Dyspnoea management can be achieved by approaching this issue from a multi-disciplinary stance. Physiotherapists are skilled in teaching patients breathing techniques and chest clearance, provision of walking aids, relaxation and managing the activities of daily living. Specialist nurses act as referral agents, providing help with anxiety management and psychological support. In addition to these interventions, patients require practical support, advice about energy conservation during panic attacks and pacing activity. Bredin et al. (1999) demonstrated in a multicentre randomised control trial that patients' breathing improved significantly with a multidisciplinary approach to managing this symptom, which also had an impact on their performance status, physical symptoms and levels of anxiety.

PRESCRIBING PRACTICE IN PALLIATIVE CARE

CONTROLLED DRUGS

The controlled drugs listed in Table 9.8 are routinely used for the relief of symptoms in palliative care patients.

Medication administered by routes other than listed in the table would be beyond the drug licence. An example of this practice is adding diamorphine to intrasite gel to apply to painful wounds, a practice used in some centres.

Anxiety still exists for the professional and the public around the issue of prescribing strong opioids. It is important for practitioners to remember that they are treating the patient and their carer as well as the pain, particularly when people have severe pain.

When a strong opioid is prescribed, the practitioner must remember to make time to explain to the patient and their family why a particular drug such as morphine has been chosen and to answer their questions and fears about this step.

It is important to anticipate and explain possible side effects, for instance nausea, and treat them prophylactically. In addition to this, it is wise to encourage the patient to report any reactions. Ensure that other staff do not hold any misconceptions about morphine and why it is being prescribed (Stannard and Booth, 2004).

Table 9.8 Details of the appropriate routes of administration

Substance	Route of administration
Diamorphine hydrochloride	Oral and parenteral
Fentanyl	Transdermal administration in palliative care
Morphine sulphate	Oral, parenteral and rectal
Morphine hydrochloride	Rectal
Oxycodone hydrochloride	Oral and parenteral administration in palliative care
Diazepam	Oral, parenteral and rectal
Lorazepam	Oral and parenteral
Midazolam	Parenteral
Codeine phosphate	Oral
Dihydrocodeine tartrate	Oral

Some common misconceptions relating to morphine prescribing include the following:

- *Morphine can be addictive*. This is a drug commonly abused outside the medical setting, but there is no evidence to suggest that opioids given for medical reasons cause addiction (Heath, 1997; McCaffery et al., 1990).
- *The dose needs to be constantly increased*. After initial titration the dose usually remains stable until the disease progresses. True pharmacological tolerance to morphine is rare.
- *If morphine is used too early there will be nothing available when the pain severity increases*. This is a common view among patients. There is no upper limit of morphine dose as long as the benefits outweigh any adverse effects.
- *Morphine is only used in dying patients*. Morphine can be used by patients for pain of any origin. People can take it for many years and live a normal life.
- *The use of morphine will shorten a patient's life*. There is evidence to say that adequate pain relief will extend life. The former practice of only prescribing morphine for dying people has led to this misplaced association with impending death (Stannard and Booth, 2004).
- *Parenteral morphine is more effective than oral morphine*. If the patient can take drugs by mouth then an oral preparation should be used. There is no evidence to show that parenteral morphine is more effective than oral morphine in comparable doses, although it is often tried if all other options have failed.

In practice, patients who are hesitant about taking oral morphine will often accept morphine therapy if it is given by an alternative route and is not obviously viewed by them as morphine, for example transdermal preparations such as fentanyl (Stannard and Booth, 2004).

UNLICENSED PRESCRIBING

A survey of prescribing by specialists in palliative care found that approximately 25 % of prescriptions were outside the drug licences – that is, were for unlicensed indications or were administered by an unlicensed route. This number of prescriptions affected 66 % of patients (Pavis and Wilcock, 2001).

It can be seen, therefore, that the use of drugs outside the drug licence is an accepted practice in palliative care. The use of drugs in this way for the control of pain and other symptoms is often referred to as off label, beyond label or beyond licence.

Using medications outside their licences often occurs when knowledge and experience increase, frequently as a result of experience in the use of a drug, but the terms of the original licence have not been extended. Failure to extend a product licence usually occurs because of the costs, the size of the therapeutic group who would benefit and the low perceived return on further investment.

It is rare, however, for drugs that have not been granted a licence to be used in palliative care. It is far more common for licensed drugs to be used in palliative care for unlicensed indications, by unlicensed routes and in unlicensed doses.

The terms of the product licence granted for a drug by the Medicines Control Agency (MCA) will indicate the age group, clinical condition, dose range, route or method of administration for which a particular drug can be used. In palliative care situations in the UK a doctor may legally prescribe a drug outside the licence. The General Medical Council and medical defence organisations expect the doctor to base such clinical decisions on a duty of care. The doctor must act in a responsible way: patients should be given information relating to the nature and risks of such treatment, because these factors will not be explained in the patient information leaflet (PIL).

It is important to note that if an unlicensed medicine is administered to the patient, the manufacturer has no liability for any harm that may ensue. The person who prescribes the medication carries the liability. If a medicine is unlicensed, it should only be administered to a patient against a patient-specific prescription and not against a patient group direction. However, medication that is licensed but used outside its licensed indications may be administered under a patient group direction if such use is exceptional, justified by best practice and the status of the product is clearly described. In addition, the nurse must be satisfied that they have sufficient information to administer the drug safely and, wherever possible, that there is acceptable evidence for the use of that product for the intended indication (Nursing and Midwifery Council, 2004). This duty of care also exists in the case of a licensed drug by an unlicensed route, such as by a feeding tube or subcutaneous injections when the route the medication is licensed for is intramuscular or intravenous, for example metoclopramide.

Table 9.9 illustrates the use of medication beyond the licence.

The practice of using drugs beyond their licence is widespread in palliative care. Physicians have gained vast experience of working in this way, in addition to this practice being documented in standard textbooks. As a result of this, a hierarchy of factors influencing the reasonableness of prescribing decisions has developed. Informed written consent is felt to be impractical in the palliative care setting. Concern was expressed in the UK survey undertaken by Pavis and Wilcock (2001) that not only would it be impractical to seek informed consent on every occasion, but also it would be burdensome for the patient. It would increase anxiety and may deter the patient from accepting beneficial treatment. The use of licensed drugs by unlicensed routes and for unlicensed indications and in unlicensed doses is so common in palliative care that the Association for Palliative Medicine and the British Pain Society prepared the guidance outlined in Table 9.10.

ANTICIPATORY PRESCRIBING

Evidence suggests that while the majority of patients wish to spend their final days at home, many do not get to do so and they spend their last days within

Table 9.9 Medications commonly used in palliative care outside the licence

Medication	Unlicensed use	Licensed use
Hyoscine butylbromide	Drying secretions	Intestinal colic
Clonidine	Sweating	Migraine prophylaxis
Tranexamic acid	Surface bleeding from ulcerating tumours	Menorrhagia
Morphine	Dyspnoea	Pain
Clonazepam	Neuropathic pain	Epilepsy
Lorazepam	Acute agitation	Anxiety
Midazolam	Intractable hiccups	Sedation with amnesia
Olanzapine	Agitation, anti-emetic	Schizophrenia
Amitriptyline	Neuropathic pain	Depression, enuresis in children
Venlafaxine	Flushes, neuropathic pain	Depression
Nabilone	Breathlessness	Nausea and vomiting
Dexamethasone	Dyspnoea, nerve compression	Suppression of inflammatory/allergic disorders
Zoledronic acid	Bone pain	Tumour-induced hypercalcaemia
Ascorbic acid	Furred tongue	Scurvy
Baclofen	Hiccups	Painful muscle spasm

an acute hospital setting (Gomes and Higginson, 2006). Often there is a breakdown in the provision of services or the families have found difficulties in coping. However, a common reason for people with palliative care needs being admitted to hospital is the inadequate management of their symptoms. This was reinforced by a study undertaken in 2005, which showed that some of the unnecessary admissions could have been avoided with advanced planning and anticipatory prescribing (Hopkins, 2006). Anticipatory prescribing is seen as good practice within palliative care and is supported within the Gold Standards Framework for palliative care. A practical example of anticipatory prescribing is the use of 'just in case' boxes.

Just in Case Boxes

In 2003, the Mount Vernon Cancer Network initiated a pilot study, with the aim being to anticipate pharmaceutical needs stemming from new or worsening symptoms, and prescribing medicines to be used on a 'just in case' basis. It was envisaged that this activity would minimise the distress caused by poor access to palliative care medication, particularly out of hours (Amas and Allen, 2005)

Having experienced similar difficulties within East Lincolnshire, a project was initiated there (Hopkins, 2006). The aim of the project is to avoid unnecessary distress caused by inadequate access to medication out of hours.

Table 9.10   Association for Palliative Medicine and the British Pain Society guidance

- The use of drugs beyond licence should be seen as a legitimate aspect of clinical practice.
- The use of drugs beyond licence in palliative care and pain management practice is currently both necessary and common.
- Choice of treatment requires partnership between patients and healthcare professionals, and informed consent should be obtained, whenever possible, before prescribing any drug. Patients should be informed of any identifiable risks and details of any information given should be recorded. It is often unnecessary to take additional steps when recommending drugs beyond licence.
- Patients, carers and healthcare professionals need accurate, clear and specific information that meets their needs. The Association for Palliative Medicine and the British Pain Society should work in conjunction with pharmaceutical companies to design accurate information for patients and their carers about the use of drugs beyond licence.
- Health professionals involved in prescribing, dispensing and administering drugs beyond licence should select those drugs that offer the best balance of benefit against harm for any given patient.
- Health professionals should inform, change and monitor their practice with regard to drugs used beyond licence in the light of evidence from audit and published research.
- The Department of Health should work with health professionals and the pharmaceutical industry to enable and encourage the extension of product licences where there is evidence of benefit in circumstances of defined clinical need.
- Organisations providing palliative care and pain management services should support therapeutic practices that are underpinned by evidence and advocated by a responsible body of professional opinion.
- There is urgent need for the Department of Health to assist healthcare professionals to formulate national frameworks, guidelines and standards for the use of drugs beyond licence. The British Pain Society and the Association for Palliative Medicine should work with the Department of Health, NHS trusts, voluntary organisations and the pharmaceutical industry to design accurate information for staff, patients and their carers in clinical areas where drugs are used off label. Practical support is necessary to facilitate and expedite surveillance and audit which are essential to develop this initiative (British Pain Society, 2005).

The objectives of the project are to ensure that:

- Common symptoms experienced at the end of life are anticipated (e.g. pain, nausea, excessive secretions and agitation).
- Small quantities of appropriate medicines are prescribed for the patient and stored in a special container, within the patient's home.
- Carers and patients are reassured that the prescribed medicines have been prescribed 'just in case', and may not be needed.

There are few identified risks, as decision making is made within the multidisciplinary team (MDT), however:

- As with all drugs open to abuse, medicine supplies in patients' houses may be subject to misuse.
- Patients and/or carers may misinterpret anticipatory prescribing as provision for euthanasia, or it may cause increased anxiety that death is near.

Nevertheless, it is felt that good communication, action planning and explanatory leaflets will allay fears.

Recommended drugs, sufficient supply to cover at least a weekend, are:

- Diamorphine for pain, e.g. 10 mg × 5 ampoules.
- Cyclizine, haloperidol or levomepromazine for nausea and vomiting.
- Midazolam for agitation.
- Glycopyrrolate or hyoscine hydrobromide for respiratory secretions.
- Oral lorazepam tablets.

However, it is important to recognise that prescriptions and the medicines supplied should reflect the individual needs of each patient. For example, in the case of a patient with a potential intestinal obstruction, metoclopramide could be prescribed in anticipation of vomiting without colic.

A three-step process for issuing and using a 'just in case' box has been identified:

Step 1 – Prescribing

- The district nurse/specialist palliative care nurse and GPs will identify relevant patients ahead of need.
- The prescribing practitioner will prescribe appropriate medications on form FP10, highlighting that they are for a 'just in case box'.
- A sufficient supply of drugs should be prescribed to cover a weekend and bank holiday.
- The prescriber will write the drugs up in the patient's notes and on the drug administration sheet.
- The district nurse/GP/specialist nurse will explain the purpose of the just in case box, stating that all items are for professional use only.
- The prescription will be dispensed by the pharmacy or the dispensing GP according to accepted dispensing practice.
- The prescription will need to be collected by the patient/carer or patient's representative in the usual way.

Step 2 – Use of the box and safekeeping

- The prescribed medications, information leaflets and symptom-control guidelines will be packed in the patient's home by the district nurse.
- Receipt of the just in case medication will be recorded by the district nurse in the patient's notes to inform other visiting health professionals.
- The district nurse will complete an out-of-hours handover form, if necessary, stating that a just in case box has been placed in the home.
- A note will also be placed at the patient's medical practice highlighting that the drugs are situated in the home.

- The district nurse will check the contents of the box and all expiry dates monthly, or more frequently if visiting on a regular basis.
- Patients' needs are subject to change, therefore a review must take place monthly, or after any change in condition.
- If any items are used, the healthcare professional should make a record in the patient's notes.
- If any items are used, the GP must be informed – this will activate a review of the patient and of the patient's prescription needs.
- A pro forma should be completed when items are used from the box to record purposes. The data could be used in future audits.

Step 3 – Safe disposal

- Following the patient's death, the GP or district nurse must inform the relevant dispensing pharmacy.
- All unused drugs should be returned to the pharmacy by the family/carer.
- The box should be returned to the district nursing team.
- Any controlled drugs from the just in case box should be handled according to local policy.

Once the project has been piloted and evaluated, it is envisaged that just in case box schemes will be introduced throughout Lincolnshire

ACCOUNTABILITY IN PRACTICE

Accountable practice is the bedrock on which professional nursing is based. Registered nurses are guided and have to abide by the Code of Professional Conduct (Nursing and Midwifery Council, 2002) in all areas of practice. The NMC is considering the benefits of a stand-alone booklet detailing new legislation around controlled drugs, following the fourth report of the Shipman Inquiry (2004), *The Regulation of Controlled Drugs in the Community*. The NMC recognises that certain areas of practice potentially present a greater risk to the public; one of these high-risk areas is palliative care.

The Nursing and Midwifery Council is an integral part of the Drugs Advisory Group, which has been set up to advise the Department of Health (England) and the Home Office on implementing the government's response to the Shipman Inquiry and the impact this will have on prescribing controlled drugs. The Drugs Advisory Group's responsibilities are provided in Table 9.11.

PALLIATIVE CARE TODAY

Multidisciplinary working is a key component of effective palliative care, reinforced by the National Council for Hospices and Specialist Palliative Care Services (1995) in their publication entitled *Information Exchange*.

Table 9.11   The Drugs Advisory Group's responsibilities

- Overseeing the controlled drugs work programme.
- Advising on how best to involve stakeholders with the implementation.
- Advising on how to encourage and implement change.
- Identifying the key challenges for the implementation of the government's response and recommending ways of addressing these.
- Identifying how best to communicate the progress of this work to stakeholders.

The most important benefit of multidisciplinary working is that it promotes enhanced clinical standards through the facilitation of the exchange of knowledge, experiences and views (Woolf et al., 2005). Team working in palliative care also provides mutual support for individuals working in an area of care that can be very draining, especially when caring for high numbers of dying people.

In delivering high-quality palliative care, all departments or team members need to work seamlessly to ensure that a quality service is provided. The benefits of close team working cannot be overemphasised when caring for vulnerable people with distressing conditions. When people are diagnosed with cancer or other life-limiting illness, they are frequently required to take regular medication to control their symptoms. This can be quite an onerous task for someone when they are feeling unwell due to a variety of symptoms, which may include anxiety, pain, nausea and vomiting and fatigue. Generally people take analgesia infrequently for headaches or musculo-skeletal problems.

When a person has a chronic symptom such as pain with acute exacerbations, there is a need to educate and inform them to take their analgesia regularly rather than intermittently; this may be outside their normal mode of practice or under-standing. Clear explanations, reassurance, close monitoring and support ensure that new ways of taking medication are maximised to their full benefit.

Prescribing for this group of patients should be undertaken by skilled team members with the appropriate qualifications and a robust level of underpinning knowledge based on education, experience and a comprehensive assessment of the individual patient.

CONCLUSION

As we move to a more patient-led NHS, it is imperative that we continue to develop a service that is flexible and responsive to the individual. At the same time, it needs to be realised that developing a cost-effective service, lowering morbidity, reducing hospital admissions and the length of hospital stays are all part of the NHS reforms. All of these factors are the drivers of non-medical prescribing in palliative care.

People with palliative care needs are at their most vulnerable and we must ensure as nurses that their experiences are as positive as they can possibly be.

Moreover, good practice in palliative care needs to continually expand to encompass patients with diseases other than cancer. This has implications for developing a more sophisticated approach to the management of pain and other symptoms. An approach that encompasses clinical skills built on solid foundations of knowledge, research and experience in association with non-medicinal prescribing expertise will result in a practitioner who will benefit patients with palliative care needs.

REFERENCES

Ahmedzai, S, Bennett, M, & Hardman, C (2002) Scientific evidence and expert clinical opinion for the use of off-licence agents. In Hillier, R, Finlay, I & Miles, A (eds) *The Effective Management of Cancer Pain* (2nd edition). London: Aesculpius Medical Press.

Amas, C & Allen, M (2005) How a just in case approach can improve out of hours palliative care. *The Pharmaceutical Journal* **275**(7356): 22–23.

Back, I (2001) *Palliative Medicine Handbook* (3rd edition). Cardiff: BPM Books.

Barton, R (2005) Managing complications in cancer. In Faull, C, Carter, Y & Daniels, L (eds) *Handbook of Palliative Care*. Oxford: Blackwell Science.

Bell, L & Sikora, K (1996) Complementary therapies and cancer care. *Complementary Therapies in Nursing and Midwifery* **2**: 57–58.

Bennett, M, Forbes, K & Faull, C (2005) The principles of pain management. In Faull, C, Carter, Y & Daniels, L (eds) *Handbook of Palliative Care*. Oxford: Blackwell Science.

Bredin, M, Corner, J, Krishnasamy, M, Plant, H, Bailey, C & A'Hern, R (1999) Multicentre randomised control trial of nursing intervention for breathlessness in patients with lung cancer. *British Medical Journal* **318**(7188): 901–904.

British Pain Society (2005) *The Use of Drugs Beyond Licence in Palliative Care and Pain Management*. www.palliative-medicine.org. [accessed 4 March 2006]

Cancer Research UK (2006) http://www.cancerhelp.org [accessed 20 April 2006].

Castledine, G (1992) The advanced practitioner. *Nursing* **5**(7): 14–15.

Clarke, D, Seymour, J, Douglas, H, Bath, P, Beech, N, Corner, J, Halliday, D, Hughes, P, Haviland, D, Hughes, P, Haviland, J, Normand, C, Marples, R, Skilbeck, J & Webb, T (2002) Clinical nurse specialists in palliative care. Part 2: Explaining diversity in the organisation and costs of Macmillan nursing services. *Palliative Medicine* **16**: 375–385.

Cutts, B (1999) Autonomy and the developing role of the clinical nurse specialist. *British Journal of Nursing* **8**(22): 1502–1506.

Daut, RL, Cleeland, CS & Flanery, RC (1983) Development of the Wisconsin Brief Pain Questionnaire to assess pain in cancer and other diseases. *Pain* **17**: 197–210.

Davies, A (2002) The assessment and measurement of physical pain. In Hillier, R, Finlay, I & Miles, A (eds) *The Effective Management of Cancer Pain* (2nd edition). London: Aesculpius Medical Press.

Doyle, D (1997) *Dilemmas and Directions: The Future of Specialist Palliative Care*. London: National Council for Hospices and Specialist Palliative Care Services.

Fishman, B, Pasternak, S, Wallenstein, SL, Houde, RW, Holland, JC & Foley, KM (1987) The Memorial Pain Assessment Card: A valid instrument for the evaluation of cancer pain. *Cancer* **60**: 1151–1158.

Froggatt, K (2000) *Palliative Care Education in Nursing Homes*. London: Macmillan Cancer Relief.

Gomes, B & Higginson, J (2006) Factors influencing death at home in terminally ill patients with cancer; systematic review. *British Medical Journal* **332**(7540): 515–521.

Heath, ML (1997) The use of pharmacology in pain management. In Thomas, VN (ed.) *Pain, its Nature and Management*. London: Baillière Tindall.

Hopkins, Y (2006) *Accessing Palliative Care Medication*. East Lincolnshire Primary Care Trust. Unpublished paper.

Hoskin, PJ (2004) Radiotherapy in symptom management. In Doyle, D, Hanks, G, Cherny, N & Calman, K (eds) *Oxford Handbook of Palliative Medicine*. Oxford: Oxford University Press.

Kohn, M (1999) *Complementary Therapies in Cancer Care*. London: Macmillan Cancer Relief.

Latter, S, Maben, J, Myall, M, Courtenay, M, Young, A, & Dunn, N (2004) *An Evaluation of Extended Formulary Independent Nurse Prescribing*. London: Policy Research Programme, Department of Health.

McCaffery, M, Ferrell, B, O'Neil-Page, E & Lester, M (1990) Nurses' knowledge of opioid analgesic drugs and psychological dependence. *Cancer Nursing* **13**(1): 21–27.

McQuay, HJ, Tramer, M, Nye, BA, Carroll, D, Wiffen, PJ & Moore, RA (1996) Pain. In Back, I (ed.) *Palliative Medicine Handbook* (3rd edition). Cardiff: BPM Books.

Melzac, R (1975) The McGill Pain Questionnaire: major properties and scoring methods. *Pain* **1**: 277–299.

Merrison, A (1979) *Royal Commission on the National Health Service*. London: The Stationery Office.

National Council for Hospices and Specialist Palliative Care Services (1995) *Information Exchange*, No. 13. London: NCHSPCS.

National Council for Hospices and Specialist Palliative Care Services (2003) *National Guidelines for the Use of Complementary Therapies in Supportive and Palliative Care*. London: The National Council for Palliative Care and The Prince of Wales Foundation for Integrated Health Care.

Nursing and Midwifery Council (2002) *Code of Professional Conduct*. London: Nursing and Midwifery Council.

Nursing and Midwifery Council (2004) *Guidelines for the Administration of Medicines*. London: Nursing and Midwifery Council.

Pavis, H & Wilcock, A (2001) Prescribing of drugs for use outside their licence in palliative care: A survey of specialists in the United Kingdom. *British Medical Journal* **323**(7311): 484–485.

Robbins, M (1998) *Evaluating Palliative Care*. Oxford: Oxford Medical Publications.

Shipman Enquiry (2004) Forth Report: The Regulation of Controlled Drugs in the Community. London: The Stationery Office.

Sinnott, C (1997) Nerve pain. In Kaye, P (ed.) *Tutorials in Palliative Medicine*. Northampton: EPL Publications.

Stannard, C & Booth, S (2004) *Pain* (2nd edition). London: Churchill Livingstone.

Syrett, E & Taylor, J (2003) Non-pharmacological management of breathlessness: A collaborative nurse–physiotherapist approach. *International Journal of Palliative Nursing* **9**(4): 150–156.

Thompson, J & Filshie, J (1993) Transcutaneous electrical nerve stimulation (TENS) and acupuncture. In Doyle, D, Hanks, G, Cherny, N & Calman, K (eds) *Oxford Handbook of Palliative Medicine*. Oxford: Oxford University Press.

Tiernan, E (1997) The use of steroids. In Kaye, P (ed.) *Tutorials in Palliative Care.* Northampton: EPL Publications.

Watson, M, Lucas, C, Hoy, A & Back, I (2005) The management of pain. In Doyle, D, Hanks, G, Cherny, N & Calman, K (eds) *Oxford Handbook of Palliative Care: Part 1.* Oxford: Oxford University Press.

Wilcock, A, Manderson, C, Weller, R, Walker, G, Carr, D, Carey, A, Broadhurst, D & Mew, J (2003) Does aromatherapy massage benefit patients with cancer attending a specialist palliative care day centre? *Palliative Medicine* **8**(4): 287–290.

Woolf, R, Carter, Y & Faull, C (2005) Palliative care: The team, the services and the need for care. In Faull, C, Carter, Y & Daniels, L (eds) *Handbook of Palliative Care.* Oxford: Blackwell Science.

10 The Mental Health Perspective

STUART KENNEDY

In keeping with the rest of this book, this chapter is designed to instil confidence in the reader as to how much they already know, while encouraging deeper reflection on some of the more troublesome elements of being a mental health non-medical prescriber.

As a mental health nurse (MHN) and non-medical prescriber, it is my intention to review best practice concisely in specific clinical areas, while examining how concordance can be maintained. As such, this should support, rather than replace, more comprehensive texts on prescribing.

Key areas covered in this chapter are depression, bipolar disorder, schizophrenia/psychosis, Alzheimer's disease and substance misuse. Medication choice is discussed, but this is not a comprehensive guide to psychotropic medication, nor a dedicated prescribing guideline. These should be sought elsewhere. Students requiring more detailed and specific exploration of individual specialities may wish to supplement this chapter with additional reading. The chapter closes with a brief examination of some of the ethical concerns that mental health prescribers may face in promoting and sustaining concordance.

THE ESSENCE OF MODERN MENTAL HEALTHCARE PRACTICE

> "Experience increases our wisdom, but doesn't reduce our follies"
>
> (Josh Billings)

There are approximately 91 million working days lost per year in the UK due to mental illness, with depression set to be the second most common disease worldwide by 2020 (Thomas and Morris, 2000). Medication for a significant number of people with mental health problems is an integral part of a treatment plan and for many is capable of providing tangible relief from often disabling symptoms.

Mental health nursing is currently a particularly heterogeneous profession, involving work in a broader range of specialities than ever before. Focus can be

Towards Prescribing Practice. Edited by J. McKinnon.
© 2007 John Wiley & Sons, Ltd.

seen on particular populations or therapeutic models, and the *NSF for Mental Health* (Department of Health, 1999) set out a wide range of proposals for mental healthcare to extend this further. These include establishing assertive outreach teams, increasing the use of psychological and psychosocial interventions, and a focus on primary care.

The past 20 years or so have seen significant steps in addressing the custodial nature of our not too distant past. Great strides are evident in terms of improving information given to clients and involving them in their care. There has also been a move towards embracing the need to clearly define and measure the success of interventions offered.

An early study by Brown and Fowler (1979) divides the work of MHNs into high- and low-visibility functions. High-visibility functions are those technical, tangible skills of value to an employer, such as the giving of medications and injections. Low-visibility functions, however, are those 'softer', less quantifiable aspects of the interpersonal relationship with the client. These are often only really noted by their absence. As such, this still remains a useful model for considering the functions of mental health nursing.

The focus of mental healthcare practice is clearly more than just the treatment of a collection of symptoms, and should seek to enable an overview of the totality of the individual, and those factors pertinent to progress and wellbeing. An awareness of the social domain, cultural factors, lifestyle choices and beliefs is necessary to any MHN offering any treatment. The phenomenological construct underpinning this is by its very nature inherently first person in focus, contrasting strongly with a third person scientific model in which diagnostic categories and prescriptive models of treatment are commonplace. Mullen, cited by Roberts (2005), argues for a more phenomenological approach to people with mental illness, pointing out that attempts to categorise mental illness often fail to take account of the subtleties and variation from patient to patient. He goes on to suggest that:

> identifying and addressing the problems that the sufferer, rather than the psychiatrist, perceives creates an understanding of each person's condition which is far more scientific, humane and effective than a blanket diagnosis.

Although a dilemma clearly exists in helping individuals who lack insight that the behaviour they exhibit is a problem to others, this quote represents a reasonable essence of MH nursing.

MH nursing has travelled quite some distance in a relatively short space of time, adapting to approaches that underline the centrality of the client in decisions about their care and treatment. The asylum system of care, the introduction of pharmacological interventions, the subsequent introduction of psychosocial models, national frameworks defining best care for key populations (NSF) and an increasing awareness of the value of practice being based on evidence are a few notable landmarks. It is against this backdrop of ideological change and rapidly changing roles that non-medical prescribing in mental health sits.

Individual mental health practitioners choosing to take up the prescribing role will encounter different issues and priorities when negotiating their first step. Empowerment, choice and involvement are undoubtedly valid guiding principles, but alone or unexplored offer little direction. Prescribing practice in mental health can be beset by many issues and potential dilemmas relating to concordance.

PRESCRIBING IN MENTAL HEALTHCARE

Everyday prescribing practice can be beset by many issues and potential dilemmas. Examples of these include the management of complex/multiple needs; the amount, type and depth of medication-related information offered to patients; and balancing patient lifestyle and choice with evidence of best practice.

The thread running through each of the subsequent therapeutic themes is that of enabling recovery or maintenance through safe, evidence-based prescribing practice against a backdrop of patient involvement and choice.

DEPRESSION

Depression can refer to a wide spectrum of mood disorders, for the most part characterised by lack of enjoyment and interest (anhedonia), low mood and often numerous biological and emotional symptoms, with daily functioning often affected. It remains the most common psychiatric disorder, with prevalence estimated (including mixed depression and anxiety) at 98/1000 (NICE, 2004). Causes are multifactorial and include gender (twice the rate in women compared to men), age (equal incidence in young adults and the old) and adverse social and economic circumstances. Pharmacological interventions for depression can be highly effective, but are crucially not the only treatments available and are not necessary in every case. Correctly used and appropriately promoted medications may enhance the effectiveness of other treatments; for example a patient too depressed to talk will derive little benefit from psychotherapy.

Drug Treatments for Depression

Antidepressant drugs fall into a number of types, such as tricyclics, SSRIs and MAOIs. Their mode of action correlates with alterations in the concentration of catecholamines and/or serotonin in the central nervous system.

The tricyclics, ostensibly imipramine and its subsequent allies, are chemically related to the neuroleptic drug chlorpromazine. Tricyclics block to varying degrees the re-uptake of serotonin and noradrenaline into the nerve cells from which they are released. Their anti-cholinergic side effects are well known, including constipation, blurred vision and dry mouth, with some studies suggesting they also affect memory, concentration and intellectual performance. Their anti-histaminic action often induces drowsiness and sedation. In addition, their adverse effect on cardiac function makes them dangerous in overdose.

For over 30 years tricyclics formed the mainstay of pharmacological treatment for depression. Selective serotonin re-uptake inhibitors (SSRIs) were introduced in the early 1990s. Serotonin plays a key role in mood, sleep, appetite, memory, sexual desire and the perception of pain. SSRIs all vary in specific chemical structure and elimination half lives, although their effects are broadly similar. Some are more likely to induce nausea (fluvoxamine), some more likely to produce sedating effects (paroxetine) and some more activating (fluoxetine). Generally, the side effect profile of SSRIs is far less unpleasant and debilitating than tricyclics. Most prominent among negative effects of this class are that libido and sexual performance may be inhibited and that some feel the effect on mood to be 'flattening'. In terms of the latter, affective flattening may be an improvement for a severely depressed person, but for a mildly depressed person is far from life enriching.

The late 1990s saw the introduction of newer agents, either targeting serotonin and noradrenaline together (SNRIs), such as venlafaxine and more recently dulox-etine, or just targeting noradrenaline (NARIs), such as reboxetine. Focusing on the noradrenergic route may produce improvement in depressed people whose main symptom is anergia or lack of drive and motivation. However, the activating effects of NARIs such as reboxetine may not always be desirable, particularly where anxiety or insomnia are key symptoms. Antidepressants such as mirtazepine, which have action on a wide range of serotonin receptors, may be useful where insomnia and/or loss of appetite are key symptoms. Venlafaxine is now avoided in people with known heart disease and only prescribed by specialist mental health professionals.

A further option for treatment-resistant or 'atypical' depression exists within the MAOI group of drugs, discovered by chance in a US veterans' hospital in the 1950s. The hypertensive effects of combining these with tyramine-rich foods are well known and need not be reiterated here. Caution should be exercised in combining MAOIs with other antidepressants, particularly SSRIs, as this increases the likeli-hood of potentially fatal serotonin syndrome. The early MAOIs have since been eclipsed by the selective and reversible moclobemide, which is reportedly useful in social phobia, irritability, panic disorder and obsessive compulsive disorder.

Treating Depression Effectively

In 2004 NICE issued guidance for the management of depression in primary and secondary care (NICE, 2004). This describes a stepped approach to recognising and treating depression. It points to the need to recognise that antidepressants are not the only treatment available for depression and to consider carefully both the severity of the condition and the patient's choice. This guidance underlines the importance of considering antidepressants for people with moderate/severe depression, but also offering psychological interventions to those who feel uncomfortable with the medication route. Taking account of patients' views when deciding treatment is essential in achieving concordance and successful outcome. Preferences may depend not only on how the prescriber presents information, but also on the patient's previous experience and views of friends, family and/or the media. A thorough assessment of a client's presenting difficulties is the baseline to discussing how these may be resolved.

For example, a person presenting with mild depression should not be offered antidepressants as first-line treatment, as the possibility of side effects may outweigh any potential advantage. Alternative sources of help should be offered first, such as brief psychological interventions, unless such approaches have already proven unsuccessful or there is a history of moderate/severe depression. Where the presentation is one of moderate depression, the potential benefits of antidepressants should be discussed frankly with the patient. NICE recommends antidepressants being offered routinely to all patients with moderate depression, as they are as effective as psychological therapies but, crucially, cheaper. Where a psychological therapy is chosen over antidepressants for moderate depression, CBT is the approach of choice as individuals completing treatment are less likely to relapse over the following year (MeReC, 2005).

Depending on the severity of the depression, follow-up should usually be within the first two weeks, continuing fortnightly for around four to six weeks. It is essential during this period not only to monitor progress and measure improvement, but also to ensure that medication is being tolerated. Adverse effects within the first two weeks, if unchecked, are likely to lead not only to poor concordance, but also to disinclination to try alternative antidepressants. Consideration is also necessary of the likelihood of a patient deciding to abruptly stop taking an antidepressant (for whatever reason).

Tricyclics are far more likely to be stopped by the patient because of side effects than are SSRIs. Tricyclics require careful, slow titration from a low starting dose if chosen, as there is a delay in achieving antidepressant effect, and it is more likely that a patient will suffer side effects before any benefit. Where a tricyclic is chosen, NICE recommends lofepramine. Clearly, where a patient is considered to be at risk of suicide tricyclics would not be considered due to toxicity in overdose. If sudden withdrawal is thought likely, some SSRIs are considered safer. These are fluoxetine and citalopram, which both carry a smaller likelihood of withdrawal effects than paroxetine. Venlafaxine now carries requirements for monitoring due to the risk to individuals with heart disease. These include ECG and BP measurement prior to starting, and BP monitoring during treatment. Venlafaxine should be avoided in patients with known cardiac problems.

Claims are often made that particular drugs will produce a faster response. Although some therapeutic effects may arise more quickly, such as the hypnotic effects of mirtazepine, there is little conclusive evidence that one antidepressant will work more quickly than another. A relevant question from anyone taking an antidepressant is how quickly they can expect to feel 'better'. According to Dunner (2003), 70 % of people can expect to feel better in some way within six to ten weeks. This is of course very subjective and does not necessarily mean symptom free.

Managing potential side effects presents a problem in many areas of mental health, not least among patients with depression. A patient who is prepared for initial side effects may be far more likely to weigh up the potential benefit and continue taking the drug. It is essential that the patient understands and is willing to endure some of the possible effects in order to improve their depression. Among the most bothersome are sexual dysfunction and weight gain. One study identified that up to 70 % of patients taking an SSRI reported sexual dysfunction (cited in Marano, 2003). This is somewhat higher than the data suggests. Some SSRIs may do better in this area, such as mirtazepine, but this, coincidentally, may also be more likely to lead to weight gain.

The mental health prescriber's skills at negotiation are key to promoting concordance with antidepressants. A patient should be informed of the delay in onset and the need to remain on the drug beyond the first three months. A first episode should be treated for four to six months after recovery before reviewing the need for continued treatment. For chronic depression (i.e. lasting more than two years) treatment may be necessary for two years after remission. Maintenance therapy is recommended in those with three or more episodes in the last five years, five or more episodes in total, and those with persistent risk factors. Maintenance treatment should be continued at the same dose used to treat the acute episode for at least five years and possibly indefinitely.

Certain populations will require special consideration. Elderly patients may be more likely to experience antimuscarinic side effects from TCAs and these may not be drugs of first choice. Likewise, those operating machinery or driving should be warned of antihistaminic effects such as sedation from TCAs. All people taking antidepressants should be advised to exercise some caution in driving, particularly during initiation and dose increases. In younger populations fluoxetine is currently considered the safest choice, with sertraline or citalopram as second-line therapies. Tricyclics are not advised in this age group due to potential side effects and toxicity in overdose. Venlafaxine, mirtazepine and paroxetine are also not recommended in this age group. Although not licensed for use in patients under the age of 18, caution is advised against prescribing for patients under the age of 18 with a major depressive disorder. The CSM advises that paroxetine, venlafaxine, sertraline, fluvoxamine, citalopram and escitalopram should not be given due to a possible increased risk of self-harm and suicidal thoughts (MHRA, 2003). Combining CBT with an antidepressant has been shown to enhance outcome.

Table 10.1   Depression: Magic bullets

- Mild depression: brief psychological interventions are preferred option (unless history of moderate/severe depression).
- Moderate depression: antidepressants and CBT show roughly equal benefit (although antidepressants are crucially cheaper).
- For 1st episode: treatment is suggested for 4–6 months post recovery, for chronic depression up to 2 years, and for 3+ episodes in 5 years or total of 5+ episodes in at least 5 years.
- SSRIs are preferred to tricyclics. Where a tricyclic is used lofepramine has best toxicity profile.
- Tricyclics should not be used where there is assessed suicide risk.
- Close monitoring during the first 2 weeks when side effects are more common may promote continued concordance.

Patient vignette Ruth

Ruth is a 42-year-old social worker, referred by her GP. She has suffered depression in the past and has returned to work after three months, having been treated with CBT offered by a GP counsellor. She has presently lost interest, become irritable and found it difficult to concentrate, and is absent from work. She complains of loss of appetite and low mood, and during the interview became tearful, stating that her sleep is very poor and that she has started drinking whisky at bedtime to help with this. A diagnosis of major depression has been made and she has been prescribed lofepramine for the past six weeks. She denies suicidal thoughts, but states that she is desperate to feel better and often wishes she were dead. What factors are relevant in reviewing and discussing treatments?

BIPOLAR DISORDER

Bipolar disorder is a term adopted in 1980 to replace what was previously referred to as manic depression. This was largely intended as a means of removing the previous associations held with psychosis, which although present in some are not necessary to confirm diagnosis. According to ICD 10 (see glossary), bipolar affective disorder is:

> characterised by two or more episodes in which the patient's mood and activity levels are significantly disturbed, this disturbance consisting on some occasions of an elevation of mood and increased energy and activity ... and on others of a lowering of mood and decreased energy and activity.

Essentially, bipolar illness is likely to be characterised by periods of both energised and depressed mood states, with fluctuation or 'cycling' between them, affecting energy levels, sleep, appetite, thinking ability and social rhythm. Bipolar disorder (type 2) has a prevalence of 1.3 % in the adult population in the UK (NICE, 2003a). The aetiology is a complex combination of psychological and biological factors, with predisposing factors such as childhood experience seen as at least partly contributory, and levels of social support and/or hostility and criticism being relevant to triggering episodes. Genetic studies have shown a strong inheritance rate with identical twins (43 % compared to 6 % in non-identical twins). The fact that this is not 100 % underlines the likelihood of other environmental and psychological factors. Mania can be triggered by giving birth, sleep deprivation and certain physical illnesses such as multiple sclerosis.

Bipolar disorder can and commonly does co-exist with other mental health problems such as anxiety, substance misuse and eating disorders. The estimates of co-existence with substance misuse vary widely depending on criteria used (abuse or dependence), and it remains unclear how much is contributory and how much is a result of the illness. People with bipolar disorder are approximately twice as likely to commit suicide as those suffering major depression. The goals of treatment are essentially to help an individual achieve the highest level of functioning possible and to minimise/avoid relapse.

Treating Bipolar Disorder Effectively

A major challenge facing the health professional in attempting to help someone with bipolar disorder is continuing to promote choice and concordance against the backdrop of changing client focus and commitment. The emphasis is on the effective long-term management of a condition and in reducing the re-occurrence of symptoms. In common with many mental health difficulties, the treatment methods incorporate both pharmacological and psychological strands. Unlike depression, however, there is a necessary and crucial dependence on medications as the primary method of symptom control, usually a mood stabiliser or an antipsychotic. The goals of the mental health professional are essentially to ensure that a strong therapeutic alliance exists, providing education, anticipating, monitoring and reducing stressors, early identification of relapse and the continued promotion of medication concordance. Although medications can reduce the duration of acute manic and depressive episodes significantly, the risk of relapse remains, and the effect of persistent symptoms on a patient's quality of life can be marked.

Bipolar disorder remains one of the least comprehensively researched areas of mental health; recruitment to trials may favour individuals with milder manifestations of the illness, limiting generalisability (Scottish Intercollegiate Guidelines Network, 2005). During a manic episode or when a person is severely depressed, the mental health professional may at times find themselves having little choice but to arrange hospital admission in order to regain stability.

Antipsychotics represent the mainstay of treatment and, as with psychosis, are generally the measure against which new agents are compared. Lithium was found to have a medical use by Australian physician John Cade, who discovered that patients with manic depressive illness experienced relief from their symptoms when treated with lithium carbonate (Cade, 1949). Its qualities in preventing recurrent manic episodes are well known and it has for many years been regarded as the 'gold standard'. RCT data supports its claimed efficacy in preventing manic and depressive relapse, both immediately post-diagnosis and prophylactically, and in reducing the rate of suicide. An essential component of lithium treatment is the maintenance of therapeutic plasma lithium concentration and the monitoring of thyroid and renal function. Usual recommendations are that lithium concentration should be maintained in the range of 0.4–1.0 mmol/L (*BNF*), monitored during maintenance every three months. The lower end of this range is advised for maintenance and elderly patients. Thyroid and renal function should be checked six monthly. Dose-related side effects include weight gain, polydipsia, polyuria, tremor and cognitive slowing.

Concordance is a crucial issue in lithium therapy, not only in terms of preventing relapse, but also because of the drug's narrow therapeutic window and potential for life-threatening toxicity (concentration over 1.5 mmol/L). In addition, recent studies suggest that withdrawal from lithium may result in a high risk of relapse (Cavanagh et al., 2004). Where patients continue to experience manic episodes despite high serum lithium levels, augmentation with an antipsychotic or additional mood stabiliser should be considered. Caution is also necessary in terms of inter-actions with sodium-depleting drugs such as diuretics (particularly thiazides). In terms of long-term use the *BNF* recommends:

> the need for continued therapy should be assessed regularly and patients should be maintained on lithium after 3–5 years only if benefit persists.

Anticonvulsant medications, particularly carbamazepine and valproic acid, are also used. Carbamazepine may be used in patients unresponsive to lithium and demonstrates good efficacy in helping patients with rapid cycling episodes. It has equivalent efficacy to lithium at preventing relapse over six weeks to three years (Lusznat et al., 1988; Okuma et al., 1990; Coxhead et al., 1992; Griel and Kliendienst, 1999; Kliendienst and Greil, 2002). Like other tricyclic compounds some adverse anticholinergic effects are possible, and there are a number of contraindications, which include anticoagulants, CNS depressants, oestrogens, vera-pamil, erythromycin, cimetidine, grapefruit juice and alcohol. The higher potential for interactions necessitates slow dose increase and/or discontinuation. Valproic acid is also licensed for the treatment of patients unresponsive to lithium. This should be avoided as much as possible in women of child-bearing potential.

Older antipsychotics such as haloperidol are often given for maintenance and prevention of bipolar disorder, although the evidence for using conventional/typical antipsychotics is weak and the likelihood of side effects high (National Collaborating Centre for Mental Health, 2006). Atypical antipsychotics, however, have demon-strated efficacy in treating both acute episodes and maintenance and may often be used in combination with a mood stabiliser to treat severe episodes. Olanzepine, risperidone and quetiapine are used, with current evidence favouring olanzepine for patients with severe manic symptoms (NICE, 2003a). Benzodiazepines are also used in the short term in acutely agitated states.

Mood stabilisers and antipsychotics are generally more effective at treating manic symptoms. Antidepressants may be used to treat periods of depression, although they do carry the danger of inducing mania. For this reason, concomi-tant treatment with mood stabilisers is strongly advised in patients with recur-rent depression (Goodwin et al., 2003). Antidepressants should be stopped after successful treatment of any depressive episode. There is little RCT data to suggest any particular antidepressant agent, but tricyclics are more likely to trigger manic episodes (Amsterdam and Brunswick, 2003; Goldberg and Truman, 2003), and the known tolerability and safety profile of SSRIs would support this as a treatment choice.

Special consideration is required for treating older people with bipolar disorder. Although the principles and goals of treatment are essentially the same, the prescriber should be mindful of the reduced capacity for drug clearance and the potential consequences of adverse effects. Close monitoring of physical state and polypharmacy is essential alongside regular review. Lower doses are often required in this population, and in terms of lithium the lower end of the serum lithium level is desirable. ECT has been used in some cases of treatment-resistant mania, but is weakly supported by evidence (NICE, 2003b).

Contraception, pregnancy and lactation also require careful management in those with bipolar disorder. Some antipsychotics with known effects on prolactin levels may reduce female fertility, while conversely women taking carbomazepine are at an increased risk of contraceptive failure, requiring further adjustment of contraceptive treatment/methods. During pregnancy the risk of foetal abnormalities is increased two- to threefold by the use of anticonvulsant drugs. The risk of the use of lithium during pregnancy is variable, with early studies pointing to increased risk of foetal abnormality, and recent evidence refuting the scale of this risk (Yonkers et al., 2004). Given the potential for major disruption of other body systems during pregnancy (vomiting, oedema, thyroid dysfunction, gestational diabetes etc.), there remains a considerable risk to the mother and careful consideration of risk/benefit is necessary. Benzodiazepines carry an increased risk during the first trimester (Dolovich et al., 1998) and should be avoided. Although the risks generally from antidepressants are probably minimal, escitalopram, venlafaxine, reboxetine and mirtazepine are not considered safe during pregnancy (Scottish Intercollegiate Guidelines Network, 2005). Both benzodiazepines and lithium are excreted in breast milk, the potential affects of lithium toxicity on an infant being possible impairment of thyroid and renal function. All forms of antipsychotic drugs are excreted in breast milk, but data thus far does not suggest risk of toxicity or impaired development (Scottish Intercollegiate Guidelines Network, 2005).

In addition to medication, certain psychosocial interventions have been shown to promote mood stability, improve social functioning and reduce hospitalisation (Huxley et al., 2000) when used in combination with patient education and mood-stabilising medications. It is difficult to gain any definitive data on specific approaches that can be generalised. Although data lacks generalisability, evidence suggests the addition of CBT to pharmacological treatment to be more beneficial than pharmacological treatment alone in bipolar type 1 disorder (National Collaborating Centre for Mental Health, 2006). There may of course be some overlap between many psychosocial interventions where the focus is on medication adherence, detection of early warning signs and seeking help (Gonzalez-Pinto et al., 2004).

There are many variables that may in part trigger severe mood changes, not least among these being altered sleep pattern. Although possibly not pertinent to all cases, mood charting as developed by Sachs (Manicdepressive.org, 2004) provides a valuable template for recording and monitoring some of the variables that may contribute to mood change. Patients and their families may also find this a valuable tool in retaining some control over the course of the illness.

Table 10.2 Bipolar disorder: Magic bullets

- For long-term treatment of bipolar disorder, lithium, olanzapine or valproate should be considered (choice dependent on previous response, known risks and patient choice).
- Plasma lithium concentrations of 0.4–1.0 mmol/L monitored 3 monthly during maintenance. Thyroid and renal function should be checked 6 monthly.
- Lithium has a narrow therapeutic window and high risk of fatal toxicity, so concordance, patient education and regular physical monitoring are essential. Use in pregnancy is not without risk to mother and it poses a risk to breast-fed infants.
- Anticonvulsant medications carbomazepine and valproic acid are useful choices for patients unresponsive to lithium, with greater evidence supporting valproate. Both carry significant risk during pregnancy.
- Antipsychotics can be used for those with severe manic symptoms or behavioural disturbance, and may augment existing mood stabilisers if presenting with severe mania. Most antipsychotics reduce fertility in women.
- Antidepressants carry potential risk of triggering manic episodes, so careful assessment is required of known patterns of mood changes. Where symptoms are predominantly depressive, consider psychological therapy before antidepressants. Where history of rapid cycling, avoid antidepressants. Commence antidepressant drug (if needed) once mood stabiliser treatment is stabilised.
- Where antidepressants are required, SSRIs are safest and best tolerated.
- Psychosocial interventions targeting medication adherence, adjustment/patient education and detection of early warning signs are probably most beneficial with evidence supporting CBT with medication.

PSYCHOSIS/SCHIZOPHRENIA

Schizophrenia as a diagnostic term can be traced back to Eugene Bleuler, who coined the phrase to more aptly describe what had previously been termed dementia praecox. It is unlikely to be a single disorder (a fact acknowledged by Bleuler, whose definition was plural rather than singular). It is a controversial disorder and many theories exist to explain the aetiology of psychosis (genetics, stress vulnerability model, social learning theories and the dopamine theory). Ultimately, it is difficult to extricate the relative effects of genes and environment and a safe assumption is that they are likely to act in combination. Effects are seen in cognition, behaviour and emotion and broadly characterised (as by Bleuler) as either positive or negative symptoms. Positive symptoms broadly refer to exaggerations of normal function such as hallucinations, delusions and thought disorder. Negative symptoms refer to loss of normal function such as emotional apathy, social withdrawal and low mood.

The DSM contains five subheadings of schizophrenia: catatonic type, disorganised type, paranoid type, residual type and undifferentiated type. It is worth noting that many of the positive symptoms of schizophrenia (psychosis) may occur in other disorders and attempts to further distinguish these have been made, most notably by Kurt Schneider (Schneider, 1959). His first-rank symptoms generally refer to positive symptoms of external control or thought broadcast. Prevalence is thought to be in the region of 0.5–1 % of the general population, with a slightly higher incidence in men. A small number will experience a single acute episode, and up to a quarter may recover completely (Wiersma et al., 1998).

Diagnosis may be complicated by concurrent drug or alcohol misuse, mania, depression, or where symptoms are transient, and remains a particularly contentious area. The anti-psychiatry movement, spearheaded by individuals such as Thomas Szasz and RD Laing, purporting that treatment of 'different' behaviours is essentially social control, gained some momentum in the 1970s, and although seen by some as essentially on the fringe, may have contributed to a questioning of some of the worst psychiatric abuses.

The dopamine theory is largely due to the work of Arvid Carlsson, a Swedish scientist whose discovery of dopamine in the 1950s led to L-dopa being used to enhance the effects of dopamine in Parkinson's disease, earning him the Nobel prize in 2000. It was, however, several years after the first antipsychotic was used that it was discovered that the antipsychotic effects were due to dopamine receptor blocking in the brain, leading to the theory that schizophrenia was due to excess dopamine activity in the brain.

The dopamine theory as it is currently understood suggests there to be an excess of dopamine in the mesolimbic pathway causing distortion of perception, language and behaviour. Low amounts of dopamine in the mesocortical pathway may result in many of the negative symptoms such as withdrawal and passivity. Early studies focused largely on D2, with more recent work looking closely at the significance of other brain neurotransmitter receptors including D4 (clozapine, a highly effective antipsychotic agent, blocks D4 efficiently).

Drug Treatments for Psychosis

Antipsychotics can be divided into two broad categories, typical (traditional, conventional) and atypical, although the exact definition of atypical is neither clear nor absolute (NICE, 2002; Drugs and Therapeutics Bulletin, 2004). Typical antipsychotics refer to drugs such as chlorpromazine, thioridazine, haloperidol and trifluperazine; atypical antipsychotics include clozapine, risperidone, olanzepine, quetiapine and amisulpiride.

The first antipsychotic drug, chlorpromazine, was discovered by chance by French anaesthesiologist and surgeon Henri Laborit, who was seeking a better pre-anaesthetic calming agent. The anti-histaminic effects he sought did indeed exist, but at the expense of unfortunate hypotensive properties, causing the drug to be abandoned as a pre-anaesthetic agent, but leading Dr Leborit to suggest that it might be of value in calming psychiatric patients. It was subsequently tested by Leborit in 1951 on psychotic patients, and fairly quickly declared a success. Agitation was noticeably reduced and thought processes were reportedly less chaotic. At a time when lobotomy had been common, this was initially seen as a great step forward, before ultimately being described as 'the chemical lobotomy'. Attempts to improve on chlorpromazine led to the development of imipramine, a structural analogue of chlorpromazine subsequently discovered to have antidepressant effects. Chlorpromazine, like many related tricyclic antidepressants, produced unwanted pharmacological actions, in turn leading to undesirable side effects. Pharmaceutical companies worked to develop further variations such as thioridazine.

Typical antipsychotics are commonly divided into low potency and high potency. These initial antipsychotics were labelled 'low potency' (potency referring to the ability to bind to a dopamine receptor) and tended to require relatively high doses to produce antipsychotic effects. While the antipsychotic effects were low potency, the anticholinergic and antihistaminic effects were high potency, tending to affect cognition, specifically concentration and memory. Generally high-potency typical antipsychotics are more likely to produce extrapyramidal side effects (EPS), but less likely to cause anticholinergic and antihistaminic effects. Low-potency antipsychotics conversely tend to produce less EPS, but more muscarinic effects. Therapeutically there is little to suggest vastly different profiles, but side effects do vary with each. Most common side effects among this group are dry mouth, EPS, muscle stiffness and cramps, tremors and weight gain. Despite being largely eclipsed by the newer agents, traditional antipsychotics have demonstrable efficacy at reducing psychotic symptoms in about 75 % of patients with acute schizophrenia, but have little effect on negative symptoms (Drugs and Therapeutics Bulletin, 1995; Kerwin, 1994).

There are a number of definitions of the term atypical, ranging from inability to produce catalepsy in lab animals, degree of selectivity for D2 and/or ratio of 5HT2:D2 blocking, and claimed benefits at treating negative symptomatology. The consensus seems to be that most of the drugs in this class are less likely to produce EPS or tardive dyskinesia, many do not raise prolactin levels (which all typicals do), and most reduce negative symptoms to a greater extent (Stahl, 1999).

The first atypical (clozapine) was produced in 1961 and provided the starting point for several subsequent atypicals. Clozapine was introduced in Europe in the 1970s and in 1975 voluntarily withdrawn by the manufacturer following reports of neutropenia and agranulocytosis. It was not seen again for a further 10 years, following a major study (Kane et al., 1988) when it was approved for use in treatment-resistant schizophrenia, requiring regular compulsory haematological monitoring. During the 1990s olanzapine, risperidone and quetiapine were introduced. Although all atypical by definition, their specific receptor-binding properties vary, possibly explaining much of the variation in clinical efficacy and side effect profile. The evidence largely suggests that atypicals have less affinity towards D2 and a greater affinity to D4, also affecting cholinergic and histaminic receptors.

The atypicals were variously hailed as 'wonder drugs' and as seeming to have less of a propensity for EPS and be better tolerated by patients. There are, however, documented metabolic effects such as weight gain and diabetes, although this is clouded somewhat by the increasing incidence of diabetes in the general population. Clozapine obviously carries a specific side effect of blood dyscrasias, which is well documented and integrated into monitoring programmes. Whether atypicals really are a superior solution compared to older antipsychotics remains difficult to answer definitively. Data certainly supports claims of reduced incidence of EPS and tardive dyskinesia, but this has to be balanced against the limited amount of long-term data (tardive dyskinesia may take many years to develop). Furthermore, as NICE (2002) points out, many trials used haloperidol (high potency for D2 so high EPS) as the comparison, and the populations studied limit generalisability. Newer agents have also been associated with a higher incidence of diabetes, hyperglycaemia and excessive weight gain. Finally, the most recent of the atypicals is aripiprazole, a partial dopamine agonist. Data thus far suggests it to be well tolerated, with no evidence of significant EPS, metabolic effect, hyperprolactinaemia or cardiac rhythm disturbance.

Patient vignette James

James is 26 years old and has been diagnosed with schizophrenia. While at university he began to hear voices telling him that he was 'bad'. He returned home, cutting short his degree programme, and subsequently began to believe that his father was bugging his room. His parents, oblivious to the problem, encouraged him to seek employment and he gained a job with a recruitment agency handling enquiries. He was unable to hold down the job beyond two months, believing that he was being constantly watched, and was sacked after shouting abusively at staff members. He was eventually admitted to hospital under the Mental Health Act and was successfully treated with haloperidol, but developed side effects and withdrew treatment within months of returning home. He has been hospitalised four times following discontinuation of antipsychotic medication, and has most recently been treated with trifluperazine. He has now been discharged home with trifluperazine and during your follow-up visit is talking about not wanting to take tablets any more because of the side effects. His family are insisting that you make sure he is 'treated'.

You have a clinical management plan signed by James while in hospital allowing prescribing and titration of 'antipsychotic medication'. As a non-medical prescriber, what issues are relevant to your prescribing in this case?

Treating Psychosis Effectively

Patients with schizophrenia often have a particularly negative attitude towards the antipsychotic drugs they are prescribed. Although lack of insight may be a factor, it cannot be ignored that much of this reflects either the unpleasant side effects that accompany treatment, or a perceived lack of improvement in areas of difficulty that matter most. Extrapyramidal side effects and emotional blunting/dysphoria are unlikely to promote a positive attitude towards treatment or maintain concordance.

The recommendations of NICE (2002) are that oral atypical antipsychotics are considered:

- 'In the choice of first-line treatments for individuals with newly diagnosed schizophrenia.'
- Where a traditional antipsychotic is producing unpleasant side effects, despite adequate symptom control.
- For patients experiencing a relapse who previously had poor symptom control or suffered side effects.

NICE further recommends that amisulpiride, olanzepine, quetiapine, risperidone and zotepine are considered first line in people newly diagnosed with schizophrenia.

These recommendations reflect the current evidence that atypical antipsychotics are generally less likely to produce EPS than their traditional counterparts, and carry a lower incidence of tardive dyskinesia. NICE also underlines the importance of involving the patient as much as possible in decisions about treatment, and providing clear information that is not jargonistic and promotes informed choice. Additionally, advanced directives can be discussed with a patient and inserted in their case notes, indicating their views should they become unable to be fully involved in treatment decisions.

Information alone, however, may not improve concordance and prevent relapse significantly, since it often fails to address the reasons why people stop taking their medications. Up to 50 % of service users will have stopped taking antipsychotics within one year and 75 % within two years (Weiden and Olfson, 1995). Historically this might have been given the patronising label of non-compliance, suggesting that the patient is failing to follow the advice given by an expert. It is worth noting that such high rates of stopping medications can also be seen in many fields of physical medicine such as diabetes, asthma and hypertension, and as such should perhaps not be seen as unnatural behaviour. One method promoted by Gray (2001) is concordance training based on a motivational interviewing approach. This attempts to encourage the patient to take a more active role in illness monitoring and treatment negotiation.

Providing help early is an essential part of any mental health service for this client group. Even with the next generation of antipsychotics, the social and physical consequences of non-treatment can be very poor, particularly during the first five years (Jablensk et al., 1992). Suicide rates are disconcertingly high at 1 in 10 of people with severe mental illness, two-thirds of whom are seen within the first five years of treatment (Wiersma et al., 1998). Naturally, the subtle nature of symptoms during this prodromal phase can make it very difficult to identify those in need. It is essential to involve the family in decisions concerning treatment and care planning. It is worth noting, however, that the emotional investment of a family coming to terms with such a diagnosis is high, and a poor response to initial treatment or unexpected/unexplained or marked side effects can easily destroy the relationship the prescriber has with the patient and family. Individuals presenting with a first-episode psychosis may be far more susceptible to adverse effects (NICE, 2002), and when symptom control is not reached speedily may be subjected to continued dose increases. The likelihood of developing potentially irreversible side effects is thus increased, and future concordance very likely threatened.

Antipsychotic medications, like antidepressants, take on average a few weeks to achieve any positive benefit, and the temptation to increase doses too quickly should be avoided, employing where possible the minimum effective dose and considering switching to another where little efficacy is achieved. Medication is, however, a component of the treatment of schizophrenia, and not the only treatment. As such, it should be considered carefully and discussed honestly with the patient. NICE (2002) underlines the fact that treatment should involve a comprehensive care package that aims to address all of the patient's clinical, emotional and social needs. This is particularly relevant in first-episode psychosis, where the likelihood of compulsory admission to hospital under the Mental Health Act is high. In a NIMHE review of available research on early intervention and psychosis, it was found that people with prodromal symptoms who received a combination of CBT and atypical antipsychotic plus care from a specialist team were far less likely to develop psychosis by the six-month follow-up than those receiving medication and specialist team follow-up alone (McGorry et al., 2002).

Individuals with schizophrenia may have over a period of time become accustomed to unpleasant side effects, perhaps even considering them 'normal', or quite possibly failing to notice their existence. This is demonstrated by a Dutch outpatient study in which objective side effects observed in 94% did not correlate with the 60% of patients who felt they had side effects (Gerlach and Larsen, 1999). Generally individuals with schizophrenia will list the most troublesome side effects to be EPS, weight gain, sexual dysfunction and sedation.

There may be a temptation to switch patients from typical antipsychotics to atypicals. This is only recommended where poor symptom control exists or unacceptable side effects are experienced. Where a typical antipsychotic is chosen for acute episodes the dose should be within 300–1000 mg chlorpromazine equivalent per day for a minimum of six weeks. Loading doses are not necessary or beneficial. Where no improvement is seen within six to eight weeks of therapeutic dose, consideration should be given to switching to another. Where failure to improve is due to non-concordance with medication, it is important to clarify if this is due to the individual experiencing side effects, and if so to discuss the option of switching with the patient. Depot medication should only be considered where all other avenues for concordance have been exhausted. A person not responding to a second antipsychotic medication (at least one of which should be atypical) should be considered for clozapine (NICE, 2002).

As with antidepressants, the question of maintenance doses is relevant. It is thought that approximately 20% of people will experience only one episode of psychosis in their lifetime. A small number will, however, suffer relapse. It is almost impossible to predict who will fall into each category and in most cases maintenance therapy should be considered and discussed with all involved. Where the decision to withdraw antipsychotic medication is reached, it may be necessary to monitor for relapse for at least two years, as the relapse rate is high (National Collaborating Centre for Mental Health, 2006). Clearly, all antipsychotics are capable of controlling positive symptoms. Atypicals are on balance slightly more effective at treating some negative symptoms, but in terms of overall efficacy they are thought to be broadly equivalent (Tandon and Jibson, 2005).

The list of potential side effects from antipsychotic medications provides daunting reading. The typical/conventional antipsychotics carry the greatest risk, in particular of dystonic reactions, pseudo-Parkinsonism, akathisia and tardive dyskinesia. Dystonic reactions such as oculogyric crisis are seen in approximately 10 % of patients on older antipsychotics, and most likely in the early stages or after a dose increase. Akathisia, a type of motor restlessness, is also seen in older antipsychotics, potentially as frequently as in 20–25 % of cases. Unlike dystonia, this generally responds poorly to anticholinergics. Pseudo-Parkinsonian side effects (tremor, rigidity, bradykinesia) can be seen in as many as 20 % of patients on older antipsychotics, and should be treated with anticholinergics. Tardive dyskinesia is due to prolonged therapy with any dopamine-blocking drug, and has a complex aetiology. Where this occurs, antipsychotic doses should be reduced where possible to the minimum effective dose and consideration given to switching to an atypical. When switching to an atypical a number of factors will influence choice, not least of which is patient choice.

Weight gain is a potential side effect of all antipsychotics and should be reviewed with the patient and advice given both on individual antipsychotic choices and lifestyle. The most likely to cause weight gain are olanzapine and clozapine, least likely to cause weight gain are risperidone and amisulpiride. The association with diabetes remains unclear, with a possible increased risk but no causal relationship demonstrated to date. Clozapine and olanzapine are possibly the greatest in terms of potential risk in this area (Henderson et al., 2005). Risperidone and amisulpiride are both potent elevators of serum prolactin. The risk of postural hypotension is found in clozapine, olanzapine, quietiapine and the first dose of risperidone. Although tolerance often develops, patients should be carefully monitored. In terms of anticholinergic effects, chlorpromazine and clozapine are probably worst, olanzapine is also likely to cause this, with amisulpiride being relatively free.

All antipsychotics carry the risk of altering cardiac conduction and of potentially fatal arrhythmias, and co-prescribing with other drugs known to affect QT interval should be avoided (e.g. tricyclic antidepressants). Zotepine and sertindole should not be used, with amisulpiride being the safest in people with arrhythmias. Risperidone and olanzapine may increase the risk of stroke in the elderly. Zotepine, risperidone and quetiapine should all be avoided in people with angina or previous myocardial infarction; the safest choice is likely to be olanzapine in such cases (Taylor et al., 2005). All antipsychotic drugs can lower the seizure threshold, and it is therefore sensible to use low starting doses and increase them slowly in patients with epilepsy. The lowest incidences of seizures in clinical trials are seen in olanzapine, risperidone and quetiapine. Neuroleptic malignant syndrome (NMS) is rare, but life threatening, and although more common with haloperidol can occur with any antipsychotic. Symptoms of NMS include hyperthermia, muscle rigidity and fluctuating consciousness.

Special consideration should be given in prescribing antipsychotics in the elderly. There is a higher risk of postural hypotension, EPS and antimuscarinic effects, especially at initiation of treatment. Starting with a low dose and increasing slowly are necessary.

Ultimately, it remains crucial to encourage any person with psychosis to be as actively involved in decisions about treatment as possible. The high incidence of side effects possible with both typical and atypical antipsychotics, and the potential (if not entirely proven) link with the development of other physical illness, places the non-medical prescriber in a central position to ensure that individuals are properly informed and that they understand the consequences of both non-concordance and concordance.

Table 10.3   Psychosis/schizophrenia: Magic bullets

- Atypical antipsychotics to date demonstrate good efficacy in the treatment of positive symptoms with a reduced likelihood of EPS and tardive dyskinesia. Several demonstrate some effect on many, if not all, negative symptoms.
- The efficacy of atypicals for positive symptoms is broadly equal.
- For a first episode of psychosis an atypical should be chosen.
- Change from typical to atypical where a patient experiences unacceptable side effects or poor symptom control.
- Aim to use the minimum effective dose, and avoid unnecessarily high doses.
- Non-concordance is a complex combination of factors, but may be a result of unacceptable side effects.
- All carry the potential for side effects, there are no 'clean' antipsychotics.

SUBSTANCE MISUSE

Substance misuse (or drug abuse) is a broad label with definitions mostly referring to the misuse or overuse of a psychoactive or performance-enhancing drug, which is not for prescribed therapeutic or medical effect. The common categorisation would be stimulants that increase alertness and activity (amphetamines, cocaine and perhaps caffeine), depressants that depress the central nervous system (alcohol, barbiturates, tranquillisers), analgesics such as morphine, heroin and codeine, and hallucinogens that alter perception of senses such as mescaline, LSD and ecstasy. These are, however, sometimes misleading distinctions, as the effects of some drugs may not necessarily match the categorisation, and different effects may be observed depending on both quantity used and duration of dependence. Alcohol, for instance, may be classed as a depressant, but may be commonly observed as a disinhibitor.

The consequences of drug misuse may include health problems, physical dependence, psychological addiction and social difficulties. For the most part this is true of all drugs that are misused, the degree often depending on not only the drug but also the extent, frequency and duration of misuse. Commonly drugs of abuse affect the central nervous system, leading to changes in mood, awareness, perceptions and sensations. Beyond the potential harm to the individual user, there are of course wider public health concerns such as the spread of blood-borne infections, driving the pragmatic policy approach of harm reduction. This paradigm views drug misuse (and many other lifestyle choices) as a public health issue rather than a criminal one.

Substance misuse is common in the general population, with for instance alcohol consumed above recommended limits by approximately eight million people in the UK (Department of Health, 2005a). The prevalence, however, among people with mental health problems is perhaps surprisingly high. According to the COSMIC study in 2003, 40 % of CMHT (community mental health team) patients reported problem drug/alcohol use during the past year (Weaver et al., 2003). Dual diagnosis, although possibly a misleading term as there are often multiple symptoms and needs in this context, refers to the coexistence of a mental health problem and substance misuse. This is according to some evidence showing a considerable increase in incidence of 60 % over the past five years (Frisher et al., 2004). As with the general population, people with mental health problems may misuse substances for a variety of reasons, which may possibly include attempts to self-medicate and relieve unpleasant symptoms.

Individuals who abuse substances are often difficult to access, may lead chaotic and highly mobile lifestyles, and may be difficult to engage in traditional treatment services. As a consequence they may be far more likely to commit self-harm or be admitted to hospital (Hunt et al., 2002). Drug treatment services are provided by a variety of agencies and organisations through primary and secondary care, specialist clinics and voluntary and charitable organisations. Treatment teams, it seems, have traditionally been split into two almost mutually exclusive groups. Mainstream mental health services may either have failed to diagnose substance misuse problems or deferred treatment of mental health problems until the patient was no longer 'using'. This may lead to individuals experiencing significant delay in accessing treatments, with CMHTs often viewing the misuse of a substance as a stumbling block to offering treatment for a mental health problems. Services targeting substance misuse, however, might traditionally have focused on this to the exclusion of coexisting mental health problems. Following Department of Health recommendations in 2002, dual diagnosis has become a focus for local services to ensure a more integrated service model.

Treatments for Substance Misuse

Separation of services across the UK has largely been along the lines of alcohol or drug teams and mental health teams. Classification may often be mental illness with a secondary substance misuse problem, or a primary substance misuse problem with a secondary mental health problem. Clearly, such a variable approach will lead to people slipping through the net, particularly when set against the backdrop of the often chaotic lifestyles of these individuals who are less likely to seek help or engage in treatment.

Although the structure of mental health services for substance misuse varies across the UK, many local services are developing in line with the Department of Health document *Models of Care* (Department of Health, 2002). This involves services being delivered in a tiered approach, ranging from health promotion and advice at tier one to specialist acute inpatient services, such as inpatient detoxification, at tier four. The recently released Models of Care for Alcohol Misusers (MOCAM) continues in a similar vein, underlining integrated local treatment systems and the tiered framework. Treatments for substance misuse (if we exclude tobacco) are primarily either concerned with alcohol dependence or opioid dependence.

Alcohol Dependence

Alcohol produces a range of pleasant reinforcing effects through regular consumption, including mild euphoria and anxiolytic effects. These are, of course, accompanied by some less desirable effects such as loss of inhibitions, balance and coordination, along with slurred speech and blurred vision. Long-term effects may include liver failure, heart failure, epilepsy, hypertension, obesity, gastritis, pancreatitis, vitamin deficiency, infertility, impotence, neurological disorders and mental health problems. Physically alcohol is implicated in 400 cases of pancreatitis and 137 deaths from cardiomyopathy per annum (Office for National Statistics, 2000). Alcohol-related liver disease is responsible for approximately 80 % of liver admissions in the UK (British Liver Trust, 2000), with 4700 deaths from alcohol-related liver disease in 1999 (Office for National Statistics, 2000). Wernicke's encephalopathy, a deficiency of thiamine, occurs in the general population in about 2 % of the population, but is present in 12.5 % of dependent drinkers, with 20 % of these dying and 80 % going on to develop Korsakoff's psychosis (Cook and Thompson, 1997). Heavy drinking also contributes to many mental health problems such as anxiety and depression, often accelerating a possible predisposition to psychosis, and is linked to 65 % of suicides (Department of Health, 1993) and one in three elderly suicides (Hislop et al., 1995). Socially it is also heavily related to crime and accidents, as many as 40 % of violent crimes (Kershaw et al., 2000) and one in six road traffic accidents (Department of Transport, 2002).

Alcohol dependence is thought to be present when three of the following exist (World Health Organization, 2005a):

- Strong desire or compulsion to use alcohol.
- Difficulty controlling alcohol use.
- Withdrawal symptoms (anxiety, sweating tremors) when drinking is ceased.
- Tolerance.
- Continued use despite harmful consequences.
- Neglect of other activities.

Community alcohol teams offer treatment to those with a physical dependency on alcohol or significant alcohol-related difficulties. Service models vary and attempts to map service provision across the UK have proved problematic. Alcohol Concern reported on the mapping of alcohol services (Alcohol Concern, 2002) but faced relatively poor response rates, limiting the confidence of generalisation. Support may often be (although not exclusively) intensive and short in duration, leading to the person regaining some control before being referred to mainstream services for long-term support. Programmes may be offered around detoxification at home with daily reviews and support. Inpatient detoxification programmes now appear to be the exception rather than the norm, with most detoxified with a good outcome as outpatients/at home. Inpatient detoxification may be necessary where significant risk exists such as history of delirium tremens (DTs), heavy use and high tolerance, significant polydrug use, benzodiazepine dependence, severe medical/psychiatric disorder, and for those who pose a significant suicide risk. Again, it is difficult to generalise over any common format, and residential rehabilitation services may be offered and may vary in length of stay and intensity of programme.

Pharmacological treatments consist of treatment for the management of withdrawal, essentially benzodiazepines, and disulfiram, which helps to maintain abstinence.

Benzodiazepines are used for short terms due to their dependence potential, usually for periods of between seven and fourteen days. Chlordiazepoxide is generally the drug of choice, as clomethiazole carries the risk of respiratory depression in combination with alcohol and the danger of dependence, and is not recommended in outpatient settings. A common chlordiazepoxide regime (depending on individual factors and severity of dependence) might be:

- *Days 1 and 2* 20–30 mg qds
- *Days 3 and 4* 15 mg qds
- *Day 5* 10 mg qds
- *Day 6* 10 mg BD
- *Day 7* 10 mg Nocte

Detoxification regimes usually include thiamine (150 per day), prescribed concurrently to minimise the risk of Wernicke's encephalopathy. Although oral thiamine is poorly absorbed, transfer to a hospital setting and IM/IV administration is only necessary where ataxia, confusion, memory disturbance, DTs, hypothermia and hypotension, ophthalmoplegia or unconsciousness are present (World Health Organization, 2005a). Clearly, it is essential to monitor hydration and nutrition as well as signs and symptoms of withdrawal. Special consideration would be advised in older adults, using lower doses of benzodiazepines due to the risk of ataxia and confusion. If the person being treated has a diagnosis of severe hepatic impairment, it would be necessary to use a benzodiazepine that is not hepatically metabolised such as lorazepam or oxazepam. This is best carried out in a hospital setting due to the short half life of lorazepam, and the difficulty at times in controlling withdrawal.

For the maintenance of abstinence, approaches should include a greater psychosocial component, focusing on support for those affected (spouse, family), the development of coping skills and behavioural self-control training. As an adjunct to psychosocial interventions, acamprosate may be used for those who have recently completed detoxification. This may continue for up to one year, although recent US evidence casts some doubt on its efficacy (Pocock, 2006). Another adjunct to treatment is disulfiram, which produces unpleasant systemic reactions to even a small amount of alcohol (flushing of face, headache, tachycardia, nausea, vomiting). Consumption of alcohol may produce unpleasant symptoms up to two weeks after cessation of treatment. If larger amounts of alcohol are consumed effects could include arrhythmia, hypotension and collapse. It is important to ensure that any individual being treated with this is aware of the existence of alcohol in many other products such as mouthwash and colognes. Disulfiram should be avoided as much as possible in pregnancy due to its being excreted in breast milk, and caution is advisable in activities requiring alertness due to the potential for drowsiness. Caution is also necessary in patients receiving phenytoin, as it may lead to phenytoin toxicity. Oral anticoagulants may also require adjustment and closer monitoring since prothrombin times may be increased.

Opioid Dependence

Turning to other kinds of substance abuse, opium is an extract derived from the seed pods of the opium poppy *Papaver somniferum*, which can be traced back as far as the ancient civilisations of Persia, Egypt and Mesopotamia. An opioid is any agent capable of binding to opioid receptors, found typically in the central nervous system and the gastrointestinal tract. There are four broad classes: endogenous opioid peptides produced in the body; opium alkaloids, such as morphine and codeine; semi-synthetic opioids such as heroin and oxycodene; and fully synthetic opioids such as pethidine and methadone. The two principal effects of opioids are that they relieve pain and produce feelings of wellbeing, while depressing the central nervous system.

Heroin is the most widely abused and rapidly acting of the opioids (existing in the UK as the prescription drug diamorphine), with approximately 300,000 children in the UK having one or both parents addicted to it (Goswami and Brosnan, 2006). It has the dubious honour of embarrassing pharmaceutical company Bayer, who originally marketed it as a non-addictive morphine substitute, before it was discovered that heroin is converted to morphine in the liver. Its abuse is associated with serious health problems including fatal overdose, spontaneous abortion, collapsed veins and, in those who inject, infectious diseases such as HIV/AIDS and hepatitis. Treatment is generally either methadone and opioid agonist or buprenorphine, which has both opioid antagonist and agonist properties.

Methadone was developed in Germany at the end of the Second World War as a substitute for morphine (Gerlach, 2004). Methadone treatment consists of gradually increasing the dose over a six-week period for most, although it may take longer for some. It should always be prescribed in liquid form to minimise illicit use. In clinical practice this may lead to ever-increasing caseload numbers due to maintenance prescribing.

Interactions with other drugs are possible, particularly with anticonvulsants carbamazepine and phenytoin, which may accelerate the metabolism of methadone and precipitate withdrawal symptoms. Some antivirals may also be affected such as zidovudine (possible increase in its plasma concentration), ritonavir and efavirenz possibly increasing the plasma concentration of methadone. An alternative is buprenorphine, particularly for those who have experienced unwanted effects from methadone previously. This should be given at least eight hours after the last dose of heroin to avoid it precipitating withdrawal symptoms. From a starting dose of 4 mg this is titrated fairly rapidly according to clinical response up to a maximum dose of 32 mg daily. For those switching from methadone the dose should be taken down to a maximum of 30 mg before starting buprenorphine. Side effects would be similar to any other opioids, such as nausea, vomiting and constipation. Overdose with buprenorphine is problematic due to the lack of a completely effective antagonist (antidote).

Table 10.4 Substance misuse: Magic bullets

- Common categories: stimulants, depressants, analgesics and hallucinogens.
- Dual diagnosis refers to the co-existence of mental health problems and substance misuse. Traditionally such people have faced difficulties in accessing services.
- Models of care for substance misuse (Department of Health, 2002) promote tiered approach from tier 1 (advice) to tier 4 (in-patient detoxification)
- MOCAM will follow similar pattern for alcohol services.

Alcohol

- Alcohol responsible for 4700 liver disease deaths annually, 65 % of suicide (1 in 3 older adult suicides), 40 % of violent crimes, 1 in 6 road traffic accidents and 40 % of violent crimes.
- Wernicke's encephalopathy (thiamine deficiency) occurs in 12.5 % of dependent drinkers, 80 % of which will develop Korsakoffs' psychosis. Thiamine given concomitantly to reduce risk of Wernicke's encephalopathy.
- Detoxification programmes mostly at home (except when high risk such as benzodiazepine dependence, history of DTs, polydrug use, severe medical/psychiatric disorder and/or suicide risk).
- Withdrawal managed with benzodiazepines (usually chlordiazepoxide), over 7–14 days. Older adults may require lower dose.
- In severe hepatic impairment lorazepam or oxazepam favoured (generally inpatient due to short half life and difficulty managing withdrawal).
- Abstinence treatments: acamprosate and disulfiram. With disulfiram exercise caution with phenytoin, anticoagulants and in pregnancy.

Heroin

- Heroin misuse associated with fatal overdose, spontaneous abortion, collapsed veins and HIV/hepatitis when injected.
- Methadone and buprenorphine. Methadone interactions possible with carbomazepine, phenytoin and some antivirals.
- Buprenorphine used when unwanted side effects from methadone. Overdose from buprenorphine problematic due to absence of truly effective antidote.

ALZHEIMER'S DISEASE

Alzheimer's disease is the commonest form of dementia. It is slightly more common in women and is clearly most common in older people. This incidence has remained largely unaltered in recent decades, accounting for 15.5 % of people over 65 in 2000. Given, however, the projected increase in people over the age of 65 in Europe of 24.3 % by 2030 (Bowie and Takriti, 2004), the problem may well be developing epidemic proportions.

The term Alzheimer's disease can be traced back to German neuropsychiatrist Alois Alzheimer and his study of a 51-year-old woman in 1906, initially leading to the assumption that it was a disease of younger people (Sisodia, 1999). The terms senility or senile dementia were more common at this time and it was not really until the 1950s that the term Alzheimer's was widely accepted. Dementia describes a chronic progressive disorder affecting to varying degrees memory, thinking, orientation and judgement, and there are many other types, including vascular dementia (second highest incidence), frontotemporal dementia, Creutzfeldt–Jakob disease, alcoholic dementia, dementia in Parkinson's disease and dementia in Huntingdon's chorea. Given this scope, prescribing in dementia is potentially a vast field, encompassing numerous condition-specific cautions (particularly antipsychotics). This section covers Alzheimer's disease only and focuses predominantly on cognitive enhancers as the field in which many older adult nurse prescribers will be practising.

The most common form of dementia is Alzheimer's disease, which according to population data from 2002 accounts for a prevalence of 290,000 (NICE, 2005). It is commonly claimed that approximately 60 % of cases of dementia will be of the Alzheimer type, followed by vascular dementia at 20 % and Lewy body dementia at 15 % (World Health Organization, 2005b). It is distinguished from other forms of dementia largely (although not always reliably) by its insidious onset and gradual development over many years. Alongside cognitive changes functional abilities are affected, impacting a person's ability to self-care and leading to the eventual dependence on another for care. There is a great deal of variation in the pace of cognitive decline, and change is measured by a number of different rating scales, such as ADASCOG, CAMCOG, MMSE, Bristol ADL and Relatives' Stress Scale (the latter three being required by NICE to monitor the effects of acetylcholinesterase inhibitor medications).

Consensus exists that the disease can be considered in three stages: early, intermediate and late; or mild, moderate and severe. In the early stage, often lasting up to three years, prominent features might include some memory impairment and concentration problems, with possible disturbance of mood and difficulty managing daily tasks. The intermediate stage may represent both a worsening of features from the early stage and possible new symptoms, which can include hallucinations, delusions, disorientation and dysphasia. The late stage can include incontinence, seizures, loss of communication and anorexia. A diagnosis of Alzheimer's disease is often one of exclusion, systematically ruling out other possible causes and factors, although the distinction between vascular dementia and Alzheimer's is somewhat blurred by the likelihood of many suffering a combination of both. Baseline routine investigations are generally carried out, supplemented by imaging techniques (CT and MRI scans), and often neuropsychological testing to detect reversible causes and aid in diagnosis. Diagnosis generally involves close examination of the possibility of treatable causes such as delirium, acute psychosis, depression, metabolic and endocrine disorders and drug treatments.

Neuropathologically Alzheimer's disease is characterised by specific molecular changes and cellular dysfunction in the brain (distinct from the pattern of multiple small strokes found in vascular dementias). There is progressive neuronal shrinkage and death affecting multiple areas of the brain, typically leading to atrophy and dilation of the ventricles. Principal among these changes are neuritic plaques, a type of degenerating nerve cell combined with a protein called beta amyloid; and neurofibrillary tangles, a malformation of the nerve cell. Theories to explain a cause have abounded, including links with aluminium, but the Holy Grail remains elusive, at best providing intriguing findings that merit further research. Genetically some connection has been made with chromosome 21, the chromosome affected in Down's syndrome, a disorder in which a high incidence of Alzheimer's can be found. Other genetic markers of interest have been identified on chromosome 14 in certain familial types and in a small number the apolipoprotein (ApoE) found on chromosome 19. Despite these genetic links, the true extent of genetic involvement remains unclear.

The impact of caring for a person with Alzheimer's disease can be enormous, and there exists a considerable rate of depression in caregivers (Schultz et al., 2003; Shua-Haim et al., 2001). It is essential to review not only the current capabilities of the person with dementia, but also how well the carer is coping. Clear explanation of assessments and treatments should be given, as well as realistic advice on managing current and future symptoms. Drug treatments for Alzheimer's can often offer an apparent 'lifeline' of hope and it is necessary to manage these expectations realistically.

Treatments for Alzheimer's Disease

Treatments for Alzheimer's disease currently offer a valuable and variable role in managing the clinical aspects of the condition: cognitive, behavioural, functional and affective. There is clearly no current treatment that can alter the underlying neuropathological process and current strategies at best provide symptomatic relief to patients. It is widely accepted that a multifactorial approach including pharmacological and non-pharmacological methods is the best way to optimise individual quality of life.

There are several types of non-pharmacological intervention available, the most widely used probably being reality orientation (Zanetti et al., 1995; Spector et al., 2000a) and reminiscence therapy (Finnema et al., 2000). Reality orientation, which aims to orientate the person to place, time and person, may be either continuous (i.e. by staff in a care environment) or where orientation activities are offered on a regular basis to groups of people. There is some evidence that supports benefits to both cognition and behaviour (Spector et al., 2000b), but it is unclear how far beyond the end of treatment benefits continue.

Reminiscence therapy involves typically a group-based approach to encouraging individuals to recall events from the past using aids such as photos, music and video. Evidence of specific benefits is less clear, and a Cochrane review (Spector et al., 2000c) concluded there to be insufficient evidence. Benefits are, however, clearer in terms of improving wellbeing and engagement.

Similarly, validation therapy, which aims to promote communication, reduce agitation and withdrawal, and improve self-worth, has demonstrated improvements for families and caregivers, but ultimately offers insufficient evidence from which clear conclusions can be drawn (Neal and Briggs, 2000).

Memory training is aimed at helping people with mild to moderate Alzheimer's disease (Butters et al., 1997), focusing on the process of encoding and storing memories. Promising results have been demonstrated when used alongside acetylcholinesterase inhibitors with higher MMSE scores than with drugs alone (De Vreese et al., 2001).

Other treatments include music therapy, light therapy, multisensory stimulation, consideration of environment and aromatherapy. For the most part some limited benefits may be possible from these in carefully selected patients, but there is insufficient evidence at present to clearly support or refute these. As Ashina (2002) points out, however, the absence of specific research evidence does not necessarily correlate with the absence of a positive effect.

Pharmacological interventions for Alzheimer's disease essentially carry the same aims as non-pharmacological treatments in aiming to improve the quality of life for the individual and carer by slowing the progression of the underlying disease process, and therefore cognitive decline, and by managing the behavioural symptoms of the condition. The presence of behavioural symptoms such as agitation, hallucinations and sleep disturbance is not only a major source of distress to carers, but is far more likely to precipitate admission into hospital or residential care. These features, often referred to as behavioural and psychological symptoms of dementia (BPSD), have traditionally been managed using antipsychotics, anxiolytics and to a lesser extent antidepressants. Conventional antipsychotics such as chlorpromazine have been used commonly and some evidence supports good efficacy (Lanctot et al., 1998), haloperidol being widely assessed and displaying good results in the control of aggression, although side effects preclude widespread or sustained use (Devanand et al., 2003). Atypical antipsychotics have also demonstrated good evidence for the control of BPSD, in particular aggression (Davidson et al., 2000). There is little clear evidence from head-to-head trials, however, of superior efficacy over conventional antipsychotics. Olanzapine and risperidone are currently not advised by the Medicines and Healthcare Products Regulatory Agency (MHRA) due to their association with stroke. Essentially, however, all antipsychotics should be used with caution in the elderly due to an increased risk of postural hypotension and hyperthermia/hypothermia.

Acetylcholinesterase inhibitors form the mainstay of drug treatment for people diagnosed with Alzheimer's disease, gaining increasing momentum since 1997.

These treatments are based on the hypothesis that decline in cognitive function is linked to the loss of cholinergic neurotransmission in the hippocampus and cortex (Perry et al., 1978). NICE guidance was published in 2001 on the use of donepezil, rivastigmine and galantamine for the treatment of Alzheimer's disease. This brought previously inconsistent 'postcode' prescribing of these drugs under a single uniform approach, going some way to ensure equal access for all diagnosed with Alzheimer's disease. In many ways the above guidance is responsible for the growth of services across the UK set up to prescribe and monitor these drugs, often referred to as memory clinics. These memory clinics (although not exclusively medication led) have undergone significant growth, from approximately 20 in 1993 to an estimated 102 in 2000, with probably over 50 % having developed since 1997, when donepezil was first licensed in the UK (Passmore and Craig, 2004). In many areas these have become integral parts of integrated models of care for dementia sufferers, often going far beyond just prescribing.

In 2001 NICE also set out a framework for old-age services to follow in prescribing these drugs. This essentially promoted the provision of these drugs to those people with mild and moderate Alzheimer's disease, whose Mini Mental State Examination (MMSE) score is above 12 points. It further ensured diagnosis in specialist clinics, setting out standardised tests of cognitive and functional ability alongside carer perception. Standards were included to encourage review of efficacy and continued benefit at regular intervals. Although a significant proportion of these reviews are carried out within memory clinic models, often involving shared care protocols with primary care, many people have also continued to be seen solely by consultant psychiatrists.

The choice of drug can depend on a number of factors, some easier than others to reliably extricate. Simplicity of dosing currently favours donepezil, which is given once daily, and this has partly contributed to its wider use than rivastigmine and galantamine. A great deal of data exists regarding efficacy, some studies such as AD2000 suggesting that no reliable conclusions can be made. Realistically, similar efficacy is probably achieved across all three. All of the acetylcholinesterase inhibitors should be used cautiously in cardiac disease, particularly sick sinus syndrome and conduction abnormalities. In liver disease donepezil is probably a safer choice than the other two, both of which are best avoided in severe liver impairment. Dosage adjustment is necessary in moderate liver impairment and galantamine should not exceed 8 mg BD in this instance. Equally, caution is necessary in renal impairment, with galantamine avoided in severe renal impairment. Rivastigmine may require titration, depending on individual tolerability. All drugs should be used with caution in epilepsy, with galantamine possibly proving the safest, and in diabetes rivastigmine should be used with caution.

Therapeutically donepezil is generally titrated to maximum dose after one month if tolerated well, galantamine commences at 4 mg BD for 4 weeks, increasing to 8 mg BD, and on an individual basis sometimes 12 mg BD. Rivastigmine commences at 1.5 mg BD, which the most recent data suggests should be maintained for one month and then increased to 3 mg BD thereafter. The dose may remain at this point until further deterioration is evident. When switching from one to another, it is important to recognise that the half lives vary from one hour with rivastigmine to 70 hours with donepezil. Switching from donepezil due to side effects would therefore require nine days, and one day switching from galantamine. Rivastigmine would not generally require a washout period. If switching is due to lack of efficacy, however, washouts are not necessary. Most common side effects are diarrhoea, muscle cramps, nausea, vomiting, dizziness and headaches, most of which last no longer than a week.

A growing body of evidence points to a potential benefit in managing many behavioural symptoms associated with Alzheimer's disease, and in other dementia syndromes. Both donepezil and galantamine have demonstrated modest improvements in behavioural symptoms in Alzheimer's disease (Tariot et al., 2000; Feldman et al., 2001). Rivastigmine has also demonstrated positive outcomes in BPSD from mild to severe stages of Alzheimer's disease and in other dementia types, including Lewy body dementia and Parkinson's disease dementia (Rosler, 2002). Importantly, however, randomised control trials comparing these drugs are needed to confirm and quantify differences. Such 'off licence' prescribing does not fall within the 2001 NICE guidelines, nor does it find any mention in recent revisions, and therefore as such remains outside of the scope of most non-medical prescribers working within CMPs. Revisions have been made to the guidance suggesting withdrawal of these drugs (for all new patients) falling within mild stages of dementia, and recommending that treatment should only commence when MMSE falls to 20 or below. There is no ignoring the sense of outrage from Alzheimer's related groups and healthcare professionals alike at the economic decision to exclude earlier stages.

An additional drug had also been considered by NICE: memantine, developed and licensed in the US and selected European markets, is the first of a newer class of anti-Alzheimer's drugs acting on the glutaminergic system, specifically NMDA receptors. This mode of action, it is claimed, enables protection of cells by inhibiting glutamate and, therefore, overexposure to calcium that degrades nerve cells. Trials, although limited, demonstrate small positive effects on cognition and functional ability in moderate to severe Alzheimer's disease (Areosa et al., 2005).

Table 10.5   Alzheimer's disease: Magic bullets

- Most common form of dementia (approximately 60 % of cases).
- Generally considered in three stages: early, intermediate and late.
- Diagnosis confirmed by full blood workup, CT/MRI and elimination of other causes.
- Characterised by presence of neuritic plaques, neurofibrillary tangles and loss of acetylcholine. Genetic links found but true extent largely unknown.
- Non-pharmacological interventions: most evidence supports reality orientation, although long-term benefits unclear. Others (validation therapy, music, aromatherapy, reminiscence etc.) have less evidence, but may benefit some. Memory training has shown significant improvements when combined with acetylcholinesterase inhibitors.
- For BPSD antipsychotics are commonly used. Olanzapine and risperidone not advised (CSM warning) due to stroke risk.

- Acetylcholinesterase inhibitors (donepezil, rivastigmine and galantamine) inhibit breakdown of acetylcholine. Use covered by NICE guidance (TA 111) 2006, for Alzheimer's disease mild–moderate (MMSE above 12 points).
- Most common side effects diarrhoea, muscle cramps, nausea, vomiting, headaches and dizziness.
- Some evidence supports use in BPSD and other dementias, although insufficient data to date and no head-to-head trials. *Not covered by NICE guidelines.*
- Recent revision of NICE guidelines has removed treatment to people with mild Alzheimer's disease; treatment can commence when MMSE reaches 20 points or below.
- Memantine has a different mode of action with possible neuroprotective properties for moderate to severe Alzheimer's disease, but not currently part of NICE guidelines.

ETHICAL DILEMMAS OF MHN PRESCRIBING PRACTICE

There exists a potential for the MHN prescriber to face many dilemmas regarding consent, legislation and the management of complex mental health problems while promoting concordance. Pharmacological interventions for mental illness can be problematic. Side effects such as weight gain, cardiovascular events and loss of libido are often reported and patient confidence in these medications can be difficult to maintain. MHN prescribers may find themselves balancing the potential benefits of psychotropic medications against the possibility for adverse effects, and having to decide how to present this information in an honest and constructive way. Conversely, there is also the desire not to become overly dependent on a medical model of care or to frame all client problems in an overly physiological way. The potential exists for mental health nurse prescribers to both encourage and increase appropriate medication use and concordance, while where relevant reducing the unnecessary reliance on psychotropic medications.

Patients' beliefs about medications are a crucial factor in establishing concordance, as is their ability to understand the information given about medication. Clearly, many factors are relevant here, such as insight, cognition, anxiety, intoxication and the type of language used by the practitioner. The information given needs to be appropriate to the patient and the nature of the problem being treated and to be presented clearly. Information given that is inadequate may lead to a patient being unprepared for side effects and therefore unwilling to continue treatment. Conversely, information that is unnecessarily complex and detailed, listing every possible side effect, may have the same effect.

The non-medical prescriber has a legal duty to obtain consent from the client before proceeding with treatment; this consent must be based on the provision of full and factual information that the individual has the capacity to understand. Capacity to understand is legitimate if a person is able to understand or retain the information, and in weighing up the information reach a considered decision (Griffith, 2004). Relatives of an individual incapable of giving consent do not hold the authority to give consent by proxy, or to make treatment decisions on their behalf (except in the case of minors). In caring for individuals with mental health problems, there are different ways in which consent and reasoned judgement may vary. People with dementia will as the condition progresses often become less able to comprehend the same degree of information as previously or reason as efficiently as before. If consent has previously been given for a treatment that is ongoing and there is no current indication of withdrawing consent, it is generally safe to assume that treatment can continue. If, however, treatment alters, and this should include dose increases, an explanation would normally be given to the patient and attempts to gain consent for this sought. Some treatment programmes, however, may include simple titration (such as with donepezil), which may have been explained to the patient at initiation. Good practice, however, would still direct a prescriber to re-assess consent to continued treatment. Conversely, the fact that an individual once gave consent does not necessarily mean they still do; consent is a continuous process and can be withdrawn at any time.

Individuals suffering hallucinations, delusions and other psychotic symptoms are perhaps more likely to present with adherence/concordance problems. According to Kisling (1994), if patients taking antipsychotics were completely adherent with medication, relapse rates would be only 15% per annum instead of 50%. Some of this failure can clearly be attributed to unnecessary side effects caused by poor prescribing, and/or failure of clinicians to recognise and monitor side effects (Weiden et al., 1987; Gray, 2001). Side effects are not the only reason for non-concordance, and awareness of the degree of the problem/insight has a great bearing. Insight and ability to judge may vary at different stages of a psychotic condition, placing the prescriber in the invidious position of attempting to maintain concordance while respecting the individual's right to choose what they feel is right for them.

Helping an individual make a decision involves giving information about the condition being treated, the recovery rates and the likely consequences of treatment and non-treatment. Despite possible frustration at a decision to withdraw consent, undue influence cannot be levied in an attempt to regain consent to treatment. The risks to treatment should be explained as well as what to do should a side effect occur. Other factors affecting consent include the behaviour and approachability of the prescriber and the convenience of taking medication (frequency and complexity of dosing). Should an individual decide to withdraw consent to treatment, it does not necessarily follow that their condition has deteriorated. It is important to take account of other factors in their life, and to prescribe in the context of what is acceptable to the client as well as what the evidence suggests to be most effective.

In certain circumstances it is legitimate to act out of necessity in the best interest of an incapable patient. The extent of this, however, is generally limited to treatment required to save life or prevent serious deterioration in the patient's condition.

Insight in many mental health conditions can be absent or variable. Where absent (i.e. the patient lacks capacity), there is clearly a need to consider the necessity of treatment balanced against the detrimental consequences of non-treatment involving all parties before reaching a decision. Reference can also be made to wishes previously expressed or documented by the individual, particularly in the form of living wills and advance directives, as these are and remain an expression of consent/non-consent. Proposals forming part of the Mental Capacity Act include appointing

Table 10.6   Ethical issues in promoting concordance

- No person can give consent on behalf of another, but their testimony can be used in ascertaining a person's current views and previously expressed wishes.
- Consent can be withdrawn at any time.
- The provision of consent depends where necessary on an assessment of capacity.
- Living wills and advance directives should be consulted where relevant. Make every attempt to ascertain what the wishes and views of the individual are.
- IMCA may in future form part of reaching decisions about treatment.
- Utilise periods of insight and plan flexibly with the individual.

Independent Mental Capacity Advocates (IMCA) for 'those who lack capacity' to assist in making 'difficult decisions such as medical treatment or changes to residence' (Department of Health, 2005b). Currently this is defined as 'serious medical treatment' and will need further clarity in respect of medications. Implementation is planned for April 2007. Where insight is variable, attempts should be made to gear support around these variations, providing closer monitoring around periods of non-concordance while utilising windows of insight to both discuss the value of treatment and consider approaches that the client finds acceptable. It is far more beneficial to agree that a client will continue treatment for 80 % of the year than to potentially alienate an individual through over-zealous insistence on treatment. Such decisions should always form part of a client's care plan, with reviews managed around changes to condition and client wishes. Covert administration of a medication is and should remain a last resort. Where necessary, reference should be made to NMC guidelines (Nursing and Midurifey Council, 2005).

In essence, a mental health non-medical prescriber is likely to face many difficulties in promoting and maintaining concordance. It is important to remember that all capable adults have an absolute right to refuse treatment and withdraw consent. If the presumption of capacity cannot be upheld, treatment may if deemed necessary be given in the patient's best interest. In promoting (rather than paying lip service to) concordance, the responsibility remains clear to promote treatments that are not only evidence based but acceptable to the patient.

CONCLUSION

The adoption of prescribing status by mental health nurses represents an exciting opportunity to dramatically alter and improve outcomes for many patients. The phenomenological construct underpinning most practice rightly places the client at the centre of decisions about their care. MHN prescribers are well placed to implement this 'new' role in a way that goes beyond a collection of symptoms and promotes choice, empowerment and recovery. Mental health nursing is now evolving to a point where prescribing is not a threat to the essence of care, but a sensible construct to fulfil a truly holistic approach to care. The promotion of concordance correlates with providing clear factual information about treatments, and where possible tapering these to fit the client, rather than the opposite.

Prescribing practice, like most areas of mental health practice, can be beset by ethical dilemmas in complex and unpredictable situations. The ability to assess clients is only one stage in the management and treatment of co-morbidity and complex interactions. A solid evidence base to practice remains essential.

GLOSSARY

Akathisia: an unpleasant sensation of 'inner' restlessness, resulting in the inability to remain still. Common side effect to antipsychotics, tricyclics, some SSRIs and certain antihistamines.

Anti-cholinergic: a drug that inhibits or blocks the action of acetylcholine at a receptor site in the central nervous system and peripheral nervous system. Typically inhibiting one of two types of acetylcholine receptor: muscarinic receptors (antimuscarinics) and nicotinic receptors. Anticholinergic effects might include loss of coordination (ataxia), increased body temperature, double vision (diplopia), tachycardia and urinary retention.

Anti-histaminic: a drug that reduces or eliminates the effects caused by histamine, a chemical released during allergic reactions. The most common adverse effect of anti-histaminics is sedation, but may also include insomnia, nausea, constipation and diarrhoea.

Dystonia: a movement disorder involving involuntary, sustained muscle contractions. Secondary dystonia may be brought on by trauma, be a disease of the nervous system or be drug induced.

Extrapyramidal: a system of the brain involved in coordination of movement. Extrapyramidal side effects (EPS) are a number of movement disorders suffered as a result of taking dopamine agonists (usually antipsychotics).

Hyperprolactinaemia: abnormally high levels of prolactin in the blood, sometimes resulting from dopamine-blocking drugs (haloperidol, trifluperazine etc.). In women this may affect menstruation, fertility and libido. In men impotence, decreased libido, erectile dysfunction and infertility may occur.

International Classification of Diseases: a means of categorising mental illness, developed by the World Health Organization. Favoured in the UK as opposed to DSM used in America.

Mesocortical region: one of the four major dopamine pathways in the brain, thought to be involved in motivation and emotional response. This area is associated with the negative symptoms of schizophrenia.

Mesolimbic region: one of the four major pathways of the brain in which the neurotransmitter dopamine is found, and an area targeted by antipsychotic medication. Excess dopamine in this area is thought to be linked to positive symptoms of schizophrenia.

Neuritic plaques: extracellular deposits of amyloid (an insoluble fibrous protein) in the brain, occurring in high numbers in Alzheimer's disease.

Neurofibrillary tangle: aggregates of pathological protein found within the neurons in cases of Alzheimer's disease.

Oculogyric crisis: a dystonic reaction to certain medical conditions and/or drugs that include antipsychotics, benzodiazepines, carbomazepine, lithium, nifedipine and tricyclic antidepressants. Most frequently presentation is backwards and lateral flexion of the neck, widely opened mouth, tongue protrusion and ocular pain.

Prodromal: an early symptom indicating the imminent development of a specific disease, for example in schizophrenia.

Tardive dyskinesia: a movement disorder characterised by repetitive, involuntary movement (grimacing, lip smacking, rapid blinking etc.). This is caused by long-term use of dopamine agonists, usually antipsychotics.

REFERENCES

AD2000 Collaborative Group (2004) Long-term treatment in 565 patients with Alzheimer's disease (AD2000): randomised double blind trial. *Lancet* **363**: 2105–2115.

Alcohol Concern (2002) *Report on the Mapping of Alcohol Services in England.* London: Alcohol Concern.

Alcohol Education and Research Council (2002) *Researching and Developing Alcohol Policy. Response from the Alcohol Education and Research Council to the National Alcohol Harm Reduction Strategy.* London: Alcohol Education and Research Council.

Amsterdam, JD & Brunswick, DJ (2003) Antidepressant monotherapy for bipolar type 2 major depression. *Bipolar Disorder* **5**(6): 388–395.

Areosa, SA, Sherriff, F & McShane, R (2005) Memantine for dementia. *Cochrane Database Systematic Review* **3**: CD003154. PMID 16034889.

Ashina, M (2002) Non-pharmacological treatment of Alzheimer's disease. http://www.cnsforum.com/magazine/nonpharmacological_treatment/dementia/.

Birks, JS, Melzer, D & Beppu, H (2003) Donepezil for mild and moderate Alzheimer's disease (Cochrane Review). *The Cochrane Library*, Issue 1. Oxford: Update Software.

Bowie, P & Takriti, Y (2004) Epidemiology of dementia. In Curran, S & Wattis, JP (eds) *Practical Management of Dementia: A Multi-Professional Approach.* Huddersfield: Radcliffe Medical Press.

British Liver Trust (2000) *Bulletin 5.* London: British Liver Trust.

British National Formulary (2005) *British National Formulary 50.* London: BMJ Publishing Group/Royal Pharmaceutical Society of Great Britain.

Brown, M & Fowler, G (1979) *Psych-dynamic Nursing: A Biosocial Orientation.* Philadelphia PA: BB Saunder Co.

Butters, MA, Soety, E & Becker, JT (1997) Memory rehabilitation. In Nusbaum, PD (ed.) *Handbook of Neuropsychology and Aging.* New York: Plenum Press.

Cade, J (1949) Lithium salts in the treatment of psychotic excitement. *Medical Journal of Australia* **36**: 349.

Cavanagh, J, Smythe, R & Goodwin, GM (2004) Relapse into mania or depression following lithium discontinuation: A 7-year follow up. *Acta Psychiatrica Scandinavica* **109**(2): 91.

Cook, C & Thompson, A (1997) B-complex vitamins in the prophylaxis and treatment of Wernicke-Korsakoff syndrome. *British Journal of Hospital Medicine* **57**(9): 461–465.

Coxhead, N, Silverstone, T & Cookson, J (1992) Carbomazepine vs lithium in the prophylaxis of bipolar affective disorder. *Acta Psychiatrica Scandinavica* **85**(2): 114–118.

Davidson, M, Weiser, M & Soares, K (2000) Novel antipsychotics in the treatment of psychosis and aggression associated with dementia: A meta-analysis of randomized controlled clinical trials. *International Psychogeriatrics* **12** (Suppl. 1): 271–277.

Department of Health (1993) *Health of the Nation Key Area Handbook: Mental Health.* London: The Stationery Office.

Department of Health (1999) *Clinical Standards Advisory Group Report on Services for People with Depression.* London: The Stationery Office.

Department of Health (2002) *Models of Care for the Treatment of Adult Drug Misusers.* London: The Stationery Office.

Department of Health (2005a) *Boost for Alcohol Treatment Provision with Publication of Programme of Improvement.* London: The Stationery Office.

Department of Health (2005b) *Consultation on the Independent Mental Capacity Advocate (IMCA) Service 2005: Summary of Responses.* London: The Stationery Office.

Department of Health (2005c) *Alcohol Misuse Interventions: Guidance on Developing a Local Programme of Improvement. Practical Steps on Improving Screening and Brief Interventions for Problem Drinkers.* London: The Stationery Office.

Department of Transport (2002) *Local Government and the Regions. Road Accidents Great Britain 2001: The Casualty Report.* London: The Stationery Office.

Devanand, DP, Pelton, GH, Marston, K, Camacho, Y, Roose, SP, Stern, Y & Sackheim, HA (2003) Sertraline treatment of elderly patients with depression and cognitive impairment. *International Journal of Geriatric Psychiatry* **18**(2): 123–30.

De Vreese, LP, Neri, M, Fioravanti, M, Belloi, L & Zanetti, O (2001) Memory rehabilitation in Alzheimer's disease: A review of progress. *International Journal of Geriatric Psychiatry* **16**: 794–809.

Dolovich, LR, Addis, A, Vaillancourt, JM, Power, JD, Koren, G & Einarson, TR (1998) Benzodiazepine use in pregnancy and major malformations or oral cleft. Meta-analysis of cohort and case control studies. *British Medical Journal* **317**(7162): 839–843.

Drugs and Therapeutics Bulletin (1995) The drug treatments of patients with schizophrenia. *Drugs and Therapeutics Bulletin* **33**(11): Nov.

Drugs and Therapeutics Bulletin (2004) Which atypical antipsychotic for schizophrenia? *Drugs and Therapeutics Bulletin* **42**(8): Aug.

Dunner, D cited by Marano, HE (2003) How to take an antidepressant. *Psychology Today* April 4.

Feldman, H, Gauthier, S, Hecker, J, Vellas, B, Subbiah, P & Whalen, E (2001) A 24 week randomised double blind study of donepezil in moderate to severe Alzheimer's disease. *Neurology* **57**: 613–620.

Finnema, E, Droes, RM, Ribbe, M & Van Tilburg, W (2000) The effects of emotion-oriented approaches in the care for persons suffering from dementia: A review of the literature. *International Journal of Geriatric Psychiatry* **15**: 141–161.

Frisher, M, Collins, J, Millson, D & Croft, P (2004) Prevalence of co-morbid psychiatric illness and substance misuse in primary care in England and Wales. *Journal of Epidemiology and Community Health* **58**: 1036–1041.

Gerard, D, Schellengber et al. (1992) Genetic linkage evidence for a familial Alzheimer's disease locus on chromosome 14. *Science* **25** (23 October): 668.

Gerlach, J & Larsen, EB (1999) Subjective experience and mental side effects of antipsychotic treatment. *Acta Psychiatrica Scandinavica* Suppl **395**: 113–117.

Gerlach, R (2004) *The History of Methadone: A Brief Overview on the Discovery of Methadone.* INDRO e.V. Münster.

Goldberg, JF & Truman, CJ (2003) Antidepressant induced mania, an overview of current controversies. *Bipolar Disorder* **5**(6): 407–420.

Gonzalez-Pinto, A, Gonzalez, C, Enjuto, S, Fernando de Corres, B, Lopez, P, Palomo, J, Gutierrez, M, Mosquera, F & Perez de Heredia, JL (2004) Psychoeducation and cognitive behavioural therapy in bipolar disorder: an update. *Acta Psychiatrica Scandinavica* **109**: 83–90.

Goodwin, GM (2003) Evidence-based guidelines for treating bipolar disorder: Recommendations from the British Association of Psychopharmacology. *Journal of Psychopharmacology* **17**: 149–173.

Goswami, N & Brosnan, G (2006) Over 20,000 children are hooked on heroin. *The Daily Telegraph*: 5 February.

Gray, R (2001) A randomised controlled trial of medication management training for CPNs. PhD thesis. London: Institute of Psychiatry, University of London.

Gray, R, Robson, D & Bressington, D (2002) Medication management for people with a diagnosis of schizophrenia. *Nursing Times* **96**.

Griffith, R (2004) Consent to examination and treatment 1: The capable adult patient. *Nurse Prescribing* **2**(4): 177–179.

Henderson, DC, Cagliero, E, Copeland, P, Barb, C, Euins, E, Hayden, D, Neber, MT, Anderson, EJ, Alison, DB, Daley, TB, Schoenfeld, D & Goff, DC (2005) Glucose metabolism in patients with schizophrenia treated with atypical antipsychotic agents. *Archive of General Psychiatry* **62**(1): 19–28.

Hislop, LJ, Wyatt, JP, McNaughton, GW, Ireland, AJ, Rainer, TH, Olverman, G & Laughton, LM (1995) Urban hypothermia in the west of Scotland. *British Medical Journal* **311**: 725–730.

Hunt, GE, Bergen, J & Bashir, M (2002) Medication compliance and co-morbid substance misuse in schizophrenia: Impact on community survival 4 years after relapse. *Schizophrenia Research* **54**: 253–264.

Huxley, NA, Parick, SV & Baldessarini, RJ (2000) Le psicoterapie nel disturbo bipolare: Lestatto attuale. No'os: Aggioramenti. *Psychiatria* (Rome) **1**: 77–101.

Jablensk, A, Sortorius, N, Ernberg, G et al. (1992) Schizophrenia: Manifestations, incidence and course in different cultures: A World Health Organization 10 country study. *Psychological Medicine* **20**: 1–97.

Kane, J, Honigfield, G, Singer, J, Meltzer, HY & the Clozaril Collaborative Study Group (1988) Clozapine for the treatment-resistant schizophrenic. A double blind comparison with chlorpromazine. *Archive of General Psychiatry* **45**: 789–796.

Kershaw, C, Budd, T, Kinshott, G, Mattinson, J, Mayhew, P & Myhill, A (2000) *The 2000 British Crime Survey, England and Wales.* London: Home Office Research, Development and Statistics Directorate.

Kerwin, RW (1994) The new atypical antipsychotics. A lack of extrapyramidal side effects and new routes in schizophrenia research. *British Journal of Psychiatry* **164**: 141–148.

Kisling, W (1994) Compliance, quality assurance and standards for relapse prevention in schizophrenia. *Acta Psychiatrica Scandinavica* **89** (supplement 382): 16–24.

Lanctot, KL, Best, TS, Mittmann, N, Liu, BA, Oh, PI, Einarson, TR, et al (1998) Efficacy and safety of neuroleptics in behavioral disorders associated with dementia. *Journal of Clinical Psychiatry* **59**(10): 550–563.

Lusznat, RH, Murphy, DP & Nunn, CM (1988) Carbomazepine vs lithium in the treatment and prophylaxis of mania (comment). *British Journal of Psychiatry* **153**: 198–204.

Manicdepressive.org (2004) www.manicdepressive.org/moodchart.html.

Marano, HE (2003) How to take an antidepressant. *Psychology Today*: April 4.

McGorry, PD, Yung, AR, Phillips, LU et al (2002) Randomised controlled trial of interventions designed to reduce the progression to 1st episode psychosis in a clinical sample with subthreshold symptoms. *Archive of General Psychiatry* **59**(10): 921–928.

Medicines and Healthcare Products Regulatory Agency (2003) *Selective Serotonin Reuptake Inhibitors (SSRIs): Overview of Regulatory Status and CSM Advice Relating to Major Depressive Disorder (MDD) in Children and Adolescents Including a Summary of Available Safety and Efficacy Data.* www.MHRA.gov.uk.

MeReC (2005) Non-drug therapies for depression in primary care. *MeReC Bulletin* **16**(1).

Mullen cited by Roberts, M (2005) Madness of labelling mental illness. BBC News, BBC.co.uk.

National Collaborating Centre for Mental Health (2006) Bipolar disorder. The management of bipolar disorder in adults, children and adolescents in primary and secondary care. Draft for 2nd consultation. London: National Collaborating Centre for Mental Health.

National Institute for Health and Clinical Excellence (2001) Guidance on the use of donepezil, rivastigmine and galantamine for the treatment of Alzheimer's disease. *NICE Technology Appraisal Guidance No. 19.* http://www.nice.org.uk/pdf/ALZHEIMER_full_guidance.pdf.

National Institute for Health and Clinical Excellence (2002) *Guidance on the Use of Newer (Atypical) Antipsychotic Drugs for the Treatment of Schizophrenia.* London: National Institute for Health and Clinical Excellence.

National Institute for Health and Clinical Excellence (2003a) Clozapine and valproate semisodium in the treatment of acute mania associated with bipolar 1 disorder. *Technology appraisal 66.* London: National Institute for Health and Clinical Excellence.

National Institute for Health and Clinical Excellence (2003b) Guidance on the use of electroconvulsive therapy. *Technology Appraisal 59.* London: National Institute for Health and Clinical Excellence.

National Institute for Health and Clinical Excellence (2004) Depression. Management of depression in primary and secondary care. *Clinical Guideline 23.* London: National Institute for Health and Clinical Excellence.

National Institute for Health and Clinical Excellence (2005) *Appraisal Consultation Document: Alzheimer's disease – Donepezil, Rivastigmine, Galantamine and Memantine (Review).* www.NICE.org.uk.

Neal, M & Briggs M (2000) Validation therapy for dementia. *Cochrane Database Systematic Review.* CD001394.

Nursing and Midwifery Council (2005) *UKCC Position Statement on the Covert Administration of Medicines. Disguising Medicines in Food.* London: Nursing and Midwifery Council.

Office for National Statistics (2000) *Living in Britain: Results from the 1998 General Household Survey.* London: The Stationery Office.

Okuma, T, Yamashita, I, Takahashi, R, Itah, H, Otsuki, G, Watanabe, S, Sarai, K, Hazama, H. & Inaga, K (1990) Comparison of the antimanic efficacy of carbomazepine and lithium carbonate by double blind controlled study. *Pharmacopsychiatry* **23**(3): 143–150.

Passmore, AP & Craig, DA (2004) The future of memory clinics. *Psychiatric Bulletin* **28**: 375–377.

Perry, EK, Tomlinson, BE & Blessed, G (1978) Correlation of cholinergic abnormalities with senile plaques and mental test scores in senile dementia. *British Medical Journal* **2**: 1457–1459.

Pocock, N (2006) The COMBINE study raise questions over role of acamprosate in treatment of alcohol dependence. *Journal of the American Medical Association* **295**: 2003–2017.

Prodigy (2006) Prodigy Guidance Depression. http://www.prodigy.nhs.uk/depression/ extended_information/management_issues.

Rosler, M (2002) The efficacy of cholinesterase inhibitors in treating the behavioural symptoms of dementia. *International Journal of Clinical practice.* **Jun** (127): 20–36.

Schneider, K (1959) *Clinical Psychopathology.* New York: Grune and Stratton.

Schultz, R, Mendlesohn, Haley, W et al. (2003) End-of-life care and the effects of bereavement on family caregivers of persons with dementia. *New England Journal of Medicine* **349**(20): 1936–1942.

Scottish Intercollegiate Guidelines Network (2003) *The Management of Harmful Drinking and Alcohol Dependence in Primary Care.* Report no. 74. Scottish Intercollegiate Guidelines Network. www.sign.ac.uk.

Scottish Intercollegiate Guidelines Network (2005) *Bipolar Affective Disorder. A National Clinical Guideline, 82.* Scottish Intercollegiate Guidelines Network. www.sign.ac.uk.

Shua-Haim, JR, Haim, T, Shi, Y, Kuo, YH & Smith, JM (2001) Depression among Alzheimer's caregivers: Identifying risk factors. *American Journal of Alzheimers Disease and Other Dementias* **16**(6): 353–359.

Sisodia, SS (1999) Series introduction: Alzheimer's disease: Perspectives for the new millennium. *Journal of Clinical Investigation* **104**(9): 1169–1170.

Spector, A, Davies, S, Woods, B & Orrell, M (2000a) Reality orientation for dementia: A systematic review of the evidence of effectiveness from randomized controlled trials. *Gerontologist* **40**: 206–212.

Spector, A, Orrell, M, Davies, S & Woods, B (2000b) Reality orientation for dementia. *Cochrane Database Systematic Review.* CD001119.

Spector, A, Orrell, M, Davies, S & Woods, RT (2000c) Reminiscence therapy for dementia. *Cochrane Database Systematic Review.* CD001120.

Stahl, SM (1999) *Psychopharmacology of Antipsychotics.* London: Martin Dunitz.

Tandon, R & Jibson, MD (2005) Efficacy of newer generation antipsychotics in the treatment of schizophrenia. *Psychoneuroendocrinology* **66**(Suppl. 5): 11–16.

Tariot, PN, Solomon, PR, Morris, JC, Kershaw, P, Lilienfeld, S, Ding, D & the Galantamine USA – Study Group (2000) A 5 month randomised placebo controlled trial of galantamine in AD. The galantamine USA 10 study group. *Neurology* **54**: 2269–2276.

Taylor, D, Paton, C & Kerwin, R (2005) *The Maudsley 2005–2006 Prescribing Guidelines* (8th edition). Oxfordshire: Taylor and Francis Group.

Thomas, CM & Morris, S (2000) Cost of depression among adults in England in 2000. *British Journal of Psychiatry* **183**: 514–519.

Waller, T & Rumball, D (2004) *Treating Drinkers and Drug Users in the Community.* Oxford: Blackwell Publishing.

Weaver, T, Hadden, P, Charles, V, Stimson, G, Renton, A et al. (2003) Co-morbidity of substance misuse and mental illness in the community in the community mental health and substance misuse services (COSMIC). *British Journal of Psychiatry* **183**: 304–313.

Weiden, P & Olfson, M (1995) Cost of relapse in schizophrenia. *Schizophrenia Bulletin* **21**(3): 419–429.

Weiden, PJ, Shaw, E & Mann, J (1987) Causes of neuroleptic non-compliance. *Psychiatric Annals* **16**: 571–578.

Wiersma, D, Nienhuis, FJ, Sloof, CJ & Giel, R (1998) Natural course of schizophrenic disorders: A 15 year follow up of a Dutch incident cohort. *Schizophrenia Bulletin* **24**(1): 75–85.

World Health Organization (2005a) *Introduction to Alcohol Misuse.* London: World Health Organization UK Collaborating Centre.

World Health Organization (2005b) *Introduction to Dementia.* London: World Health Organization UK Collaborating Centre. www.Library.nhs.uk/mentalhealth.

Yonkers, KA, Wisner, KL, Stowe, Z, Leibenluft, E, Cohen, L, Miller, L et al. (2004) Management of bipolar disorder during pregnancy and the postpartum period. *American Journal of Psychiatry* **161**(4): 608–620.

Zanetti, O, Frisoni, GB, De Leo, D, Dello, BM, Bianchetti, A & Trabucchi, M (1995) Reality orientation therapy in Alzheimer disease: Useful or not? A controlled study. *Alzheimer's Disease and Associated Disorders* **9**: 132–138.

11 Prescribing in Emergency Care

IAN LOVEDAY AND RICHARD PILBERY

In order to discuss prescribing in emergency care settings, it is useful to examine the scope of practice that forms emergency care. Until relatively recently, emergency care could be easily defined and would generally have been considered to involve nurses working within accident and emergency (A&E) departments and paramedics and ambulance technicians in the pre-hospital setting. Today the range of roles for non-medical healthcare professionals is broad and new roles are developing rapidly. There are many reasons for this: emergency care has been subject to the same challenges as the rest of UK healthcare, the effects of an ageing population, changes in working patterns for doctors and perhaps most significantly the publication of the white papers *Reforming Emergency Care* (2001) and *Taking Healthcare to the Patient* (Department of Health, 2005). These policies created targets for A&E departments that could only be met with new and innovative ways of working.

One of the earliest changes was an increase in the number of emergency nurse practitioners (ENPs) working within A&E departments. The ENP role was initially developed in the UK in the early 1980s, but *Reforming Emergency Care* (2001) made the patient with minor injuries a new priority and consequently the ENP role became more common. As these changes were taking place, other developments were affecting the pre-hospital arena. New services have been aimed at avoiding admissions and ensuring previously low-priority patient groups received attention in a more timely manner (Picton, 2006). Other developments recognized the fact that many patients accessing emergency care did not have emergency conditions; rather, the lack of flexibility in other services left them without another point of contact. Such patients not only represented unnecessary attendances at A&E departments, they often represented unnecessary admissions to hospital and if the pathways existed, could have been cared for in the community. To meet these needs the emergency care practitioner (ECP) role was developed.

In addition to these roles, those in NHS Direct and walk-in centres also fall under the umbrella of emergency care. The expansion of this area of healthcare was such that in 2003 the Royal College of Nursing's accident and emergency nursing forum was renamed 'Emergency Care Forum' (Lipley, 2003).

As the above roles developed, so did the legislation surrounding prescribing and drug administration. Initially most services utilized patient group directives (PGDs). While PGDs enabled drugs to be administered, they had many drawbacks, not

Towards Prescribing Practice. Edited by J. McKinnon.
© 2007 John Wiley & Sons, Ltd.

least that they were not patient centred, they were based on the area or service the practitioner worked in rather than a level of knowledge or skill. These and many other issues made the use of PGDs a poor substitute for genuine non-medical prescribing.

A vast range of drugs are in use in emergency care and this chapter aims to examine some of the commonly used agents. The drugs that have been selected for examination are not only important in the emergency care field, but they also demonstrate wider points relating to prescribing practice and provide useful studies of the type of knowledge required for safe and effective prescribing.

TETANUS

A commonly used agent within A&E departments is tetanus toxoid immunisation, or more correctly since 2003 tetanus and diphtheria immunisation (Pulse, 2003). Tetanus is not a common disease in the developed world and is rarely seen in the UK. Despite this, when it does occur it has a high mortality rate, often requiring ventilation and support in the intensive care department. The pharmacological and physiological issues related to tetanus are useful to examine, as they share important factors with other vaccines and infectious agents. Tetanus is mediated by the Gram-positive anaerobic bacteria *Clostridium tetani*, which is readily found in soil and manure and may be associated with contaminated illicit drugs (Walker, 2004). *Clostridium tetani* is closely related to *Clostridium perfringens* and *Clostridium botulism*, which are the infective agents involved in gas gangrene and botulism food poisoning.

The anaerobic nature of the bacteria means that puncture wounds present a high risk, as the bacteria can be injected via a small wound and once under the skin it thrives in a largely oxygen-free environment. As the bacteria multiply, the endotoxin tetanospasmin is released. The toxin affects the nerves of the central nervous system; typically the cranial nerves are affected first. Tetanospasmin blocks the inhibitory affects of γ (gamma) aminobutyric acid (GABA), the effect of which is uncontrolled motor activity (Thwaites and Farrar, 2003). Symptoms are first seen in the facial nerves and this gives rise to the term 'lockjaw' to describe tetanus. As the disease progresses, it affects the wider central nervous system. Ultimately, the nerves innervating the respiratory muscles are affected and if ventilation is not commenced death may result. Even where ITU care is available, mortality is high and there is a lack of evidence supporting any therapeutic intervention (Thwaites and Farrar, 2003).

In light of the discussion above, prevention of tetanus is important and two agents are available to achieve this. Tetanus toxoid is an active immunisation that can be used to enable individuals to develop immunity. Tetanus immunoglobulin is a passive agent that provides ready-formed antibodies. The pharmacological actions of the two drugs are different and offer a useful study to understand other vaccines. Tetanus toxoid is classed as an active agent because of its effect on the immune systems. The vaccine contains *Clostridium tetani* bacterium that has been deliberately killed in the production process (Prosser et al., 2000). The normal immune response is for the bacteria to be phagocytosed by cells that act as antigen-presenting cells (APCs). These cells present fragments of the vaccine on their surface bound with a major histolocompatibility complex (MHC) antigen. APCs then migrate to the lymphatic tissue, where the combination of APCs and MHCs is able to initiate the process, which triggers an antibody or cell-mediated immune response (Tortora and Derrickson, 2006). See Figure 11.1.

There are several important factors that need to be considered for this response to be effective. Subcutaneous fat contains relatively few of the cells able to function as an APC and hence the vaccine should be given intramuscularly. It is also for this reason that one of the most commonly used injection sites (the buttock) is unsuitable for administration of a vaccine (Zuckerman, 2000). The need to ensure intramuscular injection also makes the choice of needle size important; this can be difficult if only pre-filled syringes are available. One study (Poland et al., 1997)

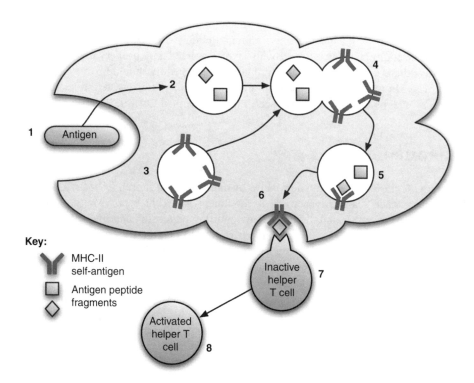

Figure 11.1 Antigen phagocytosis by antigen-presenting cells. Subsequent processing results in antigen–MHE–II complexes being inserted into the plasma membrane, which activates the T cell. (See also colour plate 23).

demonstrated that the depth of subcutaneous fat measured over the deltoid in a sample of 220 subjects would have made intramuscular injection with a 16 mm needle impossible in 17 % of men and 50 % of women. A final point to consider is that the process of the immune response outlined above is not immediate and so will not provide protection in people who have not been previously immunised. Patients who have not received previous doses of tetanus toxoid or who have wounds that present a particularly high tetanus risk require tetanus immunoglobulin.

Whereas tetanus toxoid is an active vaccine, the immunoglobulin is described as passive as its clinical effects do not depend on the production of antibodies (Prosser et al., 2000). Tetanus immunoglobulin is produced from donated blood and contains antibodies to the *Clostridium tetani* bacteria. As the immunoglobulin provides ready-formed antibodies, it gives a level of immediate immunity. This, however, is a short-term action and patients requiring immunoglobulin will also require tetanus toxoid. These will need to be administered at separate sites to avoid an immune reaction between the two agents. The recommended vaccination schedule states that five doses of tetanus toxoid at the appropriate intervals will provide lifelong immunity (Health Protection Agency, 2003) If a person sustains a tetanus-prone wound after having five doses of vaccine, they require no further treatment. If, however, the risk is particularly high, such as in the case of wounds contaminated with manure, tetanus immunoglobulin should be given to provide immediate additional cover. People who have completed their primary immunisation course and are up to date with their immunisation schedule should be treated in the same way. In the case of people who are not up to date, tetanus toxoid should be given as well as tetanus immunoglobulin (Chief Medical Officer, 2002).

THROMBOLYSIS

Cardiovascular disease is a major cause of morbidity and mortality in the UK and there have been many advances in its treatment in recent years. Many of these advances are based around therapies that control hypertension and improve cardiac function. A therapy that is particularly pertinent to emergency care is thrombolysis for the treatment of acute myocardial infarction (AMI). AMI occurs when a thrombus develops in one or more of the vessels that perfuse the myocardium. As the thrombus increases in size or deforms, the myocardium receives an inadequate blood supply. The typical effect of this is the characteristic chest pain of angina. However, if the thrombus causes a more significant occlusion, then permanent damage occurs.

The success of thrombolysis in reducing the morbidity and mortality associated with AMI was demonstrated in multicentre international trials, and thrombolysis is the principal treatment for acute AMI in most UK hospitals (Boersma et al., 1996). Initially thrombolysis was a therapy that was carried out in coronary care units, but as it became clear that the speed with which it was administered to the patient had a bearing on the outcome, it started to become common in A&E departments. In turn, it became clear that the important time span for the starting of thrombolytic therapy was not the patient's arrival at hospital, the so-called door to needle time, but rather the time since the onset of pain (Weston et al., 1994). In many cases the first healthcare professional to see the patient after the onset of chest pain is the paramedic and hence in some areas of the country thrombolysis moved into the pre-hospital setting.

There are two types of agent typically used for thrombolysis in the patient experiencing AMI. The drug that has seen the longest use is streptokinase, although the use of tissue plasminogen activating drugs (TPAs) such as alteplase and reteplase is becoming more common. TPAs have been shown to give greater benefits to the patient in some circumstances and for the pre-hospital setting; they have practical advantages in terms of ease of use as they are administered as an IV bolus rather than an infusion.

In order to understand the clinical effects of thrombolytic drugs, it is important to have an understanding of the mechanism that gives rise to the formation of thrombus in the arteries of the myocardium. Typically the cardiac arteries of patients experiencing ischaemic chest pain will contain atherosclerotic plaques, which reduce the size of the vessel lumen (Prosser et al., 2000). These plaques can occlude 75 % of the lumen without symptoms being experienced by the patient. If myocardial oxygen demand exceeds the ability of the vessel to flow blood, angina-type chest pains will result. In the case of exertional angina, this pain can be relieved by reducing the myocardium's oxygen demands by resting or with pharmacological interventions (Neal, 2002). In unstable angina, the plaque is unstable in its nature and its deformation can lead to a sudden change in the size of the lumen that may occur at rest (Prosser et al., 2000). In addition to the deformation, the plaque can rupture, releasing the 'lipid gruel' contained inside. This can result in increased aggregation of platelets and the formation of a thrombus. If the thrombus occludes the artery briefly, then the effects may be limited to an episode of angina symptoms. If, however, the occlusion remains for a significant period of time, then permanent or even fatal damage will occur to the myocardium. Typical treatment addresses both the action of platelets, which can be inhibited by aspirin, and fibrinolysis of the thrombus (Prosser et al., 2000).

The actions of the fibrinolytic and coagulation systems are interrelated and the formation of a clot triggers the fibrinolytic system to commence a process that in other circumstances would limit the size of the thrombus and ensure its destruction. The action of the fibrinolytic system involves the formation of plasmin from an inactive precursor plasminogen; this natural fibrinolytic system provides an essential function in the control of clotting generally. In the cardiac vessels, however, the destruction of the thrombus does not occur in a useful time span. This relationship between thrombus formation and fibrinolysis is summarised in Figure 11.2.

Thrombolytic drugs interact with the fibrinolytic system, causing it to lyse the forming thrombus that is threatening coronary perfusion. As with almost all drugs, the effects are not specific to the coronary vessels but affect all thrombus formations, giving rise to many of the contraindications of thrombolysis (Rang et al., 2003).

Streptokinase is the first-generation agent used for thrombolysis and is produced from the B-haemolytic streptococci. Its effects are achieved through the indirect activation of plasminogen into its active form, plasmin (Craig and Stitzel, 2004). Streptokinase has the disadvantage that it can provoke allergic or anaphylactic

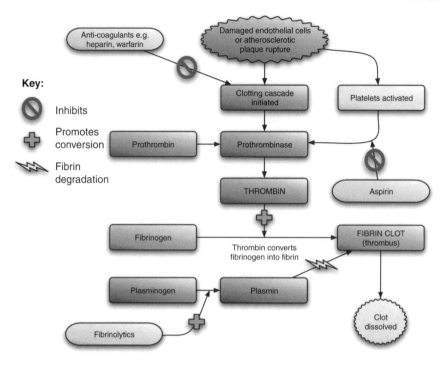

Figure 11.2 The effects of anticoagulants, aspirin and fibrinolytics on the coagulation cascade. (See also colour plate 24).

reactions, which are more likely after a first use of the drug has mediated antibody production. It is also the case that the therapeutic actions of streptokinase are blocked by the antistreptoccal antibodies that develop after first exposure (Rang et al., 2003). For these reasons patients are generally treated with streptokinase only once. Patients who require thrombolysis and have been treated with streptokinase in the past will be treated with a TPA to avoid these complications. While streptokinase has been proved to be effective and remains in common use in hospitals, it is less appropriate for use in the pre-hospital setting. Streptokinase is administered as an intravenous infusion of 1.5 M units over a one-hour period and clearly this is less than ideal when swift transport is a priority. The second-generation thrombolytics activate plasminogen more directly than streptokinase, and are more suited for use in the pre-hospital setting as they are delivered by bolus injections.

The clinical indications for thrombolytic therapy are described by the UK's Resuscitation Council (2005) as:

- ST segment elevation > 0.2 mv in 2 adjacent chest leads, or 0.1 mv in 2 or more adjacent limb leads or
- Dominant R waves and ST depression in V1–V3 (posterior infarction) or
- New onset (or presumed new onset) left bundle branch block.

The contraindications for thrombolysis arise out of the fact that thrombolytics, like all drugs, affect the whole body and thus will lyse thrombi wherever they exist; hence they put the patient at risk of bleeding. The contraindications are outlined below (Resuscitation Council, 2005: 20).

Absolute contraindications:

- previous haemorrhagic stroke
- ischaemic stroke during the previous six months
- central nervous system damage or neoplasm
- recent surgery
- active internal bleeding
- known or suspected aortic dissection
- known bleeding disorder.

Relative contraindications:

- refractory hypertension
- transient ischaemic attack in the previous six months
- oral anticoagulant treatment
- pregnancy or less than one week post-partum
- traumatic CPR
- non-compressible vascular puncture
- active peptic ulcer disease
- advanced liver disease
- infective endocarditis
- previous allergic reaction to the thrombolytic to be used.

The relative contraindications described above would in many cases not exclude the use of thrombolysis, but would require the advice of an expert clinician such as a cardiologist. While the indications listed are widely accepted, it may be the case that additional restrictions may be in place in some clinical settings. Thrombolysis by paramedics who are operating under the Joint Royal Colleges Ambulance Liaison Committee (2004) guidelines may in some cases require the electronic transmission of the ECG for analysis.

ANTIBIOTICS

Of the many types of pharmaceutical agents in common use in the care of minor injuries, antibiotics are one of the most useful and in some circumstances one of the most controversial. The range of indications for antibiotic therapy in emergency care is vast, but an indication that is particularly pertinent to non-medical prescribers is that of prophylaxis, following a bite either human or animal. Bites of this kind are very prone to infection, as the bacterial flora from the mouth is often introduced into the wound. Such wounds often occur on the hands from animals, frequently when people attempt to separate fighting dogs, or as a complication of punch injuries. Wounds to the hands present particular issues in that relatively minor injuries can prove disabling for patients, particularly when they involve structures involved with movement and sensation (Purcell, 2004). The use of antibiotics prophylactically in such circumstances is common, yet it remains controversial (Purcell, 2004).

The evidence supporting the use of prophylactic antibiotics for bite injuries is not strong and some evidence suggests that particular types of bites are more infection prone than others (Turner, 2004). Wyat et al. (2003) advocate the use of antibiotics in bites that form puncture wounds, those on hands, bites from rats and cats, in people who are immuno-compromised and in wounds that show clinical signs of infection.

While the use of antibiotic prophylaxis is controversial, the use of antibiotics to treat infected bite wounds is not. Wounds that are infected can generally be identified by the presence of erythema, the production of pus and localised heat and swelling. It is important when dealing with such infections to observe for signs of systemic infection. These include tracking, pyrexia and the patient being generally unwell. Such patients may require intravenous antibiotics and hospital admission.

The commonly used agent in patients who have sustained bites and are not allergic to penicillin is co-amoxiclav. Patients who are allergic to penicillin and its derivatives can be treated with erythromycin, however this is not effective over the same range of bacteria as co-amoxiclav (Wyat et al., 2003).

As with all drugs, antibiotics can cause a range of unwanted side effects and can potentially mediate allergies. When taking a history from a patient who has an antibiotic allergy, it is often helpful to enquire into the nature of the response. In the case of antibiotics some adverse responses can be due to pharmacological function rather than allergy. Antibiotics will act against all sensitive bacteria, including those that are not pathological. This can affect the gut and cause diarrhoea, but even in those affected it may be at a level they can accept. Some drugs use the pro-drug concept, which was discussed in Chapter 1. This process relies on the re-absorption of the drug from the gut; therefore any other drug that changes the gut's action could affect this process. There are a wide variety of pro-drugs, including some types of oral contraceptive, and so patients should be warned to use other precautions.

No discussion about side effects of antibiotics would be complete without mention of metronidazole. This is a drug that acts against protozoa and anaerobic bacteria. Metronidazole inhibits the action of the enzyme aldehyde dehydrogenase, which is involved in a range of processes including the metabolism of alcohol. The combination of alcohol and metronidazole can induce tachycardia, flushing, hyperventilation, panic and distress (Rang et al., 2003).

THE POISONED PATIENT

Poisoning is a common presentation in emergency care. It may be accidental or as part of a suicide or parasuicide attempt. The exact history and type of poisoning may be unclear, as illustrated in Table 11.1. Specific advice on the poisoned patient can be accessed from the National Poisons Information Service, either by telephone or electronically via Toxbase.

The case outlined in Table 11.1 is of a patient with a reduced level of consciousness after taking unknown drugs and alcohol. In such cases it should never be assumed that any reduction in consciousness level is due to alcohol. With no clear history of what drugs have been taken, judgements will have to be made from the patient's condition as to which drugs may be involved and which specific antidotes may be useful. In a patient with a reduced level of consciousness, opiates may be suspected, particularly if the respiratory rate is reduced and the pupils are constricted. In such cases, naloxone hydrochloride (Narcan) may be administered as it acts as an antagonist to opioid receptors. Naloxone can be given IV or IM 0.8–2 mg, which can be repeated up to a maximum of 10 mg. Naloxone has a shorter half life than all but the shortest-acting opiates that it counteracts and this can create issues when patients wish to leave hospital, particularly those who leave against medical advice (Clarke et al., 2002).

For this reason, Clarke et al. (2002) recommend that naloxone should not be administered to patients who are maintaining their own airway and have SpO_2 of > 92% and a respiratory rate of >10; rather, they should be observed for at least two hours. Those patients whose vital signs do not meet this criteria should receive naloxone and be observed. Patients who have taken long-lasting opioids may require admission. In most other cases, discharge can be safely considered after two hours (Clarke et al., 2002). It is important to note that while discharge may be considered in the case of accidental overdose, in deliberate overdose thought needs to be given to the patient's psychological health. The fact that the overdose was not lethal does not mean that it was not intended to be so. Patients who have self-harmed are at a greatly increased risk of committing suicide in the ensuing year (Norman and Ryrie, 2004).

Naloxone should be used with caution in patients who have opiate dependency, as it can induce withdrawal symptoms. Given the history, benzodiazepine overdose may be considered as this would cause drowsiness and a reduced level of consciousness. Benzodiazepines such as diazepam have active metabolites and because of this have a long half life. The drug flumazenil is able to reverse the effects of benzodiazepines, but is rarely used to do so outside of anaesthetic settings and indeed is not licensed in the UK for use in overdose. Its half life is less than that of

Table 11.1   Case study

Mandy Jones is a young woman who has been brought to A&E by concerned friends. She has been depressed for some time and has been found today in a semi-conscious state. She was found with an empty bottle of vodka and numerous empty tablet bottles, some of which are not labelled. Mandy is maintaining her own airway, has a respiratory rate of 14, pulse of 110 and blood pressure of 105/70. She is responsive to voice but is drowsy. She has no past medical history of note and it appears that the tablets may not have been hers.

its target drug and hence there is a risk of a transient recovery from the effects of the overdose. It also carries risks if used in mixed overdoses, particularly with tricyclic antidepressants, which may induce fitting. If a patient was to fit, the first-line drugs used to terminate the fit are benzodiazepines such as IV lorazepam or diazepam. After receiving treatment with flumazenil, these drugs would be rendered ineffective. Generally, people who have overdosed on benzodiazepines are observed and treated symptomatically until the effects subside.

This principle of observe and treat is a common theme in poisoning, as relatively few drugs have specific antidotes. A drug that does have a commonly used antidote is paracetamol, and while this would be unlikely to cause all the signs seen in the case study, it could have been taken in combination with other drugs. The presence of paracetamol can be demonstrated with a blood test, taken ideally four hours after ingestion. The paracetamol level is plotted on a chart, which takes into account the time that has elapsed since the overdose and the patient's level of risk. The high-risk line on the chart is used to determine the need for treatment in patients that have greater activity in their P450 oxidases (see Figure 11.3). At particular risk are patients who are malnourished, are HIV positive, have liver disease, are taking enzyme-inducing drugs or have cystic fibrosis or viral infections (Hartley, 2002).

Paracetamol can be lethal in overdose. To reduce deaths from paracetamol overdose, the number of tablets sold in a pack as a general sales list item was reduced in 1998 (Hughes et al., 2003). The dangers presented by paracetamol arise out of its route of metabolism and excretion. At normal doses most paracetamol is metabolised by the liver to glucuronide and sulphate conjugates, which are excreted with no ill effect (Hartley, 2002). A small amount of paracetamol is metabolised by P450 mixed-function oxidases to form the highly reactive metabolite N-acetyl-p-benzoquinone imine (NAPBQI). Under normal circumstances NAPBQI conjugates with glutathione, but in overdose glutathione reserves are rapidly depleted and the NAPBQI causes irreversible liver damage (Hartley, 2002).

There are two treatment options for paracetamol overdose, the intravenous agent N-acetylcysteine (parvolex) and the oral agent methionine. Parvolex is the more commonly used and there is some evidence to suggest it is more effective (Alsalim and Fadel, 2003). Parvolex is given in a weight-dependent dose, which is shown in Table 11.2.

In the past, gastric lavage has been used in patients who have overdosed, but this is now an extremely rare procedure and in the case study would require anaesthetic involvement to protect the patient's airway. Activated charcoal can be useful in many different types of poisoning and its use where possible within an hour of overdose is recommended by the European Association of Poison Centres (Karim et al., 2001). There are a range of charcoal preparations available, but most contain 50 g of charcoal that is in a form that the patient can drink. It can also be delivered via a nasogastric tube for patients who have difficulty drinking the charcoal. The patient's airway must be adequately protected before administering charcoal and in the compromised patient this may require the involvement of an anaesthetist.

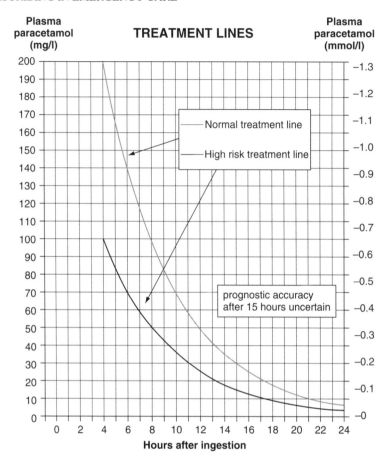

Figure 11.3 Paracetamol chart

Reproduced by permission of Professor Philip Routledge, WCM Toxicology and Therapeutics Centre, University of Cardiff

In the types of poisoning described above, specific treatments are available. However, in most poisoning instances this is not the case. All poisoned patients need careful monitoring, particularly as the exact nature of the poisoning is often unknown. The patient's clinical condition should be monitored closely. Many drugs can cause haemodynamic changes and hence ECG and blood pressure monitoring are important. Changes in the level of consciousness are common and neurological observations have a place in monitoring and identifying changes. This is important, as a fall in the level of consciousness reduces the patient's ability to maintain their own airway and thus increases the risk of aspiration.

The poisons and treatments discussed above represent some of the most common types of overdose and treatment. There are a range of other specific antidotes

Table 11.2   Parvolex dose

Adult or over 12 years

Dose	Parvolex mg/kg	Volume of 5% dextrose for dilution	Duration of infusion
1	150	200 ml	15 mins
2	50	500 ml	4 hours
3	100	1000 ml	16 hours

Child less than 12 years and over 20 kg

1	150	100 ml	15 mins
2	50	250 ml	4 hours
3	100	500 ml	16 hours

Child bodyweight less than 20 kg

1	150	3 ml/kg	15 mins
2	50	7 ml/kg	4 hours
3	100	14 ml/kg	16 hours

If for any reason dextrose is unsuitable 0.9% sodium chloride may be used

Source: Toxbase, the website of the National Poisons Information Service http://www.spib.axl. co.uk/

Table 11.3   Specific treatments

Specific treatment	Agent on which it is effective
Parvolex and methionine	Paracetamol
Naloxone hydrochloride	Opiates
Flumazenil	Benzodiazepines
Dicobalt edetate	Cyanide
Digibind	Digoxin
Glucagon	Hypoglycaemia, beta blocker overdose
Obidoxime	Organophosphates
Desferrioxamine	Iron tablets

that can used in particular circumstances and these are summarised in Table 11.3. In all cases detailed advice should be sought from the National Poisons Information Service.

LOCAL ANAESTHESIA

There are a range of procedures that require the use of local anaesthesia in emergency care. Possibly the most common is the suturing of wounds, a task performed by a variety of practitioners. The use of sutures has declined recently as the use of tissue adhesive has become more common but there many wounds where sutures are the first choice for closure (Aukerman et al., 2005). This choice is made on the basis of issues such as depth, location of the wound and the type of tissue involved.

The most commonly used agent to achieve local anaesthesia is lidocaine (formerly known as lignocaine). This is a safe and reliable drug when used appropriately, but knowledge of its actions and functions will highlight some of its contraindications and risks. There are a range of drugs used as local anaesthetics, all of which have a similar pharmacological action and relative advantages in different circumstances (Rang et al., 2003). The transmission of action potentials along nerve fibres depends on the movement of sodium across the cell membrane of the nerve cells. Lidocaine and other local anaesthetic agents are able to block the sodium channels on cell membranes and thus block the transmission of action potentials (Rang et al., 2003). The effects of local anaesthetic drugs are at their strongest in smaller diameter nerve fibres (Rang et al., 2003). The Aδ and C fibres are most affected and these are the fibres that are most involved with the transmission of pain (Tortora and Derrickson, 2006). This gives the effect of preventing painful stimuli being perceived while leaving other sensations less affected, hence the patient should be warned that while they will not feel pain during the procedure they may feel movement of the instruments.

The potential risks associated with lidocaine arise out of the fact that drugs affect the body as a whole and rarely, if ever, just the target tissue. The most important unwanted effects are on the cardiovascular and central nervous system. In excessive doses, signs and symptoms ranging from restlessness and tremor to hypotension and even cardiac arrest can occur (Rang et al., 2003). To avoid these affects when using lidocaine as a local anaesthetic, a maximum dose of 3 mg/kg is recommended or 20 ml of 1 % lidocaine in an adult (Purcell, 2004; Wyat et al., 2003). This is generally adequate for the suturing of minor cuts and lacerations. In the cases where this volume of lidocaine is inadequate, reduced concentrations such as 0.5 % lidocaine or lidocaine with epinephrine (formally known as adrenaline) can be used. It is important to note, however, that lidocaine with epinephrine should never be used in a terminal structure such as a finger or toe, as the resulting vasoconstriction can threaten the perfusion of that structure. The localised vasoconstriction that is caused by epinephrine allows a higher dose to be used, as it reduces the movement of lidocaine into the general circulation. It can also be useful in wounds, particularly scalp wounds that are bleeding heavily. The vasoconstriction reduces bleeding and once the sutures are in place the pressure that they create further reduces bleeding. The maximum recommended dose of lidocaine with epinephrine is 500 mg, which is 50 ml of 1 % lidocaine solution (Wyat et al., 2003).

PAIN

The Healthcare Commission's emergency department survey 2004/2005 identified that over two-thirds of patients who presented to an emergency department in

England were in pain. Therefore any pharmacological discussion on emergency care would not be complete without considering analgesia.

The British Association for Emergency Medicine Clinical Effectiveness Committee guidelines for the management of pain in adults and children (British Association for Emergency Medicine, 2004a, 2004b) list a number of recommended analgesic drugs, several of which are also in the Joint Royal Colleges Ambulance Liaison Committee guidelines for ambulance paramedics (Joint Royal Colleges Ambulance Liaison Committee, 2004). These broadly fall into opiates and non-steroidal anti-inflammatory drugs (NSAIDs). There are others, but the only other drug that appears in both guidelines is an analgesic gas, Entonox, which will also be considered in this section.

In order to understand how analgesic drugs work, it is necessary to understand a little more about pain. Pain is a subjective phenomenon that is difficult to define precisely, but you will almost certainly have experienced it. The International Association for the Study of Pain has provided one ubiquitous definition (Merskey and Bogduk, 1994: 210):

> An unpleasant sensory and emotional experience associated with actual or potential tissue damage, or described in terms of such damage.

Pain has many forms and can occur with no apparent traumatic cause (such as trigeminal neuralgia) and can remain long after the stimulus that was the original cause has passed, such as in phantom limb pain (Rang et al., 2003). For the sake of brevity and simplicity, the focus of this section will remain on acute pain occurring in response to tissue injury, rather than the often more problematic brain and nerve injury-induced pain, which may not respond so well to common analgesic drugs.

The first documented theory about pain transmission comes from the seventeenth century, when French philosopher René Descartes first described specific pain pathways carrying pain signals from the pain receptor in the skin to a pain centre in the brain (DeLeo, 2006). This theory remained essentially unchanged for over 300 years until 1965, when Ronald Wall and Patrick Melzack published their gate control theory of pain (Melzack and Wall, 1965). Remarkably, this theory has stood the test of time and modern science, albeit with some refinement (Dickinson, 2002).

ACUTE PAIN IN CHILDREN

Section 6 of the National Service Framework for Children recognised that pain in children is both underestimated and inadequately treated (Department of Health, 2004). There are a number of reasons for this, including the mistaken assumption that children, especially infants, do not experience pain in the same way as adults. In addition, there has been a lack of education of medical staff about paediatric pain management and measurement, and fears surrounding possible side effects and addiction of strong analgesics have tempered their use (American Academy of Pediatrics and American Pain Society, 2001).

There are numerous pain assessment tools, which take essentially one of four types. Visual analogue scales provide a straight line with no pain at one end and worst pain imaginable at the other, and the child picks the point on the line that they feel represents their pain. Similar to this are numerical scales, which consist of a straight line with numerical markers. The happy face/sad face tool provides a number of faces, usually with a happy face at one end and an unhappy, crying face at the other. These tools can generally be used with children over four years of age (Maurice et al., 2002a).

Behavioural tools can be utilised for infants and also for children who cannot understand or communicate. Scales such as the Children's Hospital of Eastern Ontario Pain Scale (CHEOPS) measure pain by assessing the child's alertness, level of agitation, respiratory response, blood pressure and facial tensions as well as several other indicators, but have the disadvantage that they are quite complicated (Royal College of Nursing, 1999). In neonates, facial scales have been validated that take account of certain facial expressions displayed by neonates in response to pain (McGrath and Unruh, 2006).

One tool described by Ball (2002) has been designed by St Bartholomew's Hospital and the London NHS Trust and utilises a combination of faces and numerical and behavioural scales to enable simple and reliable assessment of pain. Once a level of pain had been ascertained, an analgesic algorithm was used to determine appropriate treatment. During the validation of the tool, researchers found that despite the provision of the algorithm, doctors were still providing insufficient analgesia. However, the tool was sufficiently successful to be included in the latest BAEM guidelines for the management of pain in children (British Association for Emergency Medicine, 2004b). In addition, the latest edition of the JRCALC guidelines (Joint Royal Colleges Ambulance Liaison Committee, 2004) also changed its recommendation for analgesics such as morphine to be administered to children over 12 months of age, a vast improvement on the previous guidelines that did not even include morphine for paediatric administration (Roberts et al., 2005).

GATE CONTROL THEORY AND PAIN PATHWAYS

Pain is processed in three main areas, peripherally, at the spinal level and at the supraspinal level. When tissue is damaged, the sensory endings of C-polymodal nociceptors (PMN) and Aδ (A-delta) nerve fibres are stimulated. C-fibres cause dull, burning pain, whereas the Aδ fibres cause sharp and well-localised pain. There is local release of a number of chemicals including prostaglandins, which can lead to increased stimulation or sensitivity of these nerve endings. NSAIDs interfere with the action of prostaglandins and so are useful as mild analgesics (McGavock, 2005).

These afferent impulses (along with other sensory input) travel to the dorsal horn of the spinal cord, where they release peptides such as substance P and glutamate. Pain transmission is regulated within the dorsal horn by a 'gate', which consists of ascending and descending pathways as well as inhibitory interneural connections.

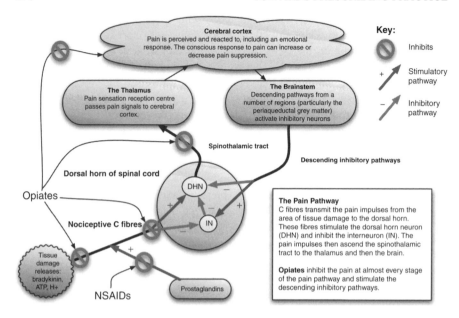

Figure 11.4 The pain pathway. Sites of action for opiates and NSAIDs are shown. (See also colour plate 25).

Figure 11.4 highlights the components of the pain pathway. The spinothalamic tract takes neural impulses from the dorsal horn up into the thalamus, where the signals are transmitted to the cortex and other areas in the brain. Inhibitory impulses arise from pathways, releasing serotonin (5HT) and enkephalins. At the spinal level, afferent impulses from Aβ (A-beta) mechanoreceptors may also stimulate inhibitory interneurons in the spinal cord, which may explain why vigorously rubbing and transcutaneous electrical nerve stimulation (TENS) appear to diminish the severity of the pain stimulus (Barlas and Lundeburg, 2006).

OPIOIDS

Probably the best-known opioid is morphine, and most notorious drug of abuse diamorphine or heroin. Opiates act in all three of the pain-processing areas, even

Table 11.4 Wind-up

Activated synapses progressively increase their action potential output with repeated C-fibre nociceptor stimulus. This results in heightened pain sensation even if the repeated stimulus is of the same intensity, and is known as 'wind-up'. This effect ceases as soon as the stimulus is removed, but highlights the importance of early administration of analgesia by healthcare professionals.

Source: Rang et al. (2003: 564)

Table 11.5   Opioid receptors and their action

Action / Receptor	μ / δ	κ	ORL
Analgesia	Supraspinal and spinal	Spinal	None
Respiratory depression	Marked	Slight	None
Pupil	Constricts	None	Dilates
Gastrointestinal motility	Reduced (constipating)	None	None
Mood / effect	Euphoria inducing and sedating	Dysphoria inducing and mildly sedating	Marked dysphoric and psychomimetic actions
Physical dependence	$+++$	$+$	None

Source: Dawson (2002: 68)

peripherally (Machelska and Stein, 2000). Along with the endogenous opioids, such as enkephalins, opiates act on four types of receptors: μ, δ, κ (mu, delta, kappa) and opioid-receptor-like (ORL). The effects of opioid on each of these receptor types are summarised in Table 11.5.

Opioids work by decreasing intracellular cyclic AMP (cAMP) and by coupling to potassium (K^+) and calcium (Ca^{2+}) channels. This inhibits presynaptic transmitter release and reduces postsynaptic excitability. Supraspinally, this results in activation of the descending (inhibitory) pathways from the periaqueductal grey matter in the brain to the dorsal horn. At the spinal level (i.e. the dorsal horn), opioids inhibit the pain impulses being transmitted up the spinothalamic pathway to the brain. Peripherally, the nociceptors' afferent impulses are also inhibited, reducing the frequency of impulses reaching the dorsal horn (Dale and Haylett, 2004).

As well as morphine's analgesic properties, it also causes euphoria, suppresses the cough reflex and inhibits enteric nerves, resulting in reduced motility and thus constipation. It also is a potent respiratory depressant, as μ-receptor activation reduces the respiratory centre's sensitivity to carbon dioxide (CO_2). Another often-cited side effect of morphine administration is nausea and vomiting. However, a recent randomised controlled trial has challenged this view, demonstrating that the incidence of nausea and vomiting following administration of morphine for acute pain is so low that prophylactic administration of anti-emetics is not justified (Bradshaw and Sen, 2006).

NON-STEROIDAL ANTI-INFLAMMATORY DRUGS

When tissue is injured, inflammation occurs as part of a protective process. There is a local release of numerous chemicals that facilitate this inflammatory process; examples include bradykinin, prostaglandins, histamine and substance P (subP).

Some of these chemicals activate nociceptors, either directly or indirectly. Others sensitise the nociceptors so that pain can be experienced even with a non-noxious level of stimulation. NSAIDs can interrupt this process by inhibiting the enzymes cyclo-oxygenase 1 (COX-1) and 2 (COX-2). This prevents the conversion of arahidonic acid to endoperoxide and subsequently into prostaglandin and thromboxane (Figure 11.5).

Prostaglandins are not just pathological, but important for the maintenance of homeostasis by regulating blood flow in the kidneys and inhibiting gastric secretion in addition to other functions. These are primarily COX-1 mediated processes and this has led to the creation of selective inhibitors for COX-2, which unlike COX-1 is only found in activated inflammatory cells. However, COX-2 inhibitors have been found to increase the risk of cardiovascular diseases such as heart attack and stroke and in 2004 (updated and confirmed in 2005), the Committee on Safety of Medicines advised patients who had established cardiovascular disease to discontinue the use of COX-2 inhibitors.

NSAIDs also have anti-pyretic properties through inhibition of E-type prostaglandins, which would otherwise reset the thermostat in the hypothalamus.

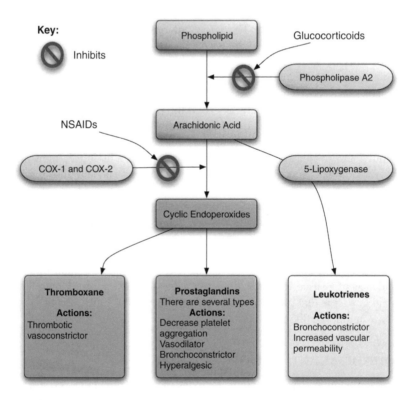

Figure 11.5 The arachidonic acid cascade and its blockade by glucocorticoids and NSAIDs (See also colour plate 26).

Unfortunately, inhibition of COX-1 and 2 can lead to increased leukotriene production, which is responsible for bronchospasm in susceptible asthmatics. Aspirin is most likely to cause this with most other NSAIDS implicated (Jenkins et al., 2004). The notable exception is paracetamol, which may rely less on COX-1 inhibition for its effect and instead inhibit COX-3, a relatively recent discovery (Schwab et al., 2003). Paracetamol certainly does not possess the anti-inflammatory effects of the other NSAIDs and is recommended in place of other NSAIDs in susceptible asthmatics (Jenkins et al., 2004).

ENTONOX

Entonox is a trade name for a self-administered gas containing 50 % oxygen and 50 % nitrous oxide. Its exact mechanism of action is still proving elusive to define. It has been suggested that nitrous oxide acts as a partial agonist at μ and κ opioid receptors, increasing the threshold for the sensation and tolerance of pain (O'Sullivan and Benger, 2003). However, studies using naloxone have shown that this is not the whole picture (Zacny et al., 1999) and animal studies have shown that nitrous oxide antagonises NMDA and benzodiazepine receptors. Irrespective, it is used extensively in the ambulance service, as well as emergency departments and labour wards. Due to its low solubility, it produces a rapid onset and offset, with analgesia typically within 3–4 minutes.

Entonox has few side effects if used for short periods of time, although vitamin B_{12} inactivation can occur with prolonged use. It is contraindicated where it may have adverse pressure effects, such as bowel obstruction or pneumothorax, and should not be used in head injuries with impaired consciousness as it can increase intracranial pressure. In decompression sickness, Entonox can increase the size of nitrogen bubbles within the bloodstream and so should not be administered to anyone who has been diving in the previous 24 hours (Joint Royal Colleges Ambulance Liaison Committee, 2004). Clinical studies have shown various degrees of pain relief when using Entonox, but it is generally accepted to be as effective as conventional medication regimens (Faddy and Garlick, 2005) and is suitable for use in children down to 3–4 years (Maurice et al., 2002b).

In conclusion, it can be seen that emergency care is a broad term that encompasses a variety of different practitioners working in different settings. Some of the drugs and issues that have been discussed are pertinent to wider healthcare, while others such as the poisoned patient are predominantly in the domain of emergency care. In all cases, however, a broad knowledge of pharmacology and pathophysiology is essential. It is always important to ensure that prescribing practice has a contemporary evidence base. In the case of poisoning, there are services dedicated to providing advice and guidance that is constantly under review. In other disease processes it is the responsibility of the practitioner to ensure that practice is informed by current evidence. This is true for all areas of prescribing practice, but particularly so in emergency care, where patients commonly present with conditions that have a high risk of mortality.

REFERENCES

Alsalim, W & Fadel, M (2003) Oral methionine compared with intravenous n-acetyl cysteine for paracetamol overdose. *Emergency Medical Journal* **20**(4): 366–367.

American Academy of Pediatrics and American Pain Society (2001) The assessment, management of acute pain in infants, children and adolescents. *Pediatrics* **108**(3): 793–797.

Aukerman, D, Sebastianelli, W & Nashelsky, J (2005) Skin adhesives offer reduced pain and less time spent closing the wound. *Journal of Family Practice* **54**(4): 378.

Ball, J (2002) Paediatric pain assessment. *Emergency Nurse* **10**(6): 31–33.

Barlas, P & Lundeburg, T (2006) Transcutaneous electrical nerve stimulation and acupuncture. In McMahon, S and Koltzenburg, M (eds) *Wall and Melzack's Textbook of Pain* (5th edition). Edinburgh: Elsevier.

Boersma, E, Maas, ACP, Deckers, JW & Simoons, ML (1996) Early thrombolytic treatment in acute myocardial infarction: Reappraisal of the golden hour. *The Lancet* **348**(9037): 771–775.

Bradshaw, M & Sen, A (2006) Use of a prophylactic antiemetic with morphine in acute pain: Randomised controlled trial. *Emergency Medical Journal* **23**(3): 210–213.

British Association for Emergency Medicine Clinical Effectiveness Committee (2004a) *Guidelines for the Management of Pain in Adults*. Available at: http://www.emergencymed.org.uk/BAEM/CEC/assets/cec_pain_in_adults.pdf [accessed 27 May 2006].

British Association for Emergency Medicine Clinical Effectiveness Committee (2004b) *Guidelines for the Management of Pain in Children*. Available at: http://www.emergencymed.org.uk/BAEM/CEC/assets/cec_pain_in_children.pdf [accessed 27 May 2006].

Chief Medical Officer (2002) Update on immunization issues. *Chief Medical Officer's Letter* August.

Clarke, S, Dargan, P & Jones, A (2002) Naloxone in opioid poisoning: Walking the tightrope. *Emergency Medicine Journal* **22**(9): 612–616.

Craig, C & Stitzel, R (2004) *Modern Pharmacology with Clinical Applications*. New York: Lippincott Williams and Wilkins.

Dale, M & Haylett, D (2004) *Pharmacology Condensed*. Edinburgh: Churchill Livingstone.

Dawson, J (2002) *Pharmacology* (2nd edn). Mosby.

DeLeo, J (2006) Basic science of pain. *The Journal of Bone and Joint Surgery* **88A**(supplement 2): 58–62.

Department of Health (2004) *National Service Framework for Children, Young People and Maternity Services*. London: The Stationery Office.

Department of Health (2005) *Taking Healthcare to the Patient: Transforming NHS Ambulance Services*. London: The Stationery Office.

Dickinson, A (2002) Gate control theory stands the test of time. *British Journal of Anaesthesia* **88**(6): 755–757.

Faddy, S & Garlick, S (2005) A systematic review of the safety of analgesia with 50 % nitrous oxide: Can lay responders use analgesic gases in the prehospital setting? *Emergency Medicine Journal* **22**(12): 901–908.

Hartley, V (2002) Paracetamol overdose. *Emergency Nurse* **10**(5): 17–24.

Health Protection Agency (2003) *Tetanus: Information for Health Professionals*. London: Health Protection Agency.

Hughes, B, Durran, A, Langford, N & Mutimer, D (2003) Paracetamol poisoning – impact of pack size restrictions. *Journal of Clinical Pharmacy and Therapeutics* **28**(4): 307–310.

Jenkins, C, Costello, J & Hodge, L (2004) Systematic review of prevalence of aspirin induced asthma and its implications for clinical practice. *British Medical Journal* **328**(7437): 434–437.

Joint Royal Colleges Ambulance Liaison Committee (2004) *UK Ambulance Service National Clinical Guidelines* (3rd edition). Available at: http://www.library.nhs.uk/emergency/ ViewResource.aspx?resID=36458&tabID=288 [accessed 27 May 2006].

Karim, A, Ivatts, S, Dargan, P & Jones, A (2001) How feasible is it to conform to the European guidelines on administration of activated charcoal within one hour of an overdose? *Emergency Medicine Journal* **18**(5): 390–392.

Lipley, N (2003) Association name change reflects EN New Workload. *Emergency Nurse* **11**(6): 2.

Machelska, H & Stein, C (2000) Pain control by immune-derived opioids. *Clinical and Experimental Pharmacology and Physiology* **27**(7): 533–536.

Maurice, SC, O'Donnell, JJ & Beattie, TF (2002a) Emergency analgesia in the paediatric population. Part I Current practice and perspectives. *Emergency Medicine Journal* **19**(1): 4–7.

Maurice, SC, O'Donnell, JJ & Beattie, TF (2002b) Emergency analgesia in the paediatric population. Part II Pharmacological methods of pain relief. *Emergency Medicine Journal* **19**(2): 101–105.

McGavock, H (2005) *How Drugs Work: basic pharmacology for healthcare professionals.* (2nd edition). Oxford: Radcliffe Publishing.

McGrath, PJ & Unruh, AM (2006) Measurement and assessment of paediatric pain. In McMahon, S & Koltzenburg, M (eds) *Wall and Melzack's Textbook of Pain* (5th edition). London: Churchill Livingstone.

Melzack, R & Wall, P (1965) Pain mechanisms: a new theory. *Science* **150**(699): 971–979.

Merskey, H & Bogduk, N (eds) (1994) *Classification of Chronic Pain* (2nd edition). Seattle: International Association for the Study of Pain Press.

Neal, M (2002) *Medical Pharmacology at a Glance.* Oxford: Blackwell Science.

Norman, I & Ryrie, I (2004) *The Art and Science of Mental Health Nursing.* Buckingham: Open University Press.

O'Sullivan, I & Benger, J (2003) Nitrous oxide in Emergency Medicine. *Emergency Medical Journal* **20**: 214–217.

Picton, C (2006) Patient choice. *Emergency Nurse* **13**(10): 1.

Poland, G, Borrund, A, Jacobsen, R, Mcdermott, K, Wollan, PC, Brackle, D & Charboneau, J (1997) Determination of deltoid fat pad thickness: Implications for needle length in adult immunization. *Journal of the American Medical Association* **227**(21): 1709–1711.

Prosser, S, Worster, B, MacGregor, J, Dewar, K, Runyard, P & Fegan, J (2000) *Applied Pharmacology: An Introduction to Pathophysiology and Drug Management for Nurses and Health Care Professionals.* London: Mosby.

Pulse (2003) Switch vaccine for diptheria. *Pulse* **63**(32): 8.

Purcell, D (2004) *Minor Injuries: A Clinical Guide for Nurses.* Edinburgh: Churchill Livingstone.

Rang, H, Dale, M, Ritter, J & Moore, P (2003) *Pharmacology.* Edinburgh: Churchill Livingstone.

Resuscitation Council (2005) *Advanced Life Support* (5th edition). London: Resuscitation Council.

Roberts, K, Jewkes, F, Whalley, H, Hopkins, D & Porter, K (2005) A review of emergency equipment carried and procedures performed by UK front line paramedics on paediatric patients. *Emergency Medicine Journal* **22**(8): 572–576.

Royal College of Nursing (1999) *Clinical Guidelines for the Recognition and Assessment of Acute Pain in Children. Implementation Guide.* London: Royal College of Nursing.

Schwab, J, Schluesener, H & Laufer, S (2003) COX-3: just another COX or the solitary elusive target of paracetamol? *The Lancet* **361**(9362): 981–982.

Thwaites, C & Farrar, J (2003) Preventing and treating tetanus. *British Medical Journal* **326**(7381): 117–118.

Tortora, G & Derrickson, B (2006) *Principles of Anatomy and Physiology*. Hoboken, NJ: John Wiley & Sons, Ltd.

Turner, T (2004) Do mammalian bites require antibiotic prophylaxis? *Annals of Emergency Medicine* **44**(3): 274–276.

Walker, B (2004) Locking down tetanus. *Nursing* **34**(9): 70–71.

Weston, CFM, Penny, WJ & Julian, DG (1994) Guidelines for the early management of patients with myocardial infarction. *British Medical Journal* **308**(6931): 767–771.

Wyat, J, Illingworth, R, Clancy, M, Munro, P & Robertson, C (2003) *Oxford Handbook of Clinical Medicine*. Oxford: Oxford University Press.

Zacny, J, Conran, A, Pardo, H, Coalson, D, Black, M, Klock, P & Klafta, M (1999) Effects of naloxone on nitrous oxide actions in healthy volunteers. *Pain* **83**: 411–418.

Zuckerman, J (2000) The importance of injecting vaccines into muscle. *British Medical Journal* **321**(7271): 1237–1238.

Index

Towards Prescribing Practice. Edited by J. McKinnon.
© 2007 John Wiley & Sons, Ltd.